Gels Horizons: From Science to Smart Materials

Series Editor

Vijay Kumar Thakur, School of Aerospace, Cranfield University, Cranfield, Bedfordshire, UK

This series aims at providing a comprehensive collection of works on the recent advances and developments in the domain of *Gels*, particularly as applied to the various research fields of sciences and engineering disciplines. It covers a broad range of topics related to *Gels* ranging from *Polymer Gels, Protein Gels, Self-Healing Gels, Colloidal Gels, Composites/Nanocomposites Gels, Organogels, Aerogels, Metallogels* & *Hydrogels* to *Micro/Nano gels*. The series provides timely and detailed information on advanced synthesis methods, characterization and their application in a broad range of interrelated fields such as chemistry, physics, polymer science & engineering, biomedical & biochemical engineering, chemical engineering, molecular biology, mechanical engineering and materials science & engineering.

This Series accepts both edited and authored works, including textbooks, monographs, reference works, and professional books. The books in this series will provide a deep insight into the state-of-art of *Gels* and serve researchers and professionals, practitioners, and students alike.

More information about this series at http://www.springer.com/series/15205

Jiya Jose · Sabu Thomas · Vijay Kumar Thakur
Editors

Nano Hydrogels

Physico-Chemical Properties and Recent Advances in Structural Designing

Springer

Editors
Jiya Jose
Mahatma Gandhi University
Kottayam, Kerala, India

Sabu Thomas
Mahatma Gandhi University
Kottayam, Kerala, India

Vijay Kumar Thakur
School of Aerospace
Cranfield University
Cranfield, UK

ISSN 2367-0061 ISSN 2367-007X (electronic)
Gels Horizons: From Science to Smart Materials
ISBN 978-981-15-7137-4 ISBN 978-981-15-7138-1 (eBook)
https://doi.org/10.1007/978-981-15-7138-1

This Springer imprint is published by the registered company Springer Nature Singapore Pte Ltd.
The registered company address is: 152 Beach Road, #21-01/04 Gateway East, Singapore 189721, Singapore

Preface

The role of nanotechnologist continues to evolve in the upcoming years as nanotechnology is an eternally growing field. In this edited book, we have addressed physicochemical properties and recent advances in structural designing of nanohydrogels by experts in the field around the globe. Hydrogels are covalently or ironically cross-linked three-dimensional networks of hydrophilic polymers. The excellent properties of nanohydrogels continue to stimulate researches in a way to tune its properties to develop novel materials. Based on the nature of the cross-linker, the polymer network can vary and significantly influence the physicochemical properties as well. So lots of interest have been focused in the tuning of physicochemical properties of nanohydrogel. Properties of synthetic hydrogels can be varied widely and also possible to tailor for specific use. In view of these, we have included chapters based on cross-linking strategies to develop hydrogels for biomedical applications, nanobased biodegradable hydrogel for biomedical application, hydrogel as bioink for organ regeneration, effect of structural properties of hydrogel in controlled drug delivery, etc. We have tried to improve it with the recent findings in the field of nanohydrogels. The focus of this book is on the formulations and physicochemical properties. We have divided the book in to 17 chapters which describes the recent developments in the structural design of nanohydrogels.

Chapter 1 deals with the three-dimensional printing of nanocellulose-based hydrogels and its applications.

Chapter 2 entitled cross-linking strategies to develop hydrogels for biomedical applications explains the different strategies of cross-linking and its advantages and disadvantages along with its biomedical applications.

Chapter 3 explains the emerging trends in the synthesis, properties and applications of nanogels derived from pullulan, collagen and gelatin.

Chapter 4 deals mainly with the biodegradable hydrogels and its biomedical applications. The chapter entitles nanobased biodegradable hydrogel for biomedical application.

Chapter 5 details about stimulus responsive hydrogels and its importance in drug delivery. The chapter entitles stimulus responsive polymers.

Chapter 6 explains about polymer water interactions in hydrogels and the importance of water ratio in a hydrogels in various applications.

Chapter 7 deals about hybrid nanohydrogels, mainly about its design and application.

Chapter 8 discusses about the cross-linking, modular design and self-assembly in hydrogels.

Chapter 9 explains the importance of bioink in organ regeneration through 3D printing. This chapter entitles hydrogel as bioink for organ regeneration.

Chapter 10 is hydrogel formulation as efficient drug carrier and delivery for selected skin diseases and explains about the formulation of hydrogels for drug delivery applications.

Chapter 11 deals with the structural properties of hydrogel in terms of controlled drug delivery. The chapter entitles effect of structural properties of hydrogel in controlled drug delivery.

Chapter 12 explains with elasticity, strength and biocompatibility of hydrogels.

Chapter 13 discusses recent developments in hydrogels and it entitles an overview of the recent developments in hydrogels.

Chapter 14 entitles self-assembled hydrogels: An overview.

Chapter 15 deals with synthesis, structural modification and physicochemical response of chitosan built nanohydrogel for control drug delivery applications.

Chapter 16 entitles novel biocompatible hydrogels via click chemistry which deals with recent developments in biocompactable hydrogels and its applications.

We hope all the scientific community and students will be benefitted by this book and we look forward to have suggestions and feedback to improve upon it.

Kottayam, India Jiya Jose
Kottayam, India Sabu Thomas
Cranfield, UK Vijay Kumar Thakur

Contents

About the Editors

Dr. Jiya Jose is a currently Postdoctoral Researcher in Mahatma Gandhi University, Kerala, India. She pursued her Ph.D. in Marine Sciences from Cochin University of Science and Technology, India. Her research interests include marine microbiology and nanobiotechnology. Dr. Jose has been the recipient of the prestigious UGC – Dr. S. Kothari Post-Doctoral Fellowship, as well as receiving many awards for the research in national and international conferences. She has served as an editor for 2 books, authored 7 book chapters and 28 research publications in international journals and conferences.

Dr. Sabu Thomas is currently Professor and Pro-Vice Chancellor at Mahatma Gandhi University, Kerala, India, in addition to being the founder director of the International and Inter University Centre for Nanoscience and Nanotechnology. After his B.Tech. in Polymer Science and Rubber Technology from the University of Cochin, he pursued his Ph.D. from Indian Institute of Technology, Kharagpur. Prof. Thomas has received many national and international awards, including Fellowship of the Royal Society of Chemistry, MRSI award, SESR award, Dr. APJ Abdul Kalam Award for Scientific Excellence, an honorary degree by Université de Lorraine, and multiple fellowships by prestigious societies and universities. Prof. Thomas' research has spanned many areas of nanocomposite and polymer science and engineering, and he has edited more than 70 books, holds 5 patents and has authored over 750 research publications.

Dr. Vijay Kumar Thakur is currently a Professor in the Biorefining and Advanced Materials Research Centre at SRUC, United Kingdom and also holds an Adjunct Professor position in the Research School of Polymeric Materials, Jiangsu University, China. He has previously held faculty positions at Cranfield University UK, Washington State University USA, Nanyang Technological University, Singapore and LHU–Taiwan. His expertise includes the synthesis of biobased monomers/ polymers and the processing of sustainable composites. He has published over 160 SCI journal articles, 2 patents, 44 books & 35 book chapters in areas concerning polymers and materials science. His research interests include the synthesis and processing of bio-based polymers, composites; nanostructured materials, hydrogels, polymer micro/nanocomposites, nanoelectronic materials, novel high dielectric constant materials, engineering nanomaterials, electrochromic materials, green synthesis of nanomaterials, and surface functionalization of polymers/nanomaterials.

Chapter 1
Three-Dimensional Printing of Nanocellulose-Based Hydrogels

Sahar Sultan and Aji P. Mathew

Abstract This chapter gives an overview of the recent developments in the field of three-dimensional (3D) printing of nanocellulose-based hydrogels. Nanocellulose has gained much attention due to its renewable sources, low toxicity, biocompatibility, good mechanical properties and availability of surface charges for further modifications as well as in situ growth of functional nanoparticles. Moreover, suitable rheological properties of nanocellulose are helpful in utilizing 3D printing technique for producing constructs with customized, controlled and complex geometries. This technique offers a high-resolution 3D constructs with precise micro- and macroscaled structures and can be extended to 3D bioprinting, where living cells are mixed in hydrogel inks. As the name suggests, nanocellulose-based hydrogel inks contain nanocellulose as reinforcement phase, while other crosslinkable biopolymers can serves as matrix phase.

1 Background

Keeping in mind the depletion of petroleum-based resources and environmental issues, cellulose is a good choice of materials for future because of its renewability, biodegradability and environmental friendliness. Cellulose is the most abundant natural biopolymer on Earth with an annual production of 10^{10}–10^{11} tons [1]. It has a variety of sources and can be extracted from a top-down approach from marine animals (e.g., tunicates) and plants (e.g., wood, cotton, wheat straw). It can also be obtained via bottom-up approach through biosynthesis such as bacteria (Acetobacter Xylinum), algae (e.g., Valonia), fungi and even amoeba (protozoa) [2]. Cellulose is a long-chain polysaccharide having a chemical formula of $(C_6H_{10}O_5)_n$ where n is the degree of polymerization depending on the sources and pretreatments of cellulose. It consists of linear chain of glucose units linked via a β-1,4 glycosidic bond [3].

S. Sultan (✉) · A. P. Mathew
Department of Materials and Environmental Chemistry, Stockholm University, Stockholm, Sweden
e-mail: sahar.sultan@mmk.su.se

J. Jose et al. (eds.), *Nano Hydrogels*, Gels Horizons: From Science to Smart Materials,
https://doi.org/10.1007/978-981-15-7138-1_1

Cellulose with at least one dimension on a nanoscale (1–100 nm) is termed as nanocellulose and can be isolated from cellulose biomass following a top-down approach (Fig. 1). Nanocellulose not only possesses the properties of cellulose, such as mechanical strength, potential for chemical modification, low toxicity, biocompatibility, biodegradable and renewability, but it also has nanoscale characteristics like high specific surface area, rheological and optical properties [4]. The family of nanocellulose is divided into three types: (i) cellulose nanofibers (CNF), (ii) cellulose nanocrystals (CNC) and bacterial cellulose (BC) (Table 1).

CNF consists of both individual and aggregated nanofibers including ordered and disordered regions, which attribute the morphology of CNF with soft and long chains [6]. For the production of CNF, mainly, mechanically induced destruction strategy is used followed by homogenization at high pressure. In this process, the individual microfibrils are delaminated from cellulosic fibers by multiple mechanical shearing actions that require high energy consumptions [7]. However, different pretreatments of cellulosic fibers can facilitate the delamination process, e.g., alkali, oxidative, enzymatic and acidic pretreatments. Alkali pretreatment removes a certain amount of lignin that interrupts its structure and weakens the bonds between lignin and carbohydrates [8]. 2,2,6,6-tetramethylpiperidine-1-oxyl radical (TEMPO)-mediated oxidation of native celluloses is also a pretreatment used for conversion of hydroxyl groups to carboxylate groups [9]. This surface treatment induces a negative charge

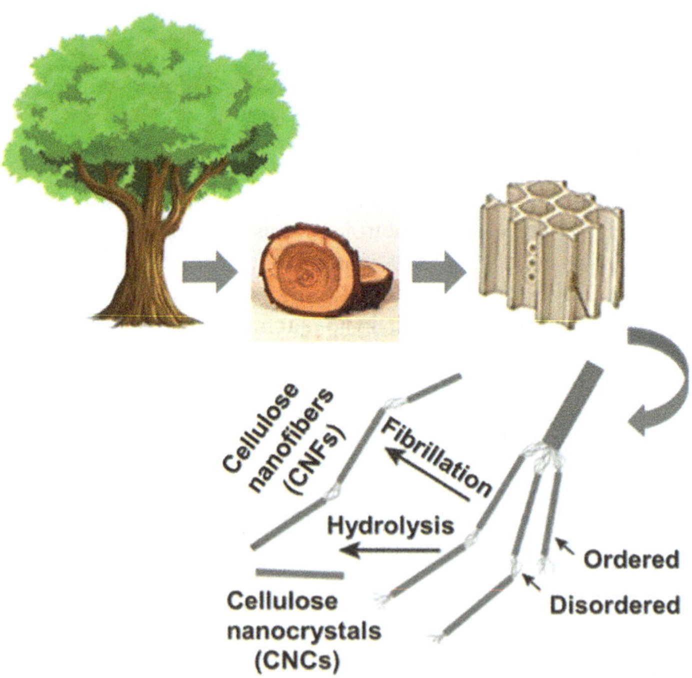

Fig. 1 Top-down approach for the production of plant-derived nanocellulose

Table 1 Family of nanocellulose [2, 5]

Types of nanocellulose	Synonyms	Typical sources	Formation and average size
Cellulose nanofibrils (CNF) 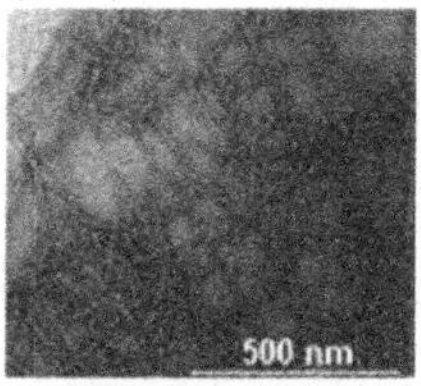	Microfibrillated cellulose, nanofibrils and microfibrils, nanofibrillated cellulose	Wood, sugar beet, potato tuber, hemp, flax	– Delamination of woodpulp by mechanical pressure before and/or after chemical or enzymatic treatment – Diameter: 5–60 nm – Length: several micrometers
Cellulose nanocrystals (CNC) 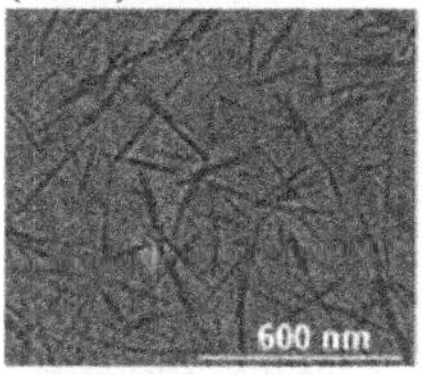	Nanocrystalline cellulose, crystallites, whiskers, rodlike Cellulose microcrystals	Wood, cotton, hemp, flax, wheat straw, mulberry bark, ramie, Avicel, tunicin, cellulose from algae and bacteria	– Acid hydrolysis of cellulose from many sources – Diameter: 5–70 nm – Length: 100–250 nm (from plant celluloses); 100 nm to several micrometers (from celluloses of tunicates, algae, bacteria)
Bacterial cellulose (BC) 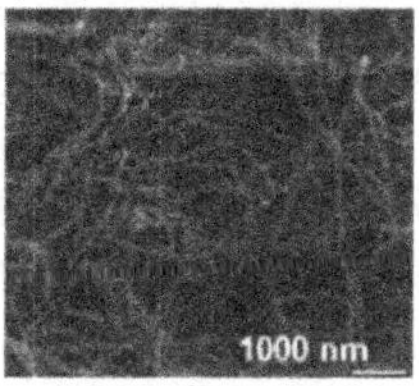	Bacterial cellulose, microbial cellulose, biocellulose	Low-molecular-weight sugars and alcohols	– Bacterial synthesis – Diameter: 20–100 nm – Different types of nanofiber networks

resulting in repulsion between cellulosic fibers, thus facilitating fibrillation process. In addition, these carboxylate group can be used for further surface attachment of other functional molecules [10]. TEMPO-CNF (TOCNF) can also be produced directly from bagasse, which is an agro-industrial residue [11]. Enzymes show strong synergistic effects to facilitate disintegration of cellulosic fibers [12]. CNF produced from enzymatically pretreated cellulosic wood fibers showed certain improvements as compared to acidic pretreatment [13], which decreases the chain length of the cellulose molecule causing embrittlement [14].

The disordered regions in the cellulosic fibers can be removed by a strong acid hydrolysis treatment resulting in crystalline rod-shaped CNCs. During this process, the hydronium ions penetrate the amorphous regions of cellulose chains, promoting the hydrolytic cleavage of the glycosidic bonds and releasing individual crystallites [15]. The commonly acid used is sulfuric acid as its reaction with the surface hydroxyl groups via an esterification process allows the grafting of anionic sulfate ester groups [16]. These negatively charged groups induce the formation of an electrostatic layer covering the nanocrystals and promote their dispersion in water [15].

During the biosynthesis of BC, the glucose chains are produced inside the bacterial body that are extruded out through pores present on the cell envelope [6]. The combination of these chains produces microfibrils that further aggregates as ribbons and generates a web-shaped network structure with BC [17]. BC has certain advantages as compared to CNF and CNC, such as better mechanical and chemical properties, high crystallinity as well as purity and control over its repeating unit and the molecular weight based on fermentation process [18, 19]. However, the relatively high cost associated with the support the growth of bacteria and low yield has limited its use if any mass production is to be considered.

2 Introduction

The research and development on the manufacturing processes to make nanocellulose into useful forms is an essential part of the development of cellulose nanocomposites. To produce cellulose nanocomposites for commercial use, the journey from laboratory to industry must contain such methods, reagents, solvents, equipments that have the potential for large-scale production.

The structure and properties of cellulose nanocomposites rely on the fiber–fiber bonding as well as fiber–matrix interfacial adhesion, which in return are dependent on the homogeneity of the nanocellulose dispersion in the matrix phase [20]. The hydrophilic nature and low thermal stability of nanocellulose limit the choice of matrix and processing techniques to form composites. The abundance of hydroxyl groups at the surface of nanocellulose makes surface functionalization possible that plays an important role to increase the surface hydrophobicity while maintaining the thermal stability [20]. The main idea behind surface functionalization is to obtain better dispersion through the introduction of stable negative or positive electrostatic charges and to tune the surface energy characteristics to improve compatibility with matrices in nanocomposites [21]. Furthermore, cationic or anionic surface charges can be incorporated, which can later be used for in situ growth of other functional molecules [22, 23].

The commonly used traditional methods for the production of cellulose nanocomposite are casting, extrusion, electrospinning and freeze-drying. The earlier publications dealing with cellulose-reinforced nanocomposites were based on casting/evaporation of an aqueous mixture of CNCs [24–26]. Nowadays, the use of the casting/evaporation technique is not limited to a water medium but is extended to organic solvents, e.g., dimethylformamide [27], pyridine [28], toluene [29] and chloroform [30]. Electrospinning is relatively a new technique and has the ability to produce three-dimensional (3D) cellulose nanocomposites with very high surface-area-to-volume ratio [31] and enhanced mechanical properties together with its electrical conductivity [22, 32]. In addition, the high surface area and microporous structure of electrospun fiber mats can absorb wound exudates, prevent excess dehydration and microbial infection as well as facilitate gas permeability. These properties make them suitable for cell attachment and proliferation in wound dressing applications [33, 34]. Freeze-drying also known as ice crystal templating offers an advantage of designing hierarchically structured composite materials by controlling the rate and direction of freezing ice [35]. CNF- and CNC-based composites can be fabricated via freeze-drying technique to have 3D scaffolds or 2D membranes [36, 37]. Another fabrication technique is melt processing in which cellulose nanomaterials are dispersed in a thermoplastic polymer melt. The first study on nanocellulose melt process reported nanocomposites developed by melt extrusion technique using a commercially available grade of microcrystalline cellulose in a biodegradable polyester matrix [38]. Later studies used polyethylene [39] and polyoxyethylene [40] as polymer matrices. However, these traditional techniques do not enable precise control of internal scaffold architecture or the fabrication of complex architectures. Moreover, they also require good fabrication skills to maintain consistency and reproducibility in the scaffold architecture.

Recently, three-dimensional (3D) printing technique has been adapted for the fabrication of 3D constructs based on the digitally controlled deposition of successive layers of material until a final structure is created with precise geometric control at macro- and microscale [41]. The process of 3D printing starts with a computer-aided design (CAD) file that can be obtained by a 3D scanner or by means of photogrammetry where the model is obtained through the combination of several images of the object taken from different positions [42]. This is an advantage in biomedical field where computed tomography (CT) or magnetic resonance imaging (MRI) of the patient can be used to create customized 3D-printed models (Fig. 2b) [43]. Currently, 3D printing techniques are classified into extrusion, powder-based, photopolymerization and lamination [42].

In case of hydrogel or paste, extrusion-based 3D printing is a popular choice as the "ink" is in a highly viscous liquid state, which is able to retain its shape after deposition (Fig. 2a) [42]. The freestanding 3D objects can be crosslinked during or after the 3D printing via ultraviolet (UV) curing or ionic crosslinking [44, 45]. However, to print hydrogel inks with high resolution is a challenge due to the swelling that occurs when viscous liquefied material is extruded through a small nozzle with high pressures. As a potential candidate for 3D printing, the rheological properties of the hydrogel ink are of prime importance. The hydrogel should have strong non-Newtonian shear thinning behavior along with viscoelastic solid-like response [44]. During extrusion, the viscosity of the hydrogel drops due to higher shear rates, but as soon as the hydrogel is extruded and shear rate drops, the viscosity of the ink increases immediately. $50\ s^{-1}$ is a typical shear rate experienced during 3D printing [46]. This shear thinning property is an important factor to make filamentary extrusion possible. To maintain the shape of the construct after 3D printing, the hydrogel should have

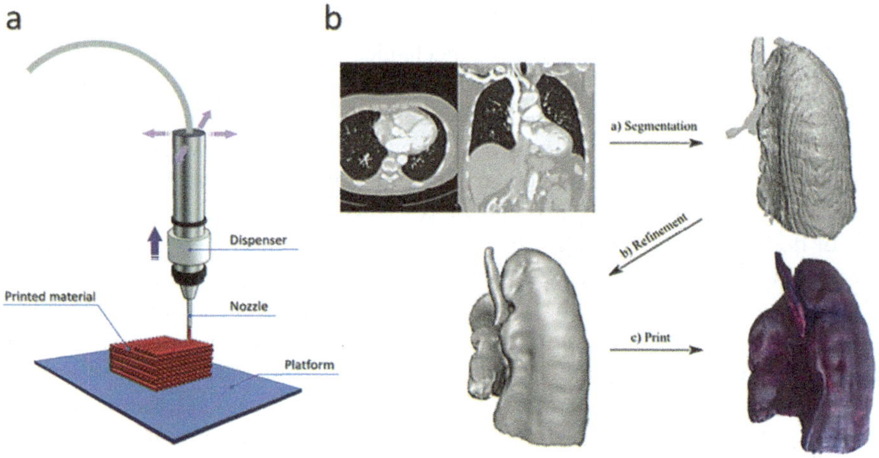

Fig. 2 **a** Schematic representation of extrusion-based 3D printing for ink and **b** work flow from medical imaging data (CT scan) to a finished 3D-printed model

a storage modulus (G′) sufficiently higher than its loss modulus (G″). This solid-like behavior of the hydrogel is highly desirable for subsequent post-treatments and handling [47].

An advancement of 3D printing is 3D bioprinting, where both living and non-living biological materials are used to fabricate 3D scaffolds, implants, engineered tissues and organs [48]. A construct is said to be 3D bioprinted when living cells, bioactive molecules, growth factors, biomaterials or cell-aggregates are mixed with the hydrogel ink or are incorporated through a separate nozzle [49]. In this way, the rejection rate of foreign objects by the human body is reduced and recovery rate is accelerated. However, extra care has to be taken when dealing with 3D printing of bioinks. Physically, the bioink should be sufficiently viscous to be dispensed as a free-standing filament but too high concentration of the bioink can negatively affect cell viability [50]. Factors such as too strong shear forces required to eject the bioink, high printing temperatures and harsh post-treatments can result in cell death. One study demonstrated an inverse relationship between extrusion pressure and cellular viability [51]. The study reveals that the high dispensing pressure and small nozzle size induce mechanical damage to cell membrane integrity causing loss in cell viability.

3 3D Printing of Nanocellulose-Based Hydrogels

The surface charges and water stability of nanocellulose allow forming hydrogels from a nanocellulose solution through physical crosslinking with inherent shear thinning property [52]. Hydrogel formation capability of nanocellulose at low concentrations (1–2 wt%) has facilitated the use of 3D printing as a fabrication technique for 2D and 3D scaffolds [53, 54]. The presence of nanocellulose is expected to enhance the elastic modulus of the nanocomposite hydrogel ink that prevents the flow and deformation of the deposited material as the shear force ceases after extrusion [47]. The presence of stiff reinforcement particles such as CNCs can introduce shear-induced alignment that is considered beneficial for inducing directionality in the 3D constructs [45]. The local orientation control of CNFs can define the elastic and swelling an isotropies for biomimetic 4D printing [55]. As compared to CNCs, CNFs readily form hydrogels at low concentration due to its long and entangled chain network. In contrast, CNCs can produce concentrated hydrogels at a given viscosity due to lower aspect ratio of CNCs than CNFs [56].

The 3D-printed structures must have fast crosslinking abilities for post-processing, handling and retaining its structure after printing. The surface charges present on nanocellulose surface can be utilized for its self-crosslinking functionalization, i.e., without the need for a matrix phase [57] or the 3D-printed constructs can directly be freeze-dried to form aerogels [58]. However, in most case alginate is a popular choice to be used as a crosslinkable matrix phase because of its bio-based origin, relatively low cost and ability of fast gelation in the presence of divalent cations [59]. In case of biomedical applications, alginate alone has low cell adhesion and cell proliferation capability, and therefore, it is often mixed with other biopolymers, such as gelatin [44]. The blends of alginate and gelatin are used to print 3D constructs for myoregenerative applications [50] or to fabricate living heterogeneous aortic valve conduits [60].

3.1 CNF-Based Hydrogels

Highlight	Composition	Post-treatment	Application	References
Human stem cell-decorated CNF threads	CNF: 1.47 (wt%)	Glutaraldehyde crosslinking	Wound dressing	[61]
Commercially available ink CELLINK	CNF/alginate 2.0/0.5 (wt%)	$CaCl_2$ crosslinking	Auricular cartilage regeneration	[62–64]
3D bioprinting human chondrocytes	CNF/alginate 2.0/0.5 (wt%)	$CaCl_2$ crosslinking	Cartilage tissue engineering	[64, 65]
Solidification of cellulose nanofibril hydrogel into controlled 3D architectures	CNF 2 wt% CNF/carbon nanotubes 2/0.2 (wt%)	$CaCl_2$ crosslinking followed by air drying/air drying with surfactants/solvent exchange/freeze drying Air drying	Diverse	[66]
Bioink: C- periodate nanocellulose substrate: TOCNF	CNF 3.9 wt%	$CaCl_2$ crosslinking followed by freeze-drying	Wound dressing	[67]
3D bioprinting of induced pluripotent stem cells (iPSCs)	CNF/alginate 60/40 (dry wt%) + iPSCs CNF/hyaluronic acid 95/5 (% volume) + iPSCs	$CaCl_2$ crosslinking H_2O_2 crosslinking	Cartilage tissue engineering	[68]
Bioink with functionalized matrix	Alginate sulfate/nanocellulose1/1.36 (%) + Passage 3 cells	$CaCl_2$ crosslinking	Cartilage Bioprinting	[69]
Biomimetic inks based on tyramine-functionalized xylan (XT)	CNF/XT 2.6–3.0/5.11–5.8 (wt%)	H_2O_2 crosslinking	Diverse	[70]
Biofunctionalization: conjugation of avidin to TOCNF hydrogel	Alginate/TOCNF 90/10 (wt%) + Water/glycerin 45/50 (v%)	$CaCl_2$ crosslinking	Biomedical devices and drug-releasing	[71]
CNF tubes as sacrificial templates	TOCNF 1 wt%	Glutaraldehyde and/or $CaCl_2$ crosslinking	Biomedical	[72]

(continued)

(continued)

Highlight	Composition	Post-treatment	Application	References
Composite microfiber based on carbon nanotube/nanofibrillated cellulose	TOCNF/CNT 1/1 (%)	Solvent exchange followed by drying under tension	Flexible electronics	[73]
Blend of CNF and lignosulfonate (LG) for 3D printing and carbonization	CNF/LG 0.25–2/20–50 (wt%)	RT drying/freeze drying followed by carbonization at 800 °C	Energy storage devices	[74]
Biomimetic 4D printing	CNF/clay/monomer/glucose 0.73/9.7/7.8/3.8(%)	Ultraviolet curing	Diverse	[55]
TOCNF aerogel	TOCNF/Kymene 2.8/0.06 (wt%)	Freeze drying followed by crosslinking at 120°	Diverse	[75]
In situ synthesis of Metal organic frameworks onto TOCNF	TOCNF/ZIF-8/Alginate/Curcumin 19.7–66.3/30.8–70.7/2.9–5.5/0–4.1 (%)	$CaCl_2$ crosslinking	Biomedical	[10]
Mechanical gradients in nanocellulose papers	TOCNF/copolymer 90–20/10–80	RT drying	Diverse	[76]
Improved rheological properties by the addition of CNF	CNF/GelMA 0–2.0/5.0 (%w/v)	Chemical crosslinking	Biomedical	[53]

Paul Gatenholm initiated the 3D printing of nanocellulose by formulating a bioink with CNF, where alginate was used as matrix [65]. Human chondrocytes in the bioink exhibited a cell viability of 73 and 86% after 1 and 7 days of 3D culture that shows the potential for cartilage tissue engineering applications. The bioink-enabled printing of 2D grid-like structures as well as 3D constructs. He also tested a commercially available ink, CELLINK with 2 wt% CNF for 3D bioprinting [62]. This ink was mixed with primary nasal chondrocytes, which upon 3D printing provides cell-laden, patient-specific auricular constructs with an open inner structure, high cell density, homogenous cell distribution and 3D culture for up to 28 days. These properties combined with 3D printability make this bioink promising for auricular cartilage applications.

Pure CNF extracted from plants can produce crosslinked threads with high mechanical strength for biomedical applications [61]. The threads were decorated with human adipose mesenchymal stem cells (hASC) which is an efficient and safe means to reduce inflammation and promote wound healing. Functionalized CNF can also be used to 3D print constructs. CNF treated with a combination of carboxymethylation and periodate oxidation was used an ink (3.9 wt%) to 3D print onto TOCNF substrate [67]. The freeze-dried 3D-printed constructs did not support bacterial growth, which can be a distinct advantage for wound dressing applications. TOCNF can be 3D printed where structures collapse upon drying, but by using different drying processes, the collapse can be controlled and the 3D structure can be preserved upon solidification [66]. TOCNF can be used to fabricate highly deformable and shape recoverable 3D-printed aerogels [75]. The surface charges present on CNF participated in crosslinking and allowed freeze-dried TOCNF aerogel to maintain structural integrity even under water and after 80% compression cycles.

The surface charges present on TOCNF can be utilized for in-situ growth of other functional materials after which the hydrogel ink can be utilized for 3D-printing scaffolds (Fig. 3) [10]. The carboxylic groups on TOCNF surface were used for in situ growth of ZIF-8. The inherent porosity of MOF was used to load curcumin, which shows pH-controlled release. This one-pot synthesis method can load up to 70% of MOF particles. The flexibility and extendibility of this system was proved by synthesizing a different MOF, MIL-100, and loading a different guest molecule, methylene blue (MB).

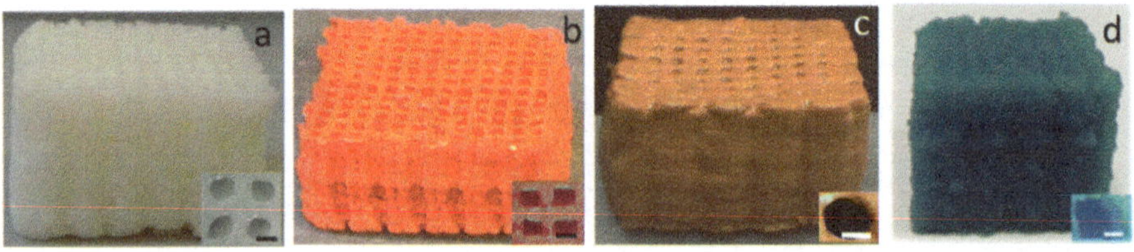

Fig. 3 In situ synthesis of metal organic frameworks onto TOCNF with and without guest molecules **a** ZIF-8@TOCNF, **b** Curcumin-ZIF-8@TOCNF, **c** Curcumin-MIL-100@TOCNF and **d** MB-ZIF-8@TOCNF. Scale bar: 1 mm

In developing cellulose-based hydrogels, instead of nanocellulose, matrix phase can also be functionalized to make its surface suitable for further attachment of growth factors that can induce cell proliferation. Muller and coworkers introduced a sulfated version of alginate, which can bind growth factors such as fibroblast growth factor (FGF), transforming growth factor (TGF) and hepatocyte growth factors (HGF) which induce potent proliferation and collagen II deposition by encapsulated bovine chondrocytes [69]. When this functionalized matrix (1%) was mixed with nanocellulose purchased from CELLINK AB (1.36%) and with passage three cells, a bioink suitable for 3D printing was developed for cartilage applications.

The hydrogel ink can be biofunctionalized by the covalent coupling of an enhanced avidin protein to TOCNF where glycerin was also used as a solvent together with water [71]. Glycerin was used to minimize excess shrinkage that will help 3D-printed samples to retain its dimensions. It was found that the 3D-printed samples without glycerin were not stable at room temperature and had to be freeze-dried; however, in the presence of glycerin, the samples were stable in room temperature after curing.

One step further, 4D biomimetic printing is achieved through the composite ink composed of stiff CNFs embedded in a soft acrylamide matrix, which mimics the composition of plant cell walls [55]. 4D-printing method relies on the ability to define the swelling anisotropies by local control of the orientation of cellulose fibers within the hydrogel composite. During printing, CNF undergoes shear-induced alignment as the hydrogel ink flows through the deposition nozzle, which induces anisotropic stiffness, and, hence, anisotropic swelling along the longitudinal printing direction. This study opens new avenues for creating designer shape-shifting architectures for tissue engineering, biomedical devices, soft robotics and beyond. In another study, TOCNF was used to fabricate a new design approach toward 4D printing, by direct filament writing of CNF-copolymer hydrogels of different composition next to each other in stripe patterns [76]. Subsequent self-healing of the hydrogels during drying leads to coherent films having linear, parabolic and striped bulk gradients leading to optimized combinations of stiffness and toughness.

Carbon nanotubes (CNTs) serve as building blocks to make mechanically robust conductive microfibers owing to their impressive mechanical and electrical properties. Both CNFs and TOCNFs have been used to make hydrogels with CNTs and 3D printed into various constructs [66, 73]. A conductive CNF-CNT hydrogel has been fabricated which demonstrate that the CNF can be functionalized by the addition of conductive CNTs, and the 3D structure can be controlled by the print design and drying mechanism. In case of 3D-printed TOCNF-CNT constructs, both the fibers were aligned in the printing direction due to shear-induced stresses. This alignment helps to improve the interaction and percolation between these two building blocks, leading to a combination of high mechanical strength and electrical conductivity. In addition, microfibrillated cellulose and lignosulfonate hydrogel were fabricated and used to fabricate carbon objects through 3D printing and carbonization [74]. The hydrogel rheological behavior was studied through flow and thixotropic modes which were further used to search for formulation/processability correlations during 3D printing.

Polylactic acid (PLA)-grafted cellulose nanofiber composite filaments were produced by melt extrusion [77]. The grafted PLA was highly crystallized which improved storage modulus of the composite filaments in both low-temperature glassy state and high-temperature rubbery state. Post-extrusion annealing treatment also had a positive effect on the tensile modulus and strength of the composite filaments. The formed composite filaments show potential to be used in 3D printing. In a similar study, polypropylene and CNF nanocomposites were also melt extruded [78].

3.2 BC-Based Hydrogels

Highlight	Composition	Post-treatment	Application	References
Dissolved BC in ionic liquid (IL)	BC: 4 wt%	Solvent exchange followed by freeze drying	regenerated cellulose structures	[79]
3D printing of bacteria	Sodium hyaluronate/fumed silica/carrageenan 1/1/1 (wt ratio) + multifunctional bacteria stem solution Bacteria + Alginate: 2.5 (wt%)	Ultraviolet curing/ Light curing $CaCl_2$ crosslinking	biotechnological and biomedical	[80, 81]

BC dissolved in an ionic liquid (1-ethyl-3-methylimidazolium acetate) was used for controlled dispensing, where water and agar aqueous gel were evaluated as coagulating solvents [79]. The highest concentration (4%) of the dissolved BC works best for printing. Water coagulation ensured good resolution but caused complications when multiple layers were extruded on top because of poor adhesion between layers. However, when dissolved BC was dispensed onto an agar gel, the print was coagulated within seconds. The agar gel diffuses through the print from the bottom up, making it possible for the next layer to adhere to the partially gelled first layer. For taller structures, vertical agar supports were used to ensure a constant and continuous coagulation of the 3D prints. This study shows that quality of the 3D-printed constructs is depended on the needle size, the viscosity of the solution, the pressure during dispensing, and the coagulation method.

A new strategy has been proposed where fully grown bacteria is embedded in a biocompatible ink which is 3D printed to produce bacteria-derived functional materials [80]. Two types of "living materials" were printed which were capable of degrading pollutants and of producing medically relevant bacterial cellulose. Bacterial cellulose films were grown in complex geometries precisely at the site of interest by locally deploying bacteria where needed. This versatile bacteria-printing platform can be used for the 3D printing of a new generation of biologically generated functional materials. In another study, 2.5 wt% alginate ink was used to deposit bacteria cells in specific three-dimensional patterns to fabricate spatially patterned materials [81].

3.3 CNC-Based Hydrogels

Cellulose nanocrystals are anisotropic particles with a high aspect ratio due to which shear-induced alignment can be expected. Siqueria and coworkers investigated and quantified the shear-induced alignment of anisotropic CNCs during 3D printing [45]. For this purpose, 20 wt% CNC aqueous ink was used which upon drying resulted in printed architectures containing 100% CNC. In the 3D-printed samples, highest degree of orientation (84%) was obtained along the longitudinal direction, i.e., the printing direction (Fig. 4b). In addition, the effect of this alignment on the mechanical properties was studied by developing composite hydrogel inks made from chemically modified CNC for ultraviolet (UV) curing. Interestingly, the mechanical tests reveal enhanced mechanical properties in the longitudinal direction likely arise due to the orientation of the CNCs along the printed filament. In our recent study, we

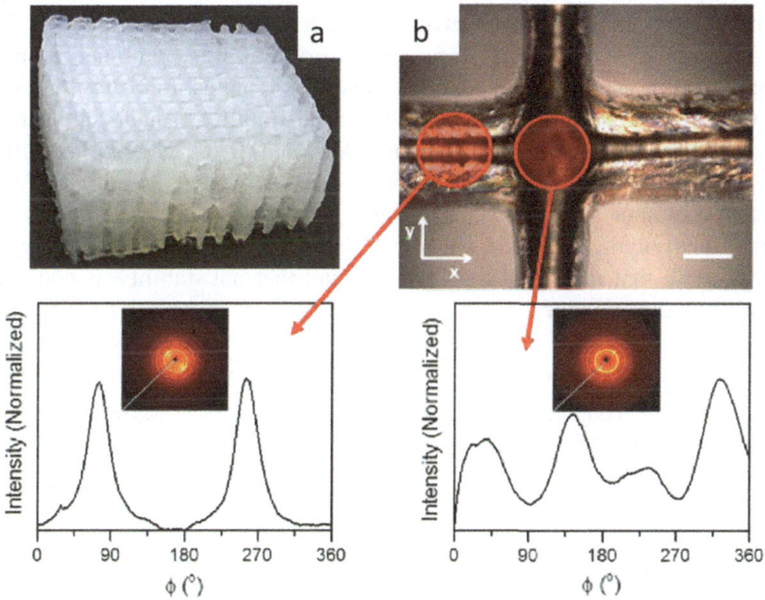

Fig. 4 Optical microscopy images of **a** 3D-printed scaffold with gradient porosity based on CNC hydrogel ink. **b** 3D-printed grids showing the positions for scattering measurements performed along axial or cross-sectional directions

took one step forward and introduced gradient porosity within one hydrogel scaffolds (Fig. 4a) [44]. A variety of 2D and 3D hydrogel scaffolds were produced with uniform and gradient porosity. The 2D wide angle X-ray scattering studies showed that the degree of orientation for CNCs varied between 61 and 76% preferably in the printing direction. This work also highlights the importance of the nozzle movement and printing pathways to obtain 3D hydrogel scaffolds with higher Z-axis while maintaining good resolution.

Pure CNC suspensions have also been used to produce 3D aerogels with controlled structures and inner pore architectures through freeze-drying [58]. An aerogel density range of 127–399 mg/cm^3 and a porosity range of 92.1–75.0% were achieved with CNC gel concentrations of 11.8–30 wt%. The preparation and extraction methods of CNCs is also a vital role in its performance and properties. CNCs when prepared through fully recyclable oxalic acid(OA) hydrolysis along with disk-milling (DM) pretreatment of bleached kraft pulp, show several advantages including large aspect ratio, carboxylated surface and excellent thermal stability along with high yield [82]. This CNC suspension was used to produce high-performance films and 3D-printed patterns which can be used for a wide variety of applications. Surface-functionalized CNCs can also be used to produce freestanding 3D-structured objects. A photoactive bis(acyl)phosphaneoxide(BAPO) derivative was directly attached to CNCs without any pretreatment, and these surface-modified CNCs were used for 3D printing [83]. This photoactive nanomaterial can be used to convert a conventional monomer into a polymeric network. The 3D-printed constructs showed a superiors welling capacity and improved mechanical properties as compared to pure CNCs.

A combination of melt extrusion and 3D printing was combined to produce CNC-reinforced acrylonitrile butadiene styrene (ABS) nanocomposites [84]. Lignin-coated CNCs were used for increased the thermal stability of nanocellulose that is considered beneficial during melt extrusion done at 180 °C. The extruded filament was used to 3D print nanocomposites that can have great potential in end-use products. In another study, melt processing of CNC-based nanocomposites with a hydrophobic polymeric matrix was done [40]. Polyoxyethylene (PEO) was used for this purpose that improved dispersibility and thermal stability as compared to neat CNC-based composites.

Highlight	Composition	Post-treatment	Application	References
Oxalic acid (OA) hydrolysis along with disk-milling (DM)	DM-OA-CNC: 15 (wt%)	Freeze drying	Diverse	[82]
Textured cellular architectures with modified CNCs	CNC: 0.5–40(wt%) CNC:10/20 (wt%) + HEMA + oligomer + photoinitiator	Ultraviolet curing	Building blocks	[45]

(continued)

(continued)

Highlight	Composition	Post-treatment	Application	References
CNCs aerogels	CNC: 11.8–30 (wt%) 2-CNC/Kymene (Kymene2 wt% based on dry cellulose mass)	Freeze drying	Diverse	[58]
3D printing of melt extruded nanocomposite filaments	Lignin-coated CNCs/ABS 0–10/100–90 (wt%)	RT drying	Diverse	[84]
Gradient porosity within one scaffold	CNC/Alginate/Gelatin 70/20/10 (Dry wt%)	$CaCl_2$ crosslinking	Biomedical	[44]
Surface modification of CNCs with bis(acyl)phosphane oxide (BAPO)	CNC-BAPO: 3.6 wt%	Photopolymerization	Diverse	[83]

4 Conclusions

The combination of 3D printing and cellulose nanomaterials has proved to be a successful step which is evident from the increased number of publications since last ten years (Fig. 5a)with Sweden being in top five countries (Fig. 5b). Cellulose nanofibers, crystals and bacterial cellulose suspensions are suitable for 3D printing due to its inherently suitable rheological properties. Either alone, functionalized or mixed with matrix phases, cellulose nanomaterials can be 3D printed for a variety of applications including biomedical applications, packaging, conduction devices, batteries, wearable electronic, etc. The presence of functional groups plays an important role in enhancing the efficiency and performance of cellulose nanomaterials. Either these functional groups can help in self-crosslinking of nanocellulose or they

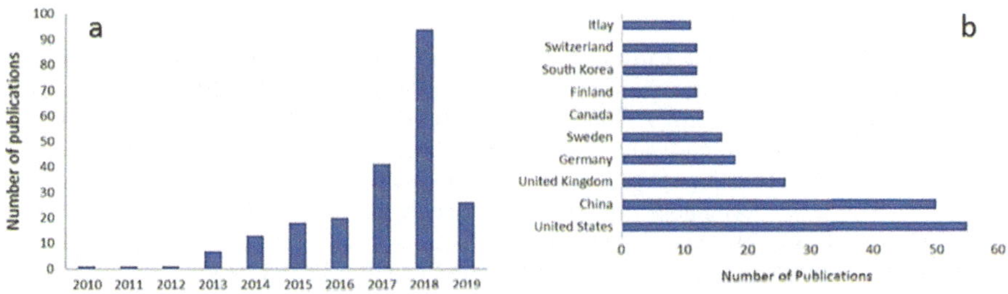

Fig. 5 Statistics from Scopus with keywords "cellulose" and "3D Printing". Number of publications versus **a** years and **b** countries

can also act as anchoring point for the in situ growth of other functional materials. After 3D printing of hydrogel ink, the scaffolds can be kept in wet state or are freeze-dried depending on its use and application area.

Being a biomaterial, nanocellulose has been a popular choice for biomedical applications. Furthermore, due the inherent shear thinning and anisotropy of nanocellulose, 3D printing has become a popular fabrication technique to produce nanocellulose-based scaffolds for biomedical applications [56, 85, 86]. 3D-printed scaffolds are commonly used in tissue engineering applications where interconnected porosity and controlled pore size have direct implications on their functionality both in vitro and in vivo. The clinical images can be used to design CAD files that allows the fabrication of 3D constructs that are customized for a particular patient, which reduces the rejection rate and speeds up the recovery [43].

The property of nanocellulose to form self-standing thermally stable films has been exploited for producing transparent and smooth substrates for 3D-printed electronics [87]. Nanocellulose can also be used as a matrix material for printing microfluidic devices [88].

Compared to traditional fabrication approaches, the 3D printing technology allows fabrication of complex and customized structures, in a layer-by-layer manner that improves the resolution and quality of the 3D construct. Moreover, untested geometric designs can be explored, for instance, a different directionality in each layer can be obtained as well as compositional and structural gradients are possible with multiple dispensing nozzles. In addition, living cells can be precisely positioned into specific locations of the scaffolds through 3D bioprinting.

Although rapid prototyping techniques may have several advantages, some challenges are there such as hydrogel swelling is an unavoidable feature that can reduce the resolution of the 3D-printed construct. Other challenges lie in CAD designing, slicing software and the nozzle movement. In our previous study, we have shown the importance of the nozzle movement [44]. It was observed that the using the same printing file, only a certain nozzle movement gave 3D cubic constructs with good print resolution.

References

1. Gupta V, Carrott P, Singh R, Chaudhary M, Kushwaha S (2016) Cellulose: a review as natural, modified and activated carbon adsorbent. Bioresour Technol 216:1066–1076
2. Moon RJ, Martini A, Nairn J, Simonsen J, Youngblood J (2011) Cellulose nanomaterials review: structure, properties and nanocomposites. Chem Soc Rev 40(7):3941–3994
3. Ummartyotin S, Manuspiya H (2015) A critical review on cellulose: from fundamental to an approach on sensor technology. Renew Sustain Energy Rev 41:402–412
4. Li M, Wu Q, Song K, Lee S, Qing Y, Wu Y (2015) Cellulose nanoparticles: Structure–morphology–rheology relationships. ACS Sustain Chem Eng 3(5):821–832
5. Guise C, Fangueiro R (2016) Biomedical applications of nanocellulose. In: Natural fibres: advances in science and technology towards industrial applications. Springer, pp 155–169
6. Lin N, Dufresne A (2014) Nanocellulose in biomedicine: Current status and future prospect. Eur Polym J 59:302–325

7. Spence KL, Venditti RA, Rojas OJ, Habibi Y, Pawlak JJ (2011) A comparative study of energy consumption and physical properties of microfibrillated cellulose produced by different processing methods. Cellulose 18(4):1097–1111
8. Wang B, Sain M (2007) Dispersion of soybean stock-based nanofiber in a plastic matrix. Polym Int. 56(4):538–546
9. Saito T, Kimura S, Nishiyama Y, Isogai A (2007) Cellulose nanofibers prepared by TEMPO-mediated oxidation of native cellulose. Biomacromol 8(8):2485–2491
10. Sultan S, Abdelhamid HN, Zou X, Mathew AP (2018) CelloMOF: nanocellulose enabled 3D printing of metal–organic frameworks. Adv Funct Mater 1805372.
11. Chinga-Carrasco G, Ehman NV, Pettersson J et al (2018) Pulping and pretreatment affect the characteristics of bagasse inks for three-dimensional printing. ACS Sustain Chem Eng 6(3):4068–4075
12. Missoum K, Belgacem M, Bras J (2013) Nanofibrillated cellulose surface modification: a review. Materials 6(5):1745–1766
13. Henriksson M, Henriksson G, Berglund L, Lindström T (2007) An environmentally friendly method for enzyme-assisted preparation of microfibrillated cellulose (MFC) nanofibers. Eur Polym J 43(8):3434–3441
14. Boldizar A, Klason C, Kubat J, Näslund P, Saha P (1987) Prehydrolyzed cellulose as reinforcing filler for thermoplastics. Int J Polym Mater 11(4):229–262
15. Dufresne A (2013) Nanocellulose: a new ageless bionanomaterial. Mater Today 16(6):220–227
16. Elazzouzi-Hafraoui S, Nishiyama Y, Putaux J, Heux L, Dubreuil F, Rochas C (2007) The shape and size distribution of crystalline nanoparticles prepared by acid hydrolysis of native cellulose. Biomacromol 9(1):57–65
17. Iguchi M, Yamanaka S, Budhiono A (2000) Bacterial cellulose—a masterpiece of nature's arts. J Mater Sci 35(2):261–270
18. Buldum G, Bismarck A, Mantalaris A (2018) Recombinant biosynthesis of bacterial cellulose in genetically modified escherichia coli. Bioprocess Biosyst Eng 41(2):265–279
19. Mishra RK, Sabu A, Tiwari SK (2018) Materials chemistry and the futurist eco-friendly applications of nanocellulose: status and prospect. J Saudi Chem Soc 22(8):949–978
20. Oksman K, Aitomäki Y, Mathew AP et al (2016) Review of the recent developments in cellulose nanocomposite processing. Compos Appl Sci Manuf 83:2–18
21. Islam MT, Alam MM, Zoccola M (2013) Review on modification of nanocellulose for application in composites. Int J Innov Res Sci Eng Technol 2(10):5444–5451
22. Thunberg J, Kalogeropoulos T, Kuzmenko V et al (2015) In situ synthesis of conductive polypyrrole on electrospun cellulose nanofibers: scaffold for neural tissue engineering. Cellulose 22(3):1459–1467
23. da Silva PM, Sierra-Avila CA, Hinestroza JP (2012) In situ synthesis of a cu-BTC metal–organic framework (MOF 199) onto cellulosic fibrous substrates: cotton. Cellulose 19(5):1771–1779
24. Favier V, Cavaille J, Canova G, Shrivastava S (1997) Mechanical percolation in cellulose whisker nanocomposites. Polym Eng Sci 37(10):1732–1739
25. Favier V, Canova G, Cavaillé J, Chanzy H, Dufresne A, Gauthier C (1995) Nanocomposite materials from latex and cellulose whiskers. Polym Adv Technol 6(5):351–355
26. Favier V, Chanzy H, Cavaille J (1995) Polymer nanocomposites reinforced by cellulose whiskers. Macromolecules 28(18):6365–6367
27. Trifol J, Plackett D, Sillard C et al (2016) A comparison of partially acetylated nanocellulose, nanocrystalline cellulose, and nanoclay as fillers for high-performance polylactide nanocomposites. J Appl Polym Sci 133(14)
28. Mariano M, El Kissi N, Dufresne A (2015) Melt processing of cellulose nanocrystal reinforced polycarbonate from a masterbatch process. Eur Polym J 69:208–223
29. Goussé C, Chanzy H, Excoffier G, Soubeyrand L, Fleury E (2002) Stable suspensions of partially silylated cellulose whiskers dispersed in organic solvents. Polymer 43(9):2645–2651
30. Xu W, Qin Z, Yu H et al (2013) Cellulose nanocrystals as organic nanofillers for transparent polycarbonate films. J Nanopart Res 15(4):1562

31. Mariano M, Dufresne A (2017) Nanocellulose: common strategies for processing of nanocomposites. Nanocelluloses Preparation Properties Appl 203–225
32. Gabr MH, Phong NT, Okubo K, Uzawa K, Kimpara I, Fujii T (2014) Thermal and mechanical properties of electrospun nano-celullose reinforced epoxy nanocomposites. Polym Test 37:51–58
33. Naseri N, Algan C, Jacobs V, John M, Oksman K, Mathew AP (2014) Electrospun chitosan-based nanocomposite mats reinforced with chitin nanocrystals for wound dressing. Carbohydr Polym 109:7–15
34. Naseri N, Mathew AP, Girandon L, Fröhlich M, Oksman K (2015) Porous electrospun nanocomposite mats based on chitosan–cellulose nanocrystals for wound dressing: Effect of surface characteristics of nanocrystals. Cellulose 22(1):521–534
35. Svagan AJ, Jensen P, Dvinskikh SV, Furó I, Berglund LA (2010) Towards tailored hierarchical structures in cellulose nanocomposite biofoams prepared by freezing/freeze-drying. J Mater Chem 20(32):6646–6654
36. Naseri N, Poirier J, Girandon L, Fröhlich M, Oksman K, Mathew AP (2016) 3-dimensional porous nanocomposite scaffolds based on cellulose nanofibers for cartilage tissue engineering: Tailoring of porosity and mechanical performance. R Soc Chem Adv 6(8):5999–6007
37. Karim Z, Mathew AP, Grahn M, Mouzon J, Oksman K (2014) Nanoporous membranes with cellulose nanocrystals as functional entity in chitosan: Removal of dyes from water. Carbohydr Polym 112:668–676
38. Oksman K, Mathew AP, Bondeson D, Kvien I (2006) Manufacturing process of cellulose whiskers/polylactic acid nanocomposites. Compos Sci Technol 66(15):2776–2784
39. De Menezes AJ, Siqueira G, Curvelo AA, Dufresne A (2009) Extrusion and characterization of functionalized cellulose whiskers reinforced polyethylene nanocomposites. Polymer 50(19):4552–4563
40. Ben Azouz K, Ramires EC, Van den Fonteyne W, El Kissi N, Dufresne A (2011) Simple method for the melt extrusion of a cellulose nanocrystal reinforced hydrophobic polymer. ACS Macro Lett 1(1):236–240
41. Gebhardt A (2012) Understanding additive manufacturing: rapid prototyping-rapid tooling-rapid manufacturing. Carl Hanser Verlag GmbH Co KG
42. Ambrosi A, Pumera M (2016) 3D-printing technologies for electrochemical applications. Chem Soc Rev 45(10):2740–2755
43. Bücking TM, Hill ER, Robertson JL, Maneas E, Plumb AA, Nikitichev DI (2017) From medical imaging data to 3D printed anatomical models. PLoS ONE 12(5):e0178540
44. Sultan S, Mathew AP (2018) 3D printed scaffolds with gradient porosity based on a cellulose nanocrystal hydrogel. Nanoscale 10:4421–4431
45. Siqueira G, Kokkinis D, Libanori R et al (2017) Cellulose nanocrystal inks for 3D printing of textured cellular architectures. Adv Func Mater 27(12):1604619–1604629
46. Compton BG, Lewis JA (2014) 3D-printing of lightweight cellular composites. Adv Mater 26(34):5930–5935
47. Studart AR (2016) Additive manufacturing of biologically-inspired materials. Chem Soc Rev 45(2):359–376
48. Zhu N, Chen X (2013) Biofabrication of tissue scaffolds. In: Advances in biomaterials science and biomedical applications. InTech
49. Lee JM, Yeong WY (2016) Design and printing strategies in 3D bioprinting of cell-hydrogels: a review. Advanced healthcare materials
50. Chung JH, Naficy S, Yue Z et al (2013) Bio-ink properties and printability for extrusion printing living cells. Biomater Sci 1(7):763–773
51. Chang R, Nam J, Sun W (2008) Effects of dispensing pressure and nozzle diameter on cell survival from solid freeform fabrication–based direct cell writing. Tissue Eng Part 14(1):41–48
52. Moberg T, Sahlin K, Yao K et al (2017) Rheological properties of nanocellulose suspensions: effects of fibril/particle dimensions and surface characteristics. Cellulose 24(6):2499–2510
53. Shin S, Park S, Park M et al (2017) Cellulose nanofibers for the enhancement of printability of low viscosity gelatin derivatives. BioResources 12(2):2941–2954

54. Lasseuguette E, Roux D, Nishiyama Y (2008) Rheological properties of microfibrillar suspension of TEMPO-oxidized pulp. Cellulose 15(3):425–433
55. Gladman AS, Matsumoto EA, Nuzzo RG, Mahadevan L, Lewis JA (2016) Biomimetic 4D printing. Nat Mater 15:413–418
56. Chinga-Carrasco G (2018) Potential and limitations of nanocelluloses as components in biocomposite inks for three-dimensional bioprinting and for biomedical devices. Biomacromol 19(3):701–711
57. Wang J, Chiappone A, Roppolo I et al (2018) All-in-One cellulose nanocrystals for 3D printing of nanocomposite hydrogels. Angew Chem Int Ed 57(9):2353–2356
58. Li VC, Dunn CK, Zhang Z, Deng Y, Qi HJ (2017) Direct ink write (DIW) 3D printed cellulose nanocrystal aerogel structures. Sci Rep 7(1):8018–8026
59. Lee KY, Mooney DJ (2012) Alginate: properties and biomedical applications. Prog Polym Sci 37(1):106–126
60. Duan B, Hockaday LA, Kang KH, Butcher JT (2013) 3D bioprinting of heterogeneous aortic valve conduits with alginate/gelatin hydrogels. J Biomed Mater Res, Part 101(5):1255–1264
61. Mertaniemi H, Escobedo-Lucea C, Sanz-Garcia A et al (2016) Human stem cell decorated nanocellulose threads for biomedical applications. Biomaterials 82:208–220
62. Ávila HM, Schwarz S, Rotter N, Gatenholm P (2016) 3D bioprinting of human chondrocyte-laden nanocellulose hydrogels for patient-specific auricular cartilage regeneration. Bioprinting 1:22–35
63. Henriksson I, Gatenholm P, Hägg D (2017) Increased lipid accumulation and adipogenic gene expression of adipocytes in 3D bioprinted nanocellulose scaffolds. Biofabrication 9(1):015022
64. Moller T, Amoroso M, Hagg D et al (2017) In vivo chondrogenesis in 3D bioprinted human cell-laden hydrogel constructs. Plast Reconstr Surg Glob Open 5(2):e1227
65. Markstedt K, Mantas A, Tournier I, Martínez Ávila H, Hägg D, Gatenholm P (2015) 3D bioprinting human chondrocytes with nanocellulose–alginate bioink for cartilage tissue engineering applications. Biomacromol 16(5):1489–1496
66. Håkansson KM, Henriksson IC, de la Peña Vázquez, Cristina et al (2016) Solidification of 3D printed nanofibril hydrogels into functional 3D cellulose structures. Adv Mater Technol 1(7):1600096
67. Rees A, Powell LC, Chinga-Carrasco G et al (2015) 3D bioprinting of carboxymethylated-periodate oxidized nanocellulose constructs for wound dressing applications. Biomed Res Int 2015(2015):925757–925764
68. Nguyen D, Hägg DA, Forsman A et al (2017) Cartilage tissue engineering by the 3D bioprinting of iPS cells in a nanocellulose/alginate bioink. Sci Rep 7(1):658
69. Müller M, Öztürk E, Arlov Ø, Gatenholm P, Zenobi-Wong M (2017) Alginate sulfate–nanocellulose bioinks for cartilage bioprinting applications. Ann Biomed Eng 45(1):210–223
70. Markstedt K, Escalante A, Toriz G, Gatenholm P (2017) Biomimetic inks based on cellulose nanofibrils and cross-linkable xylans for 3D printing. ACS Appl Mater Interfaces 9(46):40878–40886
71. Leppiniemi J, Lahtinen P, Paajanen A et al (2017) 3D-printable bioactivated nanocellulose-Alginate hydrogels. ACS Appl Mater Interfaces 9(26):21959–21970
72. Guillermo J, De L (2016) Cellulose nanofibril hydrogel tubes as sacrificial templates for freestanding tubular cell constructs. Biomacromol 17(3):905–913
73. Li Y, Zhu H, Wang Y et al (2017) Cellulose-Nanofiber-Enabled 3D printing of a carbon-nanotube microfiber network. Small Methods 1(10):1700222
74. Shao Y, Chaussy D, Grosseau P, Beneventi D (2015) Use of microfibrillated cellulose/lignosulfonate blends as carbon precursors: Impact of hydrogel rheology on 3D printing. Ind Eng Chem Res 54(43):10575–10582
75. Li VC, Mulyadi A, Dunn CK, Deng Y, Qi HJ (2018) Direct ink write 3D printed cellulose nanofiber aerogel structures with highly deformable, shape recoverable, and functionalizable properties. ACS Sustain Chem Eng 6(2):2011–2022
76. Wang B, Benitez AJ, Lossada F, Merindol R, Walther A (2016) Bioinspired mechanical gradients in cellulose nanofibril/polymer nanopapers. Angew Chem 128(20):6070–6074

77. Dong J, Li M, Zhou L et al (2017) The influence of grafted cellulose nanofibers and postextrusion annealing treatment on selected properties of poly (lactic acid) filaments for 3D printing. J Polym Sci Part B Polym Phys 55(11):847–855
78. Wang L, Gardner DJ, Bousfield DW (2018) Cellulose nanofibril-reinforced polypropylene composites for material extrusion: Rheological properties. Polym Eng Sci 58(5):793–801
79. Markstedt K, Sundberg J, Gatenholm P (2014) 3D bioprinting of cellulose structures from an ionic liquid. 3D Printing Addit Manuf 1(3):115–121
80. Schaffner M, Rühs PA, Coulter F, Kilcher S, Studart AR (2017) 3D printing of bacteria into functional complex materials. Sci Adv 3(12):eaao6804
81. Lehner BA, Schmieden DT, Meyer AS (2017) A straightforward approach for 3D bacterial printing. ACS Synth Biol 6(7):1124–1130
82. Jia C, Bian H, Gao T et al (2017) Thermally stable cellulose nanocrystals toward high-performance 2D and 3D nanostructures. ACS Appl Mater Interfaces 9(34):28922–28929
83. Wang J, Chiappone A, Roppolo I et al (2018) All-in-one cellulose nanocrystals for 3D printing of nanocomposite hydrogels. Angew Chem Int Edn. 57(9):2353–2356
84. Feng X, Yang Z, Rostom SS, Dadmun M, Xie Y, Wang S (2017) Structural, mechanical, and thermal properties of 3D printed L-CNC/acrylonitrile butadiene styrene nanocomposites. J Appl Polym Sci 134(31):45082
85. Sultan S, Siqueira G, Zimmermann T, Mathew AP (2017) 3D printing of nano-cellulosic biomaterials for medical applications. Curr Opin Biomed Eng 2:29–34
86. Xu W, Wang X, Sandler N, Willför S, Xu C (2018) Three-dimensional printing of wood-derived biopolymers: a review focused on biomedical applications. ACS Sustain Chem Eng 6(5):5663–5680
87. Hoeng F, Denneulin A, Bras J (2016) Use of nanocellulose in printed electronics: a review. Nanoscale 8(27):13131–13154
88. Shin S, Hyun J (2017) Matrix-assisted three-dimensional printing of cellulose nanofibers for paper microfluidics. ACS Appl Mater Interfaces 9(31):26438–26446

Chapter 2
Crosslinking Strategies to Develop Hydrogels for Biomedical Applications

Robin Augustine, Hashim Alhussain, Alap Ali Zahid, Syed Raza Ur Rehman, Rashid Ahmed, and Anwarul Hasan

Abstract Hydrogels can be defined as the networks of either chemically or physically crosslinked hydrophilic polymers containing large amounts of water when hydrated. They are usually used as biomaterials for various applications in the biomedical field. These applications vary from 3D cell culture and drug delivery to tissue engineering and regenerative medicine. The most important step in the development of hydrogel-based biomaterials is to make them stable under application conditions. Crosslinking of polymer chains using various approaches is utilized to stabilize the hydrogels and make them appropriate biomaterials. Mechanical and swelling characteristics of the developed materials mainly depend on the crosslinking density. Depending upon the specific requirements, different crosslinking strategies can be adopted. This chapter covers the available methods of crosslinking of polymers and preparing hydrogels. It also provides some of the advantages and disadvantages of each approach along with potential applications.

1 Introduction

Hydrogels are networks of crosslinked hydrophilic polymers with high water content when hydrated [1, 2]. They are extensively used in industrial applications including fast moving consumer goods (FMCG), cosmetics and biomaterials [3]. Due to their versatile properties and their high water-absorbing capacity, biocompatibility, temperature resistance, and sensitivity, they are used in various biomedical applications [4, 5] such as drug delivery [6, 7], wound dressings [8, 9], regenerative medicine and tissue engineering [10, 11].

R. Augustine (✉) · A. A. Zahid · S. Raza Ur Rehman · R. Ahmed · A. Hasan
Department of Mechanical and Industrial Engineering, College of Engineering, Qatar University, Doha, Qatar
e-mail: robinaugustine9@gmail.com; robin@robinlab.in

R. Augustine · H. Alhussain · A. A. Zahid · S. Raza Ur Rehman · R. Ahmed · A. Hasan
Biomedical Research Center (BRC), Qatar University, Doha, Qatar

J. Jose et al. (eds.), *Nano Hydrogels*, Gels Horizons: From Science to Smart Materials,
https://doi.org/10.1007/978-981-15-7138-1_2

Hydrogels are formed when the hydrophilic groups or segments in the polymeric network are hydrated in aqueous solutions [2]. In order to prevent the dissolution of the hydrophilic group in water or body fluid, crosslinking must be introduced between the polymer chains. Many different methods have been developed to achieve the effective crosslinking of polymers and generate hydrogels, which include physical, chemical, and natural methods. The degree of the crosslinking plays a key role in determining the physical properties of the developed hydrogel. A non-crosslinked hydrophilic polymer dissolved in solution will show a low viscosity; a limited crosslinking will result in an elastomer, whereas highly crosslinked polymers will be much more rigid [12, 13].

Biomedical applications usually require materials with sufficient mechanical properties and adequate stability in aqueous and physiological environments. Achieving such mechanical robustness while being biocompatible and biodegradable (in most cases such as tissue engineering) remains as one of the major challenges in the use of biopolymeric materials [14]. Crosslinking became the main solution to overcome this issue, as it improves the mechanical properties as well as the stability of the polymeric network by interconnecting individual macromolecular chains, and increasing the molecular weight [15]. Biodegradability is a key property that determines the application potential of many hydrogels used for therapeutic and biomedical applications [16]. To achieve this, often a labile bond which can be broken under physiological condition by enzymatic or chemical means is introduced between the polymer side chains or in the backbone of the polymer itself. The degradation products and their properties can be modulated to some extent if the hydrogel building blocks and crosslinking methods are selected properly.

In addition to the benefits, crosslinking may change the viscosity of the polymers, and the processing parameters will be different from non-crosslinked counterparts. Moreover, the crosslinked hydrogels show decreased degradability because of the reduced availability of functional groups to react with water and undergo hydrolysis [17–19]. Thus, crosslinking may sometimes lead to an increase in cytotoxicity and increased difficulties with the subsequent processing of the material [20].

The structure and properties of the hydrogel can vary depending upon crosslinking methods, duration of the crosslinking, and the conditions of crosslinking. As mentioned already, hydrogels can be crosslinked by different methods, such as physical, chemical, or biological. In the case of physical crosslinking, one or more physical interactions may exist between the polymer chains, preventing the polymeric network from dissembling in the aqueous environments. However, covalent bonds are generally formed between the different polymer chains in chemical crosslinking. Commonly used crosslinking methods for the preparation of hydrogels are described in the following sections.

2 Crosslinking by Physical Methods

Physically, crosslinked hydrogels do not require toxic chemical crosslinking agents. Such crosslinking agents can be harmful and cause several issues unless they are completely extracted from the hydrogel prior to use the use. In addition to that, chemical crosslinking agents can also affect integrity and stability of the entrapped bio-substance within the hydrogel. Due to all these disadvantages of chemical crosslinkers, physically crosslinked hydrogels received an increasing attention over the recent years.

2.1 Crosslinking by Ionic Interactions

Crosslinking of hydrogels with ionic interaction can be achieved under physiological or mild conditions at room temperature. A commonly used example of crosslinking polymers by ionic interaction is the crosslinking of polyuronates such as alginate and pectin [21]. Because of the biocompatibility and ease of gelation [22], calcium ions can be used to crosslink alginate [23]. The common biomedical applications of alginate hydrogel includes drug delivery, wound healing, tissue engineering, and it is often used as matrix for living cell encapsulation [24], and protein release [22, 23, 25]. The major advantage of this system is the possibility to generate stable hydrogels at physiological temperature and pH [26]. In this method, binding of bivalent cations such as Ca-ions to α-L-guluronic acid residues generate dimerizing junctions with other polymer chains that result in the formation of insoluble hydrogel networks. The resulting structure can be represented by the so-called eggbox model (Fig. 1). The gelation or crosslinking results in the stacking of the guluronic acid blocks of alginate chains. Further, the gel microparticles encapsulated with active agents can be stabilized by dropping a solution of sodium alginate and the protein/drug into an aqueous solution of calcium chloride. Controlled protein or drug release from the hydrogel microparticles can be achieved by coating the particles with cationic polymers such as polylysine [27] and chitosan [28, 29]. Costa et al. showed that crosslinking influences the structure and properties of alginate in terms of moisture content, solubility, mechanical properties, and water vapor permeability [30]. Crosslinking with high $CaCl_2$ concentrations resulted in the considerable increase in tensile strength.

Pectin is another natural polymer with similar chelating properties like alginate. Pectin can also be crosslinked using bivalent cations such as Ca^{2+}, Zn^{2+}, Mg^{2+}, etc. [32–35]. The interaction of ions and the carboxylate groups in pectin involves intermolecular chelate bonding of the cations, leading to the formation of macromolecular assemblies.

Plantago ovata husk mucilage (PHM)-blended Zn^{2+}-crosslinked low methoxy (LM) pectinate composite encapsulated with aceclofenac (ACF) was prepared by Guru et al. [36]. They successfully used this system for the controlled release of ACF in patients with rheumatoid arthritis and zinc deficiency. Hwang and Shin used

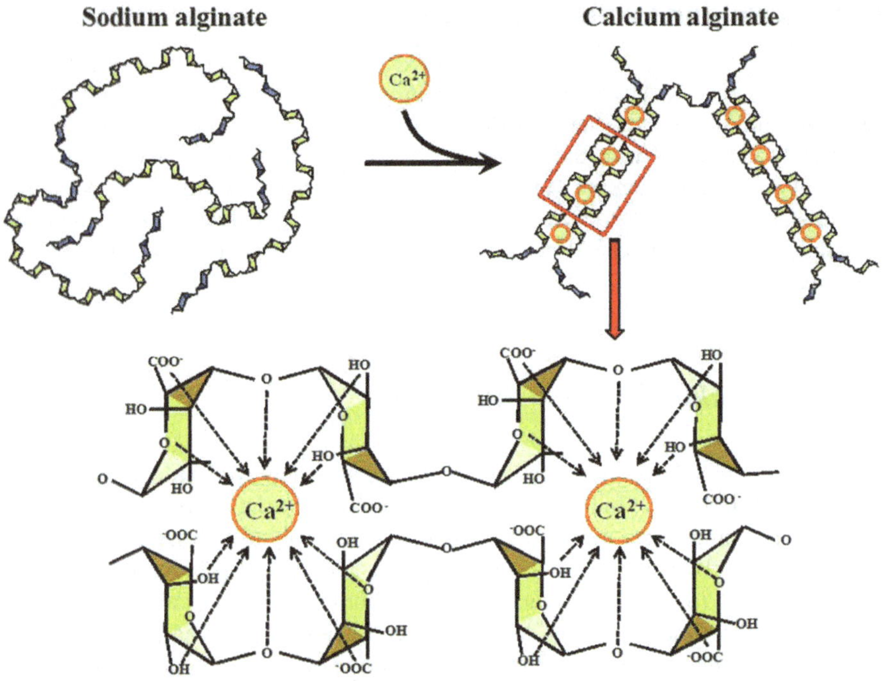

Fig. 1 Egg-box model of gelation of homopolymeric blocks of α-L-guluronic acid junction with calcium ions. Reproduced with permission from [31]

Mg^{2+} for the crosslinking of pectin; they prepared curcumin-loaded chitosan–pectin microparticles for delayed drug release [37].

Poly-[di(carboxylatophenoxy)phosphazene] (PCPP), is a synthetic polymer which is degradable under physiological condition when prepared as an ionotropic hydrogel. Similar to alginate, it can also be crosslinked with calcium ions. The degradation process can be tailored by introducing hydrolysis labile functional groups such as glycinato groups to the hydrogel [38]. The major advantage of PCPP in drug delivery is that the drug encapsulating efficiency of this polymer can reach upto 95% [39].

Chitosan is a natural biopolymer which can be obtained by chitin deacetylation [40]. It is widely used in biomedical applications such as wound dressings [41, 42], tissue engineering scaffolds [43], and drug delivery systems [44]. Crosslinking chitosan with glycerol-phosphate disodium salt is a biofriendly method to develop chitosan hydrogels. Below room temperature, chitosan solution remains aqueous in the presence of glycerol-phosphate disodium salt; however under physiological temperature (37 °C and above), it will quickly transform to a gel [45]. This transition from solution to a gel can be tuned by controlling the degree of deacetylation, which has an inverse relationship with the temperature required for sol–gel transition. The gelation time of chitosan/β-sodium glycerophosphate can be decreased, and the thermostability can be improved by introducing sodium bicarbonate to the hydrogel [46]. The major advantage of this hydrogel is its applicability as injectable thermogelling solutions containing proteins and cells which can solidify at the body temperature (37 °C). Mechanical properties of chitosan hydrogel can be further be improved by different modifications such as physical blending, chemical modification, and by using different crosslinking techniques [47]. Depending upon the crosslinking method, various viscoelastic properties such as the storage and loss modulus (G' and G'') of chitosan hydrogel may vary. Rheological study demonstrated that the gelation process appears to be governed by delicate interplay between the pH and the temperature. Rheological properties measured at low temperature (~10 °C), after the incorporation of β-GP reduced both G' and G'' compared to chitosan alone [48]. This might be due to the charge neutralization and increased flexibility of the polymer. Upon heating, from 5 to 70 °C, a rapid increase of G' indicated the gelation near 37 °C. After incubation at 37 °C for at least 60 min, rheological measurements indicated a nearly frequency independent G', while G'' increased slightly with the frequency as the general trend for hydrogel materials. Chitosan can also be crosslinked by oppositely charged low-molecular-weight anionic crosslinkers such as tripolyphosphate (TPP) [49].

Carrageenan is a natural seaweed polysaccharide which is composed of α(1–4) and β(1–3)d-galactose and different amounts of sulfate groups. This polymer can form gels in both salts containing (e.g., potassium ions) and salt-free conditions. However, gels formed in the presence of metallic ions were found to be stronger than those prepared under salt-free conditions [50]. Iota carrageenan under identical conditions of concentration and ionic strength can form gel with metal ions (K^+, Rb^+, Cs^+), and salt (NH_4^+) [51]. Swelling capacity of such hydrogels decreases with the increase of ionic salt solution in crosslinking solution [52].

Interestingly, the occurrence of cationic or anionic groups in the polymer chains is not a necessity for achieving crosslinking by ionic interaction. For instance, dextran, a polymer with no ionic binding sites for cations, can crosslink in the presence of potassium ions and form hydrogels. Watanabe et al. [53] showed that this is achieved by the formation of a cage-like structure by the oxygen atoms of glucose units of different dextran chains, and the perfect fitting of ionic radius of potassium inside this cage. However, this gel is not suitable for biomedical applications as it is relatively unstable under biological conditions.

Crosslinking anionic polymers using metallic ions is not the only way to prepare a hydrogel. Crosslinking of polyanions with polycations is another way to obtain a stable hydrogel. Chitosan-based biomaterials that are crosslinked ionically by the complex formation between chitosan and polyanions like polyphosphoric acid or dextran sulfate showed good stability under physiological conditions [54].

2.2 *Crosslinking by Crystallization*

2.2.1 Crosslinking by Crystallization in Homopolymer Systems

Polyvinyl alcohol (PVA) is a water-soluble synthetic polymer which can form hydrogels if crosslinked properly [55]. A mechanically weak gel will be gradually developed when aqueous solution of PVA is stored at room temperature. However, if the same aqueous solution underwent a freeze-thawing cycle, a strong and highly elastic gel could be formed [56]. Stability and rheological properties of PVA gel can be tuned by changing the temperature and time of the freeze-thawing cycle. Moreover, the number of freeze-thawing cycles, polymer molecular weight, and its concentration in the water influence the properties of the hydrogel. PVA crystallites formed during the freeze-thawing cycle are believed to be the reason for the gel formation by acting as a physical crosslinking centers in the polymeric network [57]. When prepared under optimum conditions, PVA hydrogel can be stable for about 6 months at 37 °C [58]. Polyvinyl alcohol/cellulose nanocrystals (PVA/CNC) prepared by freeze-thawing cycle showed an increased swelling, re-swelling, and adsorption properties which can be promising for water or fluid absorbing applications [59]. Formed protein crystals can be further crosslinked with agents such as glutaraldehyde [60]. A schematic representation of such crosslinking is given in Fig. 2.

PVA hydrogels prepared by crystallization also have important application in the biomedical field due to the lack of toxicity associated with crosslinking agents. PVA hydrogel encapsulated with bovine serum albumin (BSA) can be prepared by freeze-thawing crystallization. The protein was released by Fickian diffusion with its structure preserved [61]. Adding polymers such as alginate to the PVA solution before the freeze-thawing cycles enables the modulation of the hydrogel properties such as mechanical strength. Mechanical strength of the PVA hydrogel can be increased by increasing alginate concentration, this strengthening was associated with decreased release of drugs [62].

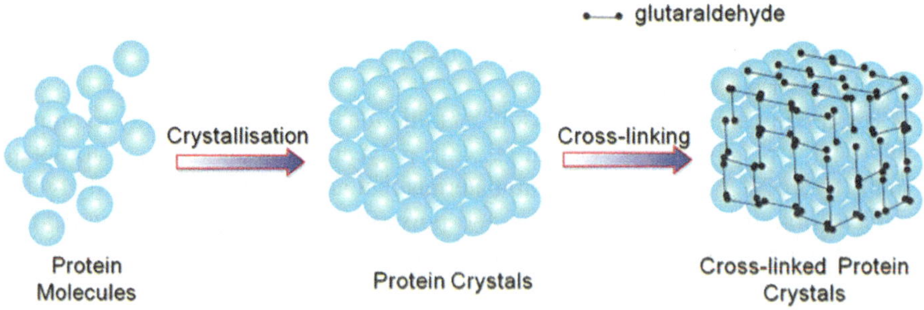

Fig. 2 A schematic illustration of the preparation process for crosslinked protein crystals. Reproduced from [60] with permission from The Royal Society of Chemistry

2.2.2 Crosslinking by Stereocomplex Formation

Stereocomplex is an intermolecular complex formed by macromolecules that share an identical chemical composition, but different configuration of repeating units [63]. Classical example of crosslinking by stereocomplex formation is the stereocomplex formation between enantiomeric PLA; poly(L-lactide) [i.e., poly(L-lactic acid) (PLLA)] and poly(D-lactide) [i.e., poly(D-lactic acid) (PDLA)]. PLLA and PDLA are semicrystalline homopolymer stereoisomers of polylactic acid. Both high molecular weight PLLA and PDLA have a melting temperature around 170 °C; however, blends of high molecular weight of the two stereoisomers have a melting temperature of 230 °C. This increase in melting temperature is ascribed to stereocomplex formation. Ikada and coworkers [64] were the first to report this ability of PLA to form stereocomplexes. Figure 3 shows the general mechanism of stereocomplex crosslinking of hydrogels.

Bare PLLA/PDLA stereocomplexes cannot be considered as hydrogels due to the low swelling behavior. However, stereocomplex formation can be established by the blends of PLLA-PEG-PLLA and PDLA-PEG-PDLA triblock copolymers which may enhance the swelling behavior. Lim and Park [65] studied BSA protein release from such triblock copolymers. They have compared the release of BSA from the microspheres of the triblock copolymers with BSA release from microspheres prepared with only one of the enantiomeric from of the triblock copolymers and with PLLA microspheres. A slightly larger burst release was observed in the stereocomplex triblock copolymer group in comparison to PLLA microsphere group. The higher water absorption capacity of the microspheres containing PEG might be the cause of the observed burst release. Lim et al. also developed another stereocomplex-based hydrogel system by grafting enantiomeric oligo(lactic acid) side chains on pHEMA (polyHEMA-g-oligo(1)lactate) [66].

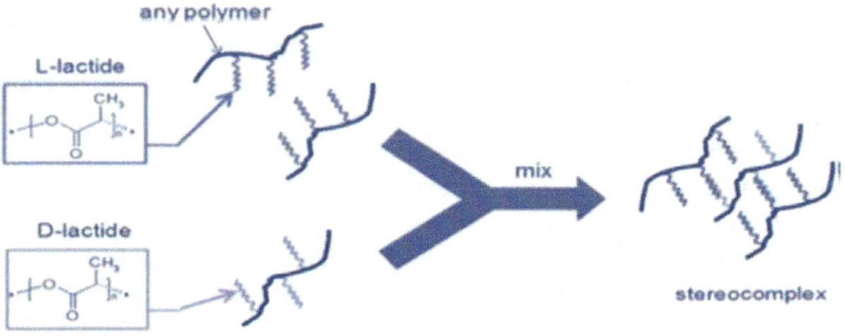

Fig. 3 Crosslinking of hydrogels by stereocomplex formation. Reproduced with permission from Taylor & Francis [67]

2.3 Physical Crosslinking of Amphiphilic Block and Graft Copolymers

In general, physically crosslinked hydrogels are assembled by graft or multi-block copolymers. Physically crosslinked thermo-responsive hydrogels are assembled via the entanglement of the polymer micelles. Such systems show higher biodegradability compared to chemically crosslinked hydrogels. Some copolymers such as graft copolymers and amphiphilic block copolymers have the ability to self-assemble in aqueous solutions to form hydrogels and other types of organized structures where the hydrophobic parts of the polymer are aggregated in the center [68]. Poly(N-isopropylacrylamide) (PNIPAM) and poly(p-phenylene oxide) (PPO) are thermoreversible polymers that are commonly used in such systems [69]. Such materials have the characteristic ability to crosslink physically and form gels near physiological temperature while maintaining low viscosity at low temperatures. PNIPAM which exhibits a lower critical solution temperature (LCST) around 33 °C remains as a transparent solution below 33 °C. They show low viscosity liquid behavior at room temperatures (below LCST); however, they can form a reversible hydrogel at body temperature. This makes them as excellent candidates for drug delivery systems [70]. PEG-PNIPAM is an example of thermosensitive physically crosslinked hydrogel based on block copolymers [71]. Linear and multi-arm PEG is the water-soluble central block whereas the thermosensitive terminal block is PNIPAM. In comparison with saline and single network delivery systems, PEG-PNIPAM double-network hydrogel showed significantly enhanced in vivo cell retention when used as the carriers of stem cells [72].

Using poly(lactic acid), glycolic acid and poly(ethylene glycol), several biodegradable block copolymers can be prepared. These copolymers can be used for drug delivery applications where the drug will be released either by passive diffusion or by degradation phenomena.

By combining two PEG–PLGA diblock copolymers, a triblock polymer can be prepared with PLGA segment which is the hydrophobic part being in the middle [70, 73, 74]. In this system, different outcomes can be achieved by varying the copolymer concentrations. They form micelles at low concentrations in water; however at higher concentrations, thermoreversible gels are formed. Upper critical solution temperature (UCST) and the critical gel concentration depend strongly on the composition of the blocks and the molecular weights.

By polycondensation of dicarboxylated PLA and PEG, multiblock copolymers of PEG and PLGA can be prepared [75, 76]. The temperature of phase transition depends on the molecular weight of PLA; polymers containing small PLA blocks show LCST behavior and are soluble in water. Some preliminary results indicated the preservation of basic fibroblast growth factor bioactivity in dried films of the multiblock copolymer as it improved wound healing in rats [76].

Feijen and team investigated multiblock copolymers of PEG and poly(butylene terephthalate) (PBT) which is another hydrophobic polyester [77–81]. These hydrogels are prepared by melt polycondensation of PEG, butanediol and dimethyl terephthalate where PBT hard domains form thermally reversible physical crosslinks. Lysozyme was loaded in the polymer as a model protein. The polymer solutions were prepared in a mixture of chloroform and hexafluoro isopropanol, followed by water-in-oil emulsion containing the protein in the aqueous phase [78]. It takes 3 days for the swelling of PEG/PBT films in water to reach equilibrium [77, 78]. Control over the release rate of the protein can be achieved by controlling the copolymer composition. Increasing molecular weight of PEG and increasing PEG/PBT weight ratio resulted in the increase of release rates. Other researchers loaded vitamin B12 (1335 Da) in multiblock copolymers composed of hydrophilic poly(ethylene glycol)-terephthalate (PEGT) blocks and hydrophobic PBT blocks [82]. The release can last from one day up to 12 weeks with a relatively constant release according to the copolymer composition. Increasing PBT content or increasing PEG molecular weight resulted in enhanced phase separation which influences the mechanical properties, degradation rates and swelling properties of the copolymers. Moreover, copolymer composition shows considerable effect on the physical properties and degradation behavior of poly(ethylene oxide) (PEO)-PBT copolymers [83].

2.4 Crosslinking of Polysaccharides by Hydrophobic Interactions

Chitosan, pullulan, carboxymethyl curdlan and dextran are some examples of polysaccharides used for assembling physically crosslinked hydrogels using hydrophobic modification approaches. Sunamoto and his group focused on cholesterol-bearing pullulan-based hydrophobized hydrogels [84–89]. Chitosan solutions containing glycerol-2-phosphate (β-GP), which undergoes temperature-controlled pH-dependent sol–gel transition at a temperature close to 37 °C, have recently been proposed by this approach [90].

For gene delivery, a modified hydrophobized glycol chitosan (HGC) was prepared by modifying a primary amine of glycol chitosan with 5β-cholanic acid [91]. DNA nanoparticles were formed spontaneously by hydrophobic interaction between HGC and hydrophobized DNA. In COS-1 cells, endocytic uptake of HGC nanoparticles was enhanced by increasing HGC content. In genetic engineering applications, HGC showed enhanced and superior transfection efficiencies both in vitro and in vivo. Another example of hydrophobic modified polysaccharide is glycol chitosan substituted with palmitoyl chains. In the presence of cholesterol, they form unilamellar polymeric vesicles [92] that are not only biocompatible, but also can entrap water-soluble drugs [93]. Upon freeze drying, a solid and highly porous material that can hydrate without swelling upto 20 times its dry weight in alkaline buffer was formed [94].

Qu et al. grafted chitosan with PLGA where the hydrophobic interactions in water resulted from the hydrophobic polyester side chains [95]. Changing the pH between 2.2 and 7.4 showed reversible water uptake. The highest swelling of this hydrogel was obtained with the lowest pH which is caused by the charge repulsion due to the protonation of the free amine groups in the polymer. Other examples of chitosan hydrogels which can respond to external conditions such as temperature and pH are poly(acrylic acid) (PAAc) [96] and poly(*N*-isopropylacrylamide) (PNIPAAm) [97]. Poly(*N*-vinylpyrrolidinone-*g*-styrene) hydrogels [98] and PMMA microemulsion particles [99] can also be developed by hydrophobic interactions.

2.5 Crosslinking by Hydrogen Bond Formation

Hydrogels physical crosslinking can also be achieved by hydrogen bonding. In this approach, by mixing two or more natural polymers, a gel-like structure can be prepared. Poly(acrylic acid) and poly(methacrylic acid) can form complexes with poly(ethylene glycol) by hydrogen bond formation between the oxygen of poly(ethylene glycol) and the carboxylic group of poly((meth)acrylic acid) [100]. Hydrogen bonding has also been observed in poly(methacrylic acid-*g*-ethylene glycol) [101, 102].

Injectable physically crosslinked hydrogels based on polymer systems such as gelatin–agar, starch–carboxymethyl cellulose and hyaluronic acid–methylcellulose can also be prepared by hydrogen bond formation. In such cases, the hydrogen bonds form only after protonation of the carboxylic acid groups which suggest a strong dependency of the swelling based on the pH. The issue with hydrogen-bonded gel-like structures is their fast collapse of gel structure which restricts their use to only relatively short acting drug release systems. Nagahara et al. made a DNA hydrogen bonding mimicking hydrogel in which crosslinking was established by hybridization [103]. To achieve this, they coupled oligodeoxyribonucleotides to a water-soluble polymer (poly(*N*, *N*-dimethylacrylamide-co-*N*-acryolyloxysuccinimide)). Xue et al. developed tissue mimicking composite hydrogels based on poly(acrylic acid)/surface-modified boron nitride nanosheets (PAA/BNNS-NH2) through molecular-scale metal coordination interaction between –COOH of PAA and Fe^{3+} and H-bond between –COOH of PAA and $–NH_2$ of BNNS-NH_2 (Fig. 4).

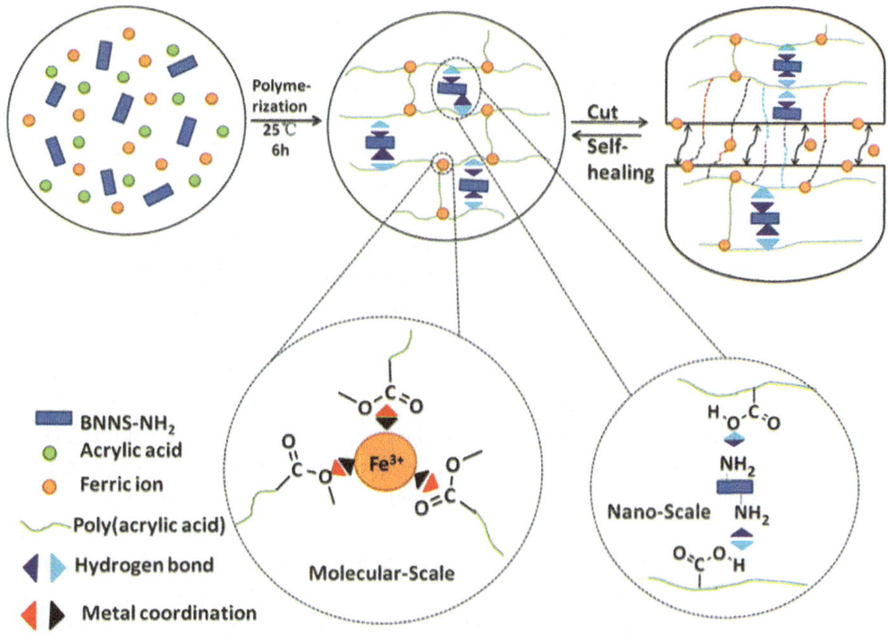

Fig. 4 Scheme illustrating the formation of a poly(acrylic acid)/surface-modified boron nitride nanosheets. Reproduced with permission from [104]

3 Crosslinking of Hydrogels by Chemical Methods

3.1 Crosslinking by Radical Polymerization

Radical polymerization method is used in the presence of suitable crosslinking agents to chemically crosslink low-molecular weight polymers like poly(2-hydroxyethyl methacrylate) (pHEMA). pHEMA was first described by Wicheterle and is a frequently studied hydrogel system in biomedical applications [105]. It can be fabricated by the polymerization of HEMA with a crosslinking agent (e.g., ethylene glycol dimethacrylate). Also, many other hydrogel system have been synthesized using this procedure [106]. Furthermore, by the addition of *N*-isopropylacrylamide (temperature-sensitive gels) [107] or methacrylic acid (pH-sensitive gels) [108], stimuli-sensitive materials can be obtained [109]. In addition to this, radical polymerization of vinyl monomers mixture, hydrogel can also be obtained by chemically crosslinking the water-soluble polymers by radical polymerization. For the design of hydrogel via this route, water soluble polymers like natural, synthetic and semi-synthetic polymers have been used. Particularly, dextran is a polysaccharide and is being used as a building block of degradable hydrogels. It consists of α-1,6 linked d-glucopyranose residues. Dextran (molecular weight between 40 and 100 kDa) has been used as a plasma expander and examined for the delivery of imaging agents, proteins and drugs. Furthermore, dextran-based gels are under investigation as a colon delivery system due to the presence of dextranase in the colon [110]. Edman et al. [111] have pioneered in the production of polymerizable dextran by reacting glycidyl acrylate with dextran dissolved in water to form a hydrogel. An initiator system consisting of ammonium peroxydisulfate and *N*, *N*, *N′N′*-tetramethylene-diamine was added to aqueous solution of the acryl dextran which contains *N*, *N*, -methylenebisacrylamide. By employing an emulsion polymerization technique, enzymes were immobilized with almost full retention of their activity in micro-spheres of polyacryldextran [112]. Using the method developed by Edman et al., some water-soluble polymers other than dextran were also functionalized with (meth)acrylic groups, e.g., hyaluronic acid [113], polyvinyl alcohol [114], poly-aspartamide [115–117], (hydroxyethyl) starch [118] and albumin [119]. Because of very low degree of substitution due to the reaction in an aqueous solution, it is difficult to control the degree of substitution due to the hydrolysis of glycidyl(meth)acrylate with water-soluble polymer before and after the reaction. Therefore, an alterna-tive method was used for the synthesis of methacylated dextran [10]. The glycidyl methacrylate functionalized dextran (Dex-GMA) were prepared by crosslinking in the presence of a crosslinker: N,N-methylene-bisacrylamide (NMBA), and a photoinitiator: 2,2-dimethoxy-2-phenyl acetophenone (DMPA) (Fig. 5) [120]. In addition to superior mechanical strength, developed Dex-GMA hydrogel exhibited good biodegradability.

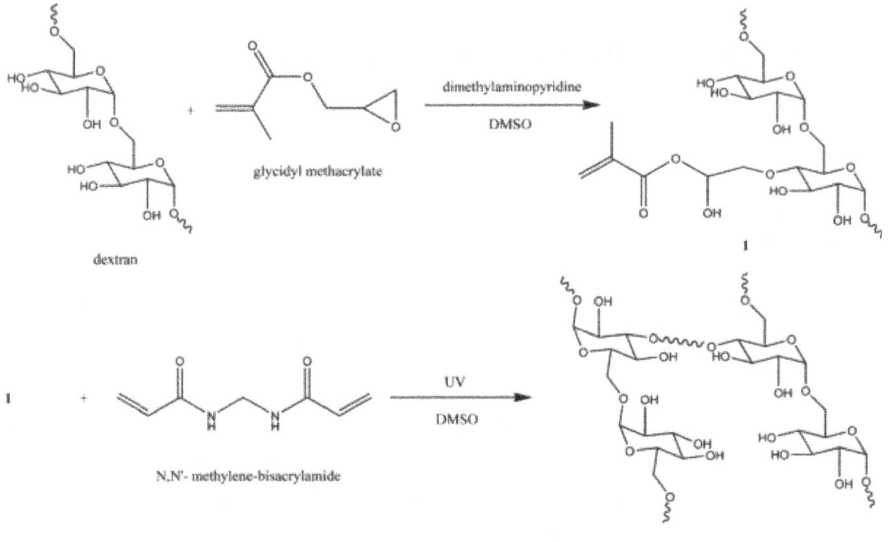

Fig. 5 Synthesis route of Dex-GMA hydrogel. Reproduced with permission from [120]

3.1.1 Free Radical Polymerization (FPR)

Free radical polymerization (FPR) is one of the most suitable polymer synthesis methods which require relatively moderate conditions and can be applied to a large number of monomers. In addition to its simple experimental setup, it has tolerance toward impurities, solvents and functional groups, and their purifying agents are easy to prepare and inexpensive. However, it is not possible to obtain polymer with narrow distribution of molecular weights and accurately defined end groups. For free radical polymerization of vinyl monomers on carbohydrate polymers, various initiation methods including thermal and photolysis, γ-radiation, Fenton's reagent, ceric ion and persulfate were examined. Ceric ion and persulfate with various organic compounds through a redox reaction create free radicals capable of initiating radical polymerization in tetravalent state (Ce^{4+}) [121–123]. γ-radiation produces macro-radicals on carbohydrate polymers using its high energy radiation [124]. In addition, Fenton's reagent generates hydroxy radicals by the redox reaction of ferrous ion (Fe^{2+}) with hydrogen peroxide [125]. Free radical polymerization of vinyl monomers can be initiated by macro-radicals on carbohydrate polymers produced by these initiation methods. However, there are some limitations associated with free radical polymerization method. FRP produces homo-polymer as a side product with attached copolymer and provides insufficient control over molecular weight distribution and molecular weight ($Mw/Mn > 2.0$) of attached vinyl polymers. Therefore, it is essential to limit those undesirable radical reactions that do not contribute in polymer chain growth in order to control the molecular structure of polymer chains. However, to control the radical polymerization, several procedures have been developed during the last 10–15 years [126].

Gelatin methacryloyl (GelMA) undergoes photoinitiated radical polymerization (i.e., under light exposure with the presence of a photoinitiator) to form covalently crosslinked hydrogels. Gelatin is the hydrolysis product of collagen and contains the key components of natural extracellular matrix like RGD (arginine-glycine-aspartic acid) peptides that enhance cell attachment [19]. GelMA can be synthesized by the substitution of the free amine groups of gelatin with methacrylate anhydride without losing the RGD sequences. Photocrosslinking of GelMA hydrogel can be done under UV light using a photoinitiator. A generalized scheme of the crosslinking process is given in Fig. 6. Hyaluronic acid methacrylate (HAMA) can be used as an optional component to make the gel more cell friendly. For crosslinking, most commonly used water-soluble initiators are lithium acylphosphinate salt (LAP) [127] and 2-hydroxy-1-[4-(2-hydroxyethoxy) phenyl]-2-methyl-1-propanone (Irgacure 2959) [128, 129]. Particularly, for photopolymerization in aqueous environments, Irgacure 2959 is being used, having higher solubility in water (up to 8.5 wt%) which is more than sufficient for the photopolymerization in aqueous environment. In addition, a water-soluble photoinitiator LAP has newly developed, which has higher molar extinction coefficient than Irgacure 2959 at 365 nm and comparable water solubility with Irgacure 2959 [28]. GelMA hydrogel has highly tunable physical properties. Some major parameters like UV exposure time, initiator concentration, degree of substitution and GelMA concentration can be changed for required physical properties

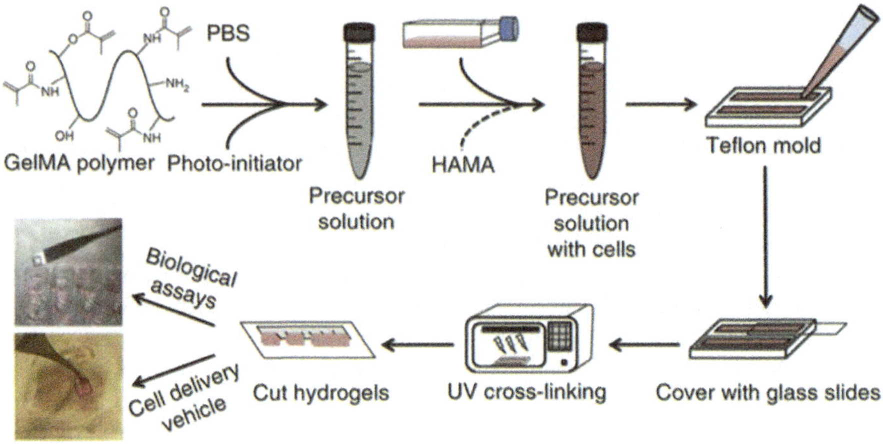

Fig. 6 Overview of the GelMA-based hydrogel preparation protocol [134]

of GelMA hydrogels. High crosslinking degree of polymer can be obtained at low concentration of photoinitiator within a minute or even second, which minimizes cytotoxicity. The proliferation and attachment of different cells in GelMA hydrogels have been widely characterized and established. GelMA hydrogels can be used in tissue engineering due to the acceptable mechanical properties, existence of bioactive peptide sequences and adequate biocompatibility [130]. For example, for the synthesis of cell-laden 3D hydrogels, cells can be suspended in GelMA prepolymer solutions and crosslinked upon exposure to UV light. Generally, in photocrosslinked cell-laden GelMA hydrogels, higher cell viability (upto 80%) was observed [131]. In a relatively similar approach, alginate hydrogels can be synthesized by the in situ photo-crosslinking of alginate polymers. Here also, polymers can be modified with functional groups (i.e., methacrylates) and then crosslinked with free radical polymerization under UV light in the presence of photoinitiator. This polymerization reaction provides an ideal environment for in situ encapsulation of cells under physiological conditions [132]. In contrast to the synthetic ethylene glycol derivatives, methacrylated alginate is more similar to the negatively charged mucopolysaccharides in cartilaginous tissues and has also been studied as platforms for tissue engineering applications [133]. Compared to ionically crosslinked alginate constructs, photocrosslinked alginate hydrogels have enhanced mechanical properties, ECM accumulation and structural integrity [132].

3.1.2 Controlled/Living Radical Polymerization

Controlled/living radical polymerization (CLRP) is a highly useful method for producing controlled molecular weight, chain architecture, polydispersity, composition and site-specific functionalities in hydrogels which cannot be generated by conventional free radical chemistries [135, 136]. All the steps in free radical polymerization reaction are also applied in controlled/living radical polymerization. However, to control the polymerization, a mediating species can be employed which in turn can aid in the formation of block copolymers, polymers with narrow molecular weight distributions and very short oligomers. Despite the successful implementation of controlled/living polymerization technique in bulk or solution polymerization, successful transmission of these polymerization reactions into aqueous dispersed phase system such as micro-emulsion, mini-emulsion and emulsion system is essential in order to produce these hydrogels at an industrially feasible scale. By employing CLRP approaches, hydrogel can be synthesized at much higher monomer and crosslinker concentrations. Due to the living nature of CRP, it is possible to achieve chain extensions after the addition of a second monomer batch. By this approach, the structural arrangement and features of the hydrogels can be controlled, and different forms of gels can be developed [137]. Moreover, the use of functional initiators facilitates the integration of functionalities in the core or at the surface of hydrogels which is not possible by conventional radical crosslinking polymerization (Fig. 7). This is particularly very useful when nano- or microgels for drug delivery applications are produced. Such surface functional groups can be used for the conjugation of biomolecules.

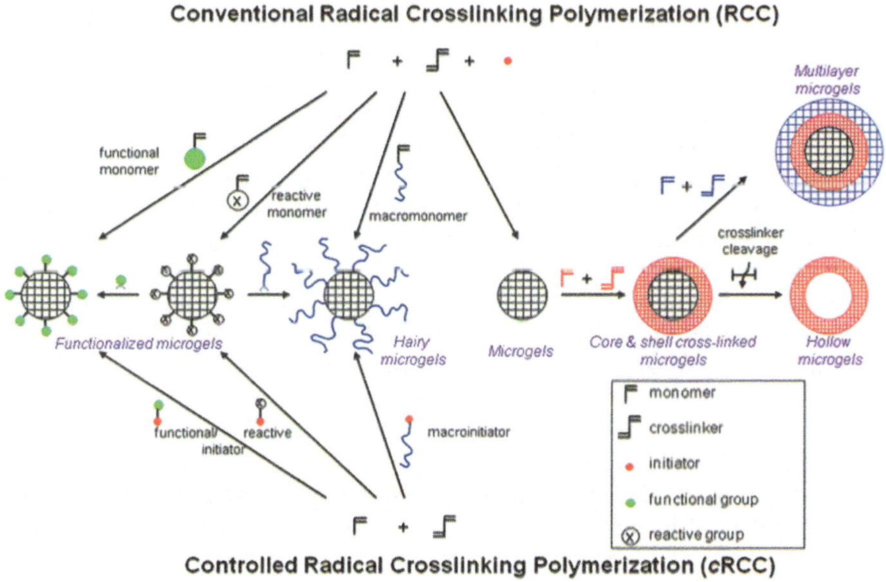

Fig. 7 Scheme showing the synthesis approaches for the preparation of nano- or microgels of different morphologies and functionalities by conventional and controlled radical crosslinking. Reproduced with permission from [137]

3.2 *Crosslinking by Chemical Reaction of Complementary Groups*

Several polymers show their aqueous solubility due to the presence of functional groups such as COOH, OH and NH_2. Covalent bonding between different polymer chains can be established by the reaction between such functional groups with complementary reactivity.

3.2.1 Crosslinking with Aldehydes

Crosslinking with aldehyde groups is a commonly used technique for the crosslinking of polymeric systems such as chitosan-PVA hydrogels. In the range of different aldehyde crosslinkers, glutaraldehyde is mostly used because it can attach with different functional groups in both proteins and carbohydrates. Glutaraldehyde crosslinking of hydrogels considerably increases the tensile strength. One of the drawbacks of glutaraldehyde crosslinked hydrogel is their higher cytotoxicity on mammalian cells. However, it can be reduced by optimizing crosslinking conditions such as pH and temperature.

Hydrogel can be prepared by the crosslinking of gelatin with polyaldehydes such as dextran dialdehydes [138]. Per-iodate oxidation of dextran (Dex) was used for the preparation of polyaldehyde derivatives. Since in dextran, the structural units contain three vicinal hydroxyl groups, the oxidation can lead to various types of aldehydes (Fig. 8a). The crosslinking was mainly due to Schiff base formation between amino groups of lysine and hydroxylysine residues of gelatin and the aldehyde (Fig. 8b). The fabricated gelatin hydrogel film was used in wound treatment where epidermal growth factor (EFG) was encapsulated to enhance wound healing. The dextran dialdehyde crosslinked hydrogels showed acceptable biocompatibility under both in vitro and in vivo conditions [139].

Partially depolymerized alginate produced by oxidation with poly(aldehyde guluronate) can be transformed into a hydrogel by crosslinking with adipic acid dihydrazide. Crosslinking with this crosslinker has improved the swelling and degradation rate of the gel [140]. Daunomycin, a cancer drug used for the chemotherapy, was incorporated in the hydrogel through covalent linkage. Because of the hydrolysis of this linkage, the drug was released in the time period between 2 days and 6 weeks [141]. Hyaluronic acid hydrogel can also be prepared by the crosslinking of hyaluronic acid with adipic dihydrazide. This reaction further proceeded with the crosslinking with a macromolecular crosslinker (poly(ethylene glycol)-propionaldehyde). The obtained hydrogels were enzymatically degradable and have shown anti-bacterial activity and manifested the controlled release of therapeutic drugs [142]. Wang developed an injectable hydrogel using a combination of hydrazine-modified elastin-like protein (ELP) and aldehyde-modified hyaluronic acid by dynamic covalent hydrazone bond formation (Fig. 9a, b) which can be performed at room temperature [143]. This hydrogel facilitated the successful

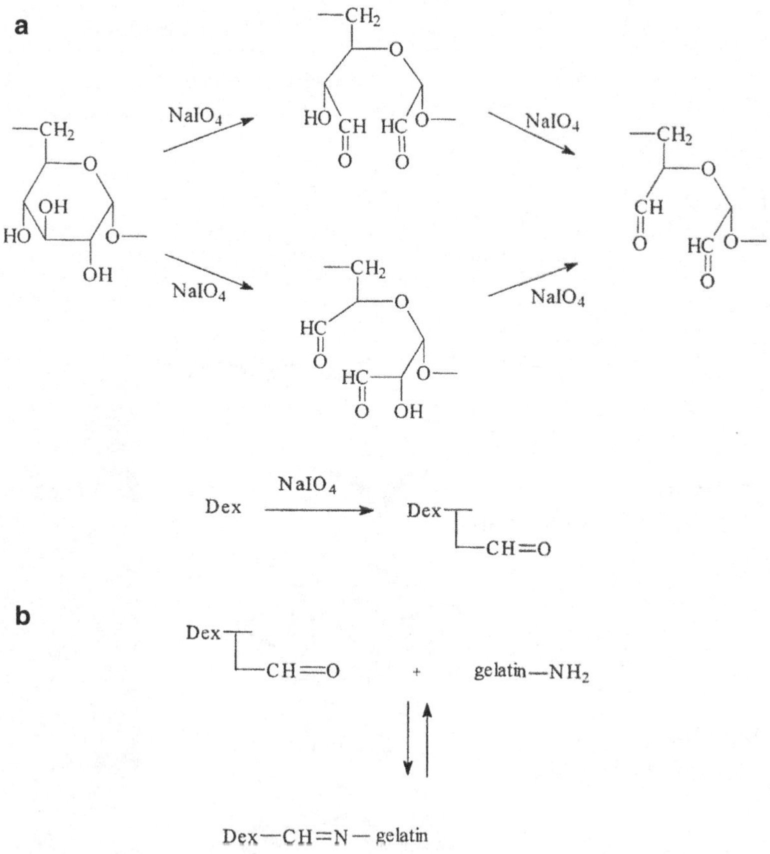

Fig. 8 Crosslinking of polymers containing gelatin dextran aldehyde. **a** Partial oxidation of dextran (Dex) for synthesizing dextran dialdehyde. **b** Crosslinking of gelatin. Reproduced with permission from [138]

injectability of stem cells (Fig. 5c). Developed hydrogels were able to support cell proliferation for three weeks post injection, and encapsulated cells maintained their ability to differentiate into multiple lineages.

3.2.2 Crosslinking by Addition Reactions

Hydrophilic polymers can be converted into hydrogels by using highly reactive crosslinking agents which react with the functional groups of polymers via addition reactions. Different crosslinkers have been used for crosslinking with polysaccharides such as 1,6-hexamethylene diisocyanate [144], divinyl sulfone [145], or 1,6-hexane dibromide [146] and many other chemicals. By using the addition reactions, the functional properties can easily be tailored by changing the concentration

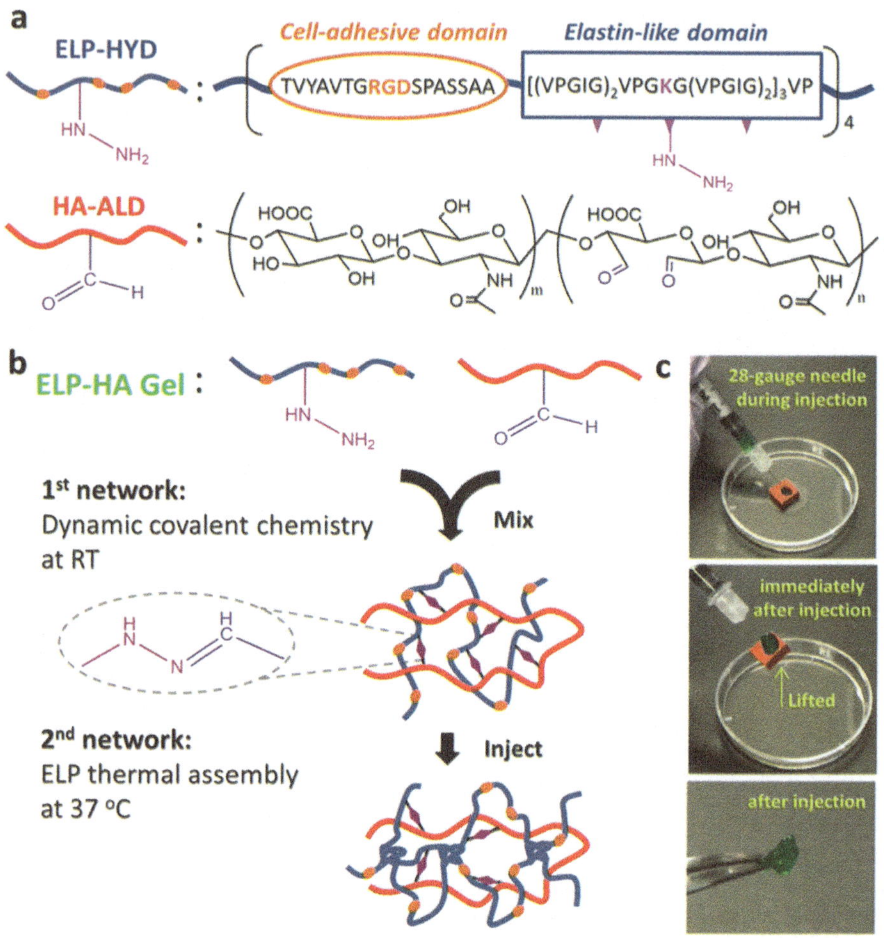

Fig. 9 **a** Elastin-like protein (ELP–HA) is composed of hydrazine-modified elastin-like protein (ELP-HYD) and aldehyde-modified hyaluronic acid (HA-ALD). **b** Schematic of ELP–HA hydrogel formation. **c** Photographs demonstrating the injectability and rapid self-healing of ELP–HA hydrogels. Reproduced with permission from [143]

of dissolved polymer and the quantity of crosslinker. Organic solvents are preferred over aqueous solutions for crosslinking to avoid the unfavorable reactions between water and crosslinker which affects polymer crosslinking. However, these organic solvents sometimes can leave their traces after the crosslinking. Therefore, it must be washed extensively to remove the unreacted traces of the crosslinker.

3.2.3 Crosslinking by Condensation Reactions

Crosslinking by condensation reactions is useful when polymer chains with hydroxyl, amines or carboxylic acid groups were used. They are commonly used for the synthesis of polymers to produce polyesters and polyamides. N,N-(3-dimethylaminopropyl)-N-ethyl carbodiimide (EDC) is one of the most frequently used crosslinkers to crosslink water-soluble polymers with amide bonds. Feijen et al. used this EDC crosslinker for the fabrication of gelatin hydrogels [147]. While the process of crosslinking incorporated *N*-hydroxysuccinimide (NHS) to reduce the possible side reactions which could give better crosslink density to the gels. This hydrogel was formulated as a drug delivery medium to provide the release of antibacterial proteins and later utilized in Dacron prosthetic valves. Moreover, the same EDC/NHS crosslinker can be used to crosslink collagen films where several fold increase in tensile strength and modulus can be achieved in crosslinked films [148]. In addition, swelling of the films was decreased significantly. In another research, Kuijpers et al. [149] have used a negatively charged polysaccharide, chondroitin sulfate to enhance the loading capacity. In earlier studies, researchers have used the ionic crosslinking approach to crosslink alginate gels to obtain better mechanical properties; however, the degree of crosslinking was limited. Then, Mooney et al. used EDC chemistry to covalently crosslink alginate and PEG diamines where the mechanical properties could be controlled by changing the quantity of PEG diamines in the gel [150].

Hydrolysable polyrotaxane have been used to crosslink PEG hydrogels where α-cyclodextrins (α-CD) were joined by a PEG chain and capped with bulky and degradable ester end groups [151]. After that, hydroxyl groups of the cyclodextrins can be activated via carbonyldiimidazole, and subsequently, PEG bisamines can be crosslinked with it. Because of the hydrolysis of the ester groups, the prepared gel was degraded steadily. However, the degradation period of the gel can be controlled by its composition. Figure 10 shows the preparation of cationic PEG hydrogels crosslinked by the hydrolysable polyrotaxane. The developed gel was used as a scaffold for soft tissue regeneration.

3.3 Crosslinking by High Energy Irradiation

High energy irradiation technique has been used widely to crosslink different polymers. Recently, collagen films with the formulation of glucose have successfully been crosslinked with UV irradiation. The idea is based on the fact that when UV irradiation hits the target sample, it can generate free radicals. This free radicals react with linear glucose molecules which could facilitate the crosslinking [148]. UV crosslinking has improved the mechanical properties and reduced enzymatic degradation of collagen [148]. Usually, high energy radiation, such as gamma and electron beam, has been used to polymerize unsaturated compounds. Furthermore, high energy irradiation was used to crosslink water-soluble polymers synthesized

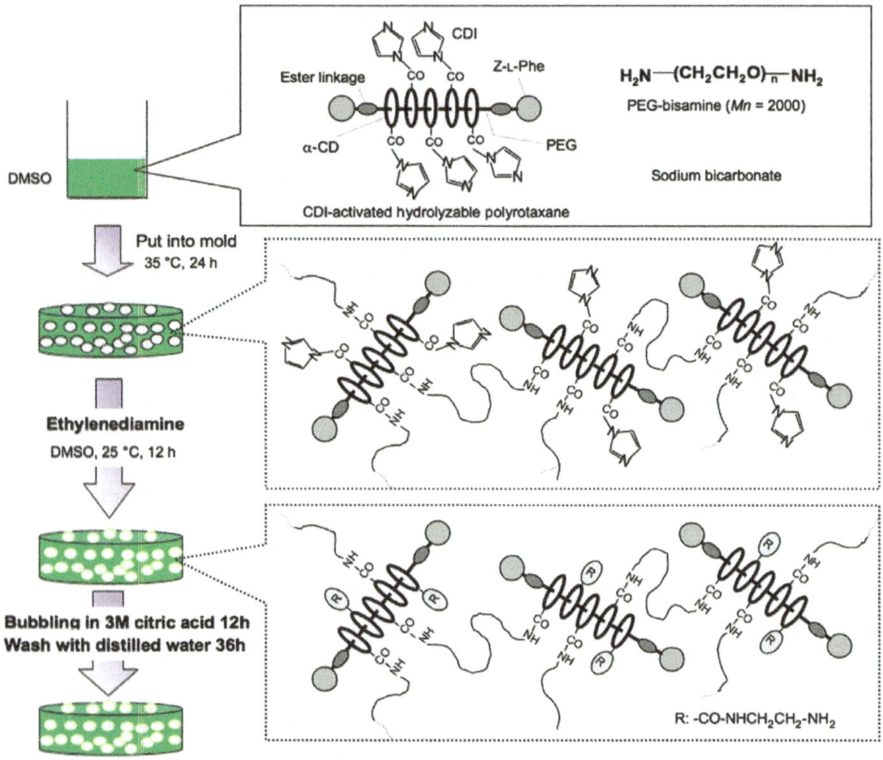

Fig. 10 Preparation of cationic PEG hydrogels crosslinked by the hydrolysable polyrotaxane. Reproduced with permission from [152]

from vinyl groups to form hydrogels [106]. It can also crosslink the water-soluble polymers in the absence of vinyl groups. PVA [153], GelMA [130], poly(acrylic acid) [154] and PEG [155–157] can be crosslinked with high energy irradiation. The swelling, degradation and other properties of the formed hydrogel are dependent on the concentration of polymer and the radiation time. In an interesting study, poly(amino acid)-based hydrogel was developed by crosslinking polypentapeptides with gamma irradiation [158]. High energy irradiation-based crosslinking can be performed in aqueous conditions at specific temperature and/or pH. In addition, the toxicity associated with chemical crosslinking agents can be avoided. However, biologically active drugs/materials can be incorporated only after the irradiation because the radicals generated during the exposure may damage the biologically active compounds.

4 Crosslinking Using Enzymes

Crosslinking of hydrogels by proteins especially by enzymes has been emerged as one of the most useful technique for developing hydrogels for biological applications. Hydrogels crosslinked with chemical agents show toxicity to the cells due to the presence of reactive free functional groups and unreacted chemicals. Another advantage of enzymatic crosslinking is that this can be performed at mild biological conditions. Crosslinking of hydrogels by enzymes such as transferases, tyrosinases and lysyl oxidases makes them excellent vehicles for controlled drug release [159]. In the presence of calcium, transglutaminase enzyme catalyzes covalent bond formation between lysine and glutamine residues in in vivo conditions during wound healing as well as extracellular matrix stabilization and organization [160]. This crosslinking potential of transglutaminase family was later employed for the synthesis of poly(ethylene glycol) hydrogel [161] and elastin-like protein polymers [162]. Transglutaminase crosslinked carboxymethyl chitosan/carboxymethyl cellulose/collagen composite membranes have shown enhanced mechanical properties and improved biodegradability [163]. Westhaus and Messersmith designed a hydrogel system [164] based on a mixture of fibrinogen and Ca-loaded liposomes which was crosslinked with Ca^{2+}-dependent transglutaminase enzyme. This remained as fluid at room temperature, but as soon as the mixture was warmed to higher temperature (37 °C only), gelling process started leading to the formation of a hydrogel. Such hydrogels may find application in thermoresponsive drug delivery systems. Sperinde and Griffith reported that addition of transglutaminase enzyme in lysine end-functionalized PEG polymers can result in the formation of hydrogels [165]. In another study, a two step crosslinking method composed of the enzymatic crosslinking and Diels–Alder (DA) click chemistry was adopted to prepare injectable hyaluronic acid/PEG (HA/PEG) hydrogel system [166]. The enzymatic crosslinking resulted in the formation of HA/PEG injectable hydrogel within short time due to faster gelation of polymers. Furthermore, use of DA click reaction attributed remarkable anti-fatigue and shape retaining properties. In addition to the improvement in mechanical strength and modulus, hydrogels displayed desirable compressive strain recovery properties.

Horseradish peroxidase (HRP) is commonly used as di-tyrosine crosslinker between silk fibroin proteins [167]. Similar method of crosslinking was used to develop tyramine-substituted hyaluronic acid (HA) bioactive hydrogels, but it possesses poor mechanical properties and stability leading to rapid degradation. Therefore, HA was covalently crosslinked with silk fibers resulting in the formations of composite hydrogels that possessed improved mechanical stability and good hydrophilicity [168]. In these HA silk fiber hydrogel assemblies, increase in HA concentration resulted in decreased gelation time and increased degradation rate. This offers controllable stiffening and elasticity characteristics which could be highly advantageous in tissue engineering applications. Yang et al. prepared gelatin hydrogels using multiple crosslinking agents comprising of genipin (GP), glutaraldehyde (GTA), 1-ethyl-3-(3-dimethyl aminopropyl) carbodiimide (EDC) and microbial transglutaminase (mTG) [169]. Hydrogels developed using GTA and GP as crosslinking agents showed very high compressive moduli, whereas EDC crosslinked sponges (hydrogels) displayed fast degradation rate. In addition, GTA and GP crosslinked sponges showed immediate rejection during in vivo trials, whereas GP crosslinked sponges showed poor growth of adipose derived stromal cells during in vitro experiments. mTG–sponge displayed desirable properties with enough porosity, durability, improved compressive modulus and good biocompatibility. In another study, transglutaminase crosslinked collagen hydrogels were fabricated to mimic native extracellular matrix architecture [170]. HRP crosslinkable injectable hydrogel based on poly(L-glutamic acid)-graft-tyramine (PLG-g-TA) was developed to explore the behaviors of BMSCs during three-dimensional (3D) culture. A fast geleation was observed after subcutaneous injection of PLG-g-TA, HRP and H_2O_2-based hydrogel. The histological analysis of the tissues at the application site after different time points demonstrated its biocompatibility [171]. Such systems may also find applications in cardiac tissue repair [172]. It can also be used as a cell carrier [173], drug delivery system and wound healing patches [174–176]. The biocompatibility of this hydrogel system is a great advantage and major factor for its potential use in biomedical applications [177, 178].

Tyrosinase (Tyr) is a copper-containing enzyme present in both plants and animal tissues that catalyze the production of pigments from tyrosine by oxidation. Tyrosinase catalyzes oxidation of phenols into activated quinones [179] in the presence of copper co-factor and O_2. These activated quinones can react with hydroxyl group or amino group of polymers by Michael-type addition reaction and form hydrogels [180]. Chen et al. [181] compared the effects of tyrosinase or transglutaminase enzymes on the formation of gelatin and chitosan hydrogels and concluded that tyrosinase induced faster gelation as compared to transglutaminase.

In another work, gelatin-based tissue adhesive hydrogels were prepared by dual-enzymatic crosslinking using HRP and Tyr (Fig. 11) [182]. Here, Tyr convert phenol groups of gelatin derivatives into *o*-quinone, which can react with amines or thiols on tissue surfaces and facilitate tissue adhesion. Incorporating tyrosinase did not affect the gelation rate or mechanical strength of HRP-crosslinked hydrogels. Importantly, the dual-enzymatically crosslinked hydrogels (GH/HRP/Tyr) exhibited significantly improved adhesive strength (34 kPa), which was superior to single HRP-crosslinked hydrogels (GH/HRP; 19 kPa) and commercially available fibrin glues (7 kPa). Thus, dual-enzymatic crosslinking of gelatin-based hydrogels could be a promising approach to develop bio-adhesives for tissue engineering or surgical applications.

5 Crosslinking by Natural Crosslinking Agents

Natural crosslinking agents not only improve the thermal stability of hydrogels but also enhance their biocompatibility with biological systems. Crosslinking of collagen films by proanthocyanidin (PA), a polyphenol found in grape seeds, not only

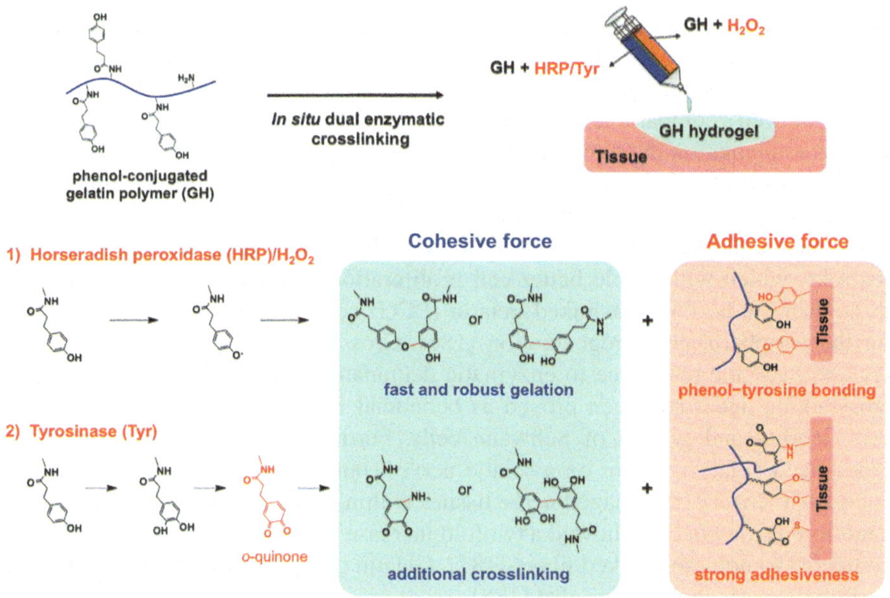

Fig. 11 Schematic showing the development of GH hydrogels by dual-enzymatic crosslinking using HRP and Tyr. Reproduced with permission from [182]

improves the thermal resistance but also enhances its resistance to enzymatic degradation without disturbing their cytocompatibility [183]. PA-crosslinked collagen membranes after several weeks of subcutaneous implantation displayed significantly greater penetration of fibroblasts without causing any damage to nearby native tissues.

Genipin can also be used for crosslinking hydrogels and making stable biomaterials. For example, genipin was used to crosslink chitosan, bovine serum albumin (BSA), and gelatin [184]. The results obtained through several spectroscopic techniques demonstrated that primary amine groups were crosslinked with two types of chemical reactions. The first reaction was a nucleophilic attack on genipin by a primary amine group of chitosan. This resulted in the formation of a heterocyclic compound of genipin that was bonded to the glucosamine residue in chitosan as well as the basic residues of gelatin and BSA. The second reaction involved a nucleophilic substitution of ester group of genipin leading to the formation of a secondary amide linkage among gelatin, chitosan and BSA. The rheological behavior of chitosan solutions changes with amount of genipin used [185]. The stress and frequency sweeps were used to find out G' of the crosslinked hydrogels. Results of this study shows that solutions of chitosan crosslinked with genipin could form strong and stable flexible gels when compared to those of pure chitosan.

Additionally, proanthocyanidin (PA) was selected as a natural crosslinking agent to crosslink biopolymers in biological tissues [183]. The evaluation of crosslinking and degradation rate besides cytotoxicity testing of PA on fixed tissues showed very interesting results. The cytotoxicity studies showed that PA crosslinked tissues are

~120 times less toxic compared to the tissues where glutaraldehyde (GA) was used as the crosslinking agent. The fixed tissues displayed marked resistance to bacterial collagenase digestion during in vitro studies. Unlike fresh tissues, PA crosslinked tissues showed a comparable stability with that of GA crosslinked tissues after subcutaneous implantation in animal models. Unlike GA counterparts, PA fixed implants started to degrade after six weeks of implantation which led to the migration and subsequent proliferation of fibroblasts into the PA fixed implants. Therefore, PA crosslinked collagen matrices could be very useful for designing tissue engineering scaffolds which will enable better cell proliferation and encourage cell ingrowth. In another study, PA crosslinked gelatin (PCG) conduit was developed and used for the peripheral nerve regeneration [186]. Crosslinking of gelatin conduit with PA improved the resistance to enzymatic degradation. In addition, use of PA as a crosslinking agent has been proved as beneficial for the enhanced cell adhesion, cell viability and growth of Schwann cells. Furthermore, the application of PA crosslinked gelatin conduit on a sciatic nerve wound (10 mm) in rat resulted in a complete recovery of damaged nerve tissues within 8 weeks. PA crosslinked gelatin nanofibrous membranes showed a twofold increase of L929 fibroblast cell adhesion compared to non-crosslinked fibers [187]. Gelatin crosslinked with PA can be used in drug delivery applications also [188].

6 Challenges in Hydrogel Crosslinking

Hydrogels provides a vast variety of biomedical applications ranging from drug delivery to tissue engineering. There are several methods used for the crosslinking of hydrogels to make them suitable for biomedical applications. However, there are many disadvantages and limitations for such methods too. The major disadvantage is that several crosslinking methods are not adequate to provide enough mechanical properties and stability under physiological conditions. For examples, they start breaking up immediately, especially when they are placed in the aqueous medium due to the collapsing of gel-like structure. This is particularly more evident in hydrogels that are crosslinked by physical methods. This is because, in physically crosslinked gels, interactions between polymers chains in amphiphilic block and graft copolymers are established by ionic and/or hydrophobic interactions, or crystallization which can be weakened under physiological conditions. In order to improve their stability and mechanical properties, crosslinking with a chemical agent is preferred to enhance their lifetime. However, cytotoxicity associated with the chemical crosslinking agents is a major disadvantage of chemically crosslinked hydrogels. Cytotoxicity of chemical crosslinkers such as glutaraldehyde is dependent on the concentration of crosslinking agents used [189]. Apart from glutaraldehyde, several other agents including epichlorohydrin, carbodiimide and sodium metaphosphate have also been used for the crosslinking of biopolymers, but they show limited improvement in properties owing to their low crosslinking efficiency. There are other methods of crosslinking of hydrogels such as those using ionic radiations. On one hand, these types of crosslinking methods have the advantage of reversibility and lack of potentially harmful chemical reactions that affect the incorporated bioactive agents or cells. On the other hand, their stability in vivo might be severely affected by biochemical as well as mechanochemical conditions. For instance, conditions including application in weight bearing regions, for example in the bone and joints, for which these gels might provide insufficient mechanical strength.

For the successful encapsulation of human cells in hydrogels, they should be completely biocompatible. Moreover, the crosslinking agents and crosslinking conditions should be cell friendly. But, most of the crosslinking agents and conditions currently used are not favorable to maintain the cells at a viable state. In addition, a quick gelation of the polymer is very important, especially when techniques like bioprinting are used [190]. Another important issue is the lack of enough porosity under swollen state where porosity is very important for the cell migration and to facilitate fluid transport.

Crosslinked hydrogels are extensively used in drug delivery applications. However, when the delivery of small hydrophilic molecules is concerned, hydrogels show a burst release of drugs which may create transient higher plasma drug concentration and results in adverse effects. So, future research should focus on the development alternative approaches to encapsulate small molecule in hydrogel network such as increasing the crosslinking density.

7 Conclusions

Hydrogels are synthesized either from natural or synthetic polymers by crosslinking with various methods such as physical, chemical and biological approaches. The physical hydrogels are developed by reversible crosslinking while chemical hydrogels are made by irreversible covalent bond formation. For the encapsulation of biomolecules such as growth factors and living cells, physically crosslinked gels are popular since it can be performed under simulated physiological conditions. However, for fabricating highly stable and rigid hydrogels for applications such as bone tissue engineering, chemical crosslinking approaches are inevitable. In order to avoid the disadvantages of chemical crosslinking agents, relatively nontoxic crosslinking agents and processes were developed. Enzymatic crosslinking uses various enzymes that can facilitate the interaction between end functional groups in polymer chains and can be performed under mild conditions. Also, natural agents might contribute to the development of nontoxic hydrogel systems and thus provide the full advantage of their application potential in health care. Finally, it can be expected that smart hydrogels which will be developed in near future in which triggered gelation and gel collapsing will find great applications in controlled drug delivery and tissue engineering.

Acknowledgements This article was made possible by the NPRP9-144-3-021 grant funded by Qatar National Research Fund (a part of Qatar Foundation). The statements made here are the sole responsibility of authors.

References

1. Hoffman AS (2012) Hydrogels for biomedical applications. Adv Drug Deliv Rev 64:18–23. https://doi.org/10.1016/J.ADDR.2012.09.010
2. Hennink WE, van Nostrum CF (2012) Novel crosslinking methods to design hydrogels. Adv Drug Deliv Rev 13–36
3. Augustine R, Rajendran R, Cvelbar U, Mozetič M, George A (2013) Biopolymers for health, food, and cosmetic applications. In: Handbook of biopolymer-based materials: from blends and composites to gels and complex networks, pp 801–849
4. Bahrami MK, Mahdavinia GR (2016) Carrageenan-based semi-IPN nanocomposite hydrogels: swelling kinetic and slow release of sequestrene Fe 138 fertilizer. Azarian J Agric 3:1–10
5. Chen S, Lu X (2016) Smart materials as forward osmosis draw solutes. In: Wang P (ed) Smart materials for advanced environmental applications. Royal Society of Chemistry, pp 19–50
6. Merino S, Martín C, Kostarelos K, Prato M, Vázquez E (2015) Nanocomposite hydrogels: 3D polymer-nanoparticle synergies for on-demand drug delivery. ACS Nano 9:4686–4697. https://doi.org/10.1021/acsnano.5b01433
7. Sosnik A, Augustine R (2016) Challenges in oral drug delivery of antiretrovirals and the innovative strategies to overcome them. Adv Drug Deliv Rev 103:105–120. https://doi.org/10.1016/j.addr.2015.12.022
8. Kamoun EA, Kenawy ERS, Chen X (2017) A review on polymeric hydrogel membranes for wound dressing applications: PVA-based hydrogel dressings. J Adv Res 8:217–233
9. Augustine R, Kalarikkal N, Thomas S (2014) Advancement of wound care from grafts to bioengineered smart skin substitutes. Prog Biomater 3:103–113. https://doi.org/10.1007/s40204-014-0030-y
10. Stapleton F, Stretton S, Papas E, Skotnitsky C, Sweeney DF (2006) Silicone hydrogel contact lenses and the ocular surface. Ocul Surf 4:24–43. https://doi.org/10.1016/S1542-0124(12)70262-8
11. Yang J, Zhang YS, Yue K, Khademhosseini A (2017) Cell-laden hydrogels for osteochondral and cartilage tissue engineering. Acta Biomater 57:1–25. https://doi.org/10.1016/j.actbio.2017.01.036
12. Zhao X (2014) Multi-scale multi-mechanism design of tough hydrogels: building dissipation into stretchy networks. Soft Matter 5:672–687. https://doi.org/10.1039/c3sm52272e
13. Li CH, Wang C, Keplinger C, Zuo JL, Jin L, Sun Y, Zheng P, Cao Y, Lissel F, Linder C, You XZ, Bao Z (2016) A highly stretchable autonomous self-healing elastomer. Nat Chem 8:618–624. https://doi.org/10.1038/nchem.2492
14. Augustine R, Kalarikkal N, Thomas S (2016) Effect of zinc oxide nanoparticles on the in vitro degradation of electrospun polycaprolactone membranes in simulated body fluid. Int J Polym Mater Polym Biomater 65:28–37. https://doi.org/10.1080/00914037.2015.1055628
15. Reddy N, Reddy R, Jiang Q (2015) Crosslinking biopolymers for biomedical applications. Trends Biotechnol 33:362–369. https://doi.org/10.1016/J.TIBTECH.2015.03.008
16. Augustine R, Nethi SK, Kalarikkal N, Thomas S, Patra CR (2017) Electrospun polycaprolactone (PCL) scaffolds embedded with europium hydroxide nanorods (EHNs) with enhanced vascularization and cell proliferation for tissue engineering applications. J Mater Chem B 5:4660–4672. https://doi.org/10.1039/c7tb00518k

17. Yu S, Zhang X, Tan G, Tian L, Liu D, Liu Y, Yang X, Pan W (2017) A novel pH-induced thermosensitive hydrogel composed of carboxymethyl chitosan and poloxamer cross-linked by glutaraldehyde for ophthalmic drug delivery. Carbohydr Polym 155:208–217. https://doi.org/10.1016/J.CARBPOL.2016.08.073
18. Holloway JL, Ma H, Rai R, Burdick JA (2014) Modulating hydrogel crosslink density and degradation to control bone morphogenetic protein delivery and in vivo bone formation. J Control Release. https://doi.org/10.1016/j.jconrel.2014.05.053
19. Bakaic E, Smeets NMB, Hoare T (2015) Injectable hydrogels based on poly(ethylene glycol) and derivatives as functional biomaterials. RSC Adv 5:35469–35486. https://doi.org/10.1039/c4ra13581d
20. Hu Y, Ren G, Deng L, Zhang J, Liu H, Mu S, Wu T (2016) Degradable UV-crosslinked hydrogel for the controlled release of triclosan with reduced cytotoxicity. Mater Sci Eng C 67:151–158. https://doi.org/10.1016/J.MSEC.2016.05.003
21. Augustine R, Venugopal B, Snigdha. S, Kalarikkal N, Thomas S (2015) Polyuronates and their application in drug delivery and cosmetics. In: Sabu Thomas JP (ed) Green polymers and environmental pollution control. CRC Press, pp 240–269
22. Lee KY, Mooney DJ (2012) Alginate: properties and biomedical applications. Prog Polym Sci 37:106–126. https://doi.org/10.1016/j.progpolymsci.2011.06.003
23. Ertesvåg H (2015) Alginate-modifying enzymes: biological roles and biotechnological uses. Front Microbiol 6:523
24. Utech S, Prodanovic R, Mao AS, Ostafe R, Mooney DJ, Weitz DA (2015) Microfluidic generation of monodisperse, structurally homogeneous alginate microgels for cell encapsulation and 3D cell culture. Adv Healthc Mater 4:1628–1633. https://doi.org/10.1002/adhm.201500021
25. Zhang Z, Zhang R, Zou L, McClements DJ (2016) Protein encapsulation in alginate hydrogel beads: effect of pH on microgel stability, protein retention and protein release. Food Hydrocoll 58:308–315. https://doi.org/10.1016/j.foodhyd.2016.03.015
26. Augustine R, Rajarathinam K (2012) Synthesis and characterization of silver nanoparticles and its immobilization on alginate coated sutures for the prevention of surgical wound infections and the in vitro release studies. Int J Nano Dimens 2:205–212. https://doi.org/10.7508/ijnd.2011.03.009
27. Ren Y, Xie H, Liu X, Bao J, Yu W, Ma X (2016) Comparative investigation of the binding characteristics of poly-L-lysine and chitosan on alginate hydrogel. Int J Biol Macromol 84:135–141. https://doi.org/10.1016/J.IJBIOMAC.2015.12.008
28. Chen H, Xing X, Tan H, Jia Y, Zhou T, Chen Y, Ling Z, Hu X (2017) Covalently antibacterial alginate-chitosan hydrogel dressing integrated gelatin microspheres containing tetracycline hydrochloride for wound healing. Mater Sci Eng C 70:287–295. https://doi.org/10.1016/J.MSEC.2016.08.086
29. Augustine R, Ashkenazi DL, Arzi RS, Zlobin V, Shofti R, Sosnik A (2018) Nanoparticle-in-microparticle oral drug delivery system of a clinically relevant darunavir/ritonavir antiretroviral combination. Acta Biomater 74:344–359. https://doi.org/10.1016/j.actbio.2018.04.045
30. Costa MJ, Marques AM, Pastrana LM, Teixeira JA, Sillankorva SM, Cerqueira MA (2018) Physicochemical properties of alginate-based films: effect of ionic crosslinking and mannuronic and guluronic acid ratio. Food Hydrocoll 81:442–448. https://doi.org/10.1016/J.FOODHYD.2018.03.014
31. Kashima K, Imai M (2012) Advanced membrane material from marine biological polymer and sensitive molecular-size recognition for promising separation technology. In: Advancing desalination
32. Penhasi A (2017) Preparation and characterization of in-situ ionic cross-linked pectin films: II. Biodegradation and drug diffusion. Carbohydr Polym 157:651–659. https://doi.org/10.1016/j.carbpol.2016.10.027
33. Bera H, Kumar S (2018) Diethanolamine-modified pectin based core-shell composites as dual working gastroretentive drug-cargo. Int J Biol Macromol 108:1053–1062. https://doi.org/10.1016/j.ijbiomac.2017.11.019

34. Bera H, Nadimpalli J, Kumar S, Vengala P (2017) Kondogogu gum-Zn^{+2}-pectinate emulgel matrices reinforced with mesoporous silica for intragastric furbiprofen delivery. Int J Biol Macromol 104:1229–1237. https://doi.org/10.1016/j.ijbiomac.2017.07.027
35. Augustine R, Augustine A, Kalarikkal N, Thomas S (2016) Fabrication and characterization of biosilver nanoparticles loaded calcium pectinate nano-micro dual-porous antibacterial wound dressings. Prog Biomater 5:223–235. https://doi.org/10.1007/s40204-016-0060-8
36. Guru PR, Bera H, Das MP, Hasnain MS, Nayak AK (2018) Aceclofenac-loaded *Plantago ovata* F. husk mucilage-Zn^{+2}-pectinate controlled-release matrices. Starch/Staerke 70:1–8. https://doi.org/10.1002/star.201700136
37. Hwang SW, Shin JS (2018) Pectin-coated curcumin-chitosan microparticles crosslinked with Mg^{2+} for delayed drug release in the digestive system. Int J Polym Sci 2018:1–7. https://doi.org/10.1155/2018/2071071
38. Ogueri KS, Ivirico JLE, Nair LS, Allcock HR, Laurencin CT (2017) Biodegradable polyphosphazene-based blends for regenerative engineering. Regen Eng Transl Med 3:15–31. https://doi.org/10.1007/s40883-016-0022-7
39. Garlapati S, Eng NF, Wilson HL, Buchanan R, Mutwiri GK, Babiuk LA, Gerdts V (2010) PCPP (poly[di(carboxylatophenoxy)-phosphazene]) microparticles co-encapsulating ovalbumin and CpG oligo-deoxynucleotides are potent enhancers of antigen specific Th1 immune responses in mice. Vaccine 28:8306–8314. https://doi.org/10.1016/j.vaccine.2010.09.080
40. Islam M, Park T-E, Reesor E, Cherukula K, Hasan A, Firdous J, Singh B, Kang S-K, Choi Y-J, Park I-K, Cho C-S (2015) Mucoadhesive chitosan derivatives as novel drug carriers. Curr Pharm Des 21:4285–4309. https://doi.org/10.2174/1381612821666150901103819
41. Ahmed R, Tariq M, Ali I, Asghar R, Noorunnisa Khanam P, Augustine R, Hasan A (2018) Novel electrospun chitosan/polyvinyl alcohol/zinc oxide nanofibrous mats with antibacterial and antioxidant properties for diabetic wound healing. Int J Biol Macromol 120:385–393. https://doi.org/10.1016/j.ijbiomac.2018.08.057
42. Zahid AA, Ahmed R, Raza ur Rehman S, Augustine R, Tariq M, Hasan A (2019) Nitric oxide releasing chitosan-poly (vinyl alcohol) hydrogel promotes angiogenesis in chick embryo model. Int J Biol Macromol 136:901–910. https://doi.org/10.1016/j.ijbiomac.2019.06.136
43. Jin RM, Sultana N, Baba S, Hamdan S, Ismail AF (2015) Porous PCL/chitosan and nHA/PCL/chitosan scaffolds for tissue engineering applications: fabrication and evaluation. J Nanomater 357372:1–8. https://doi.org/10.1155/2015/357372
44. Thakral NK, Ray AR, Majumdar DK (2010) Eudragit S-100 entrapped chitosan microspheres of valdecoxib for colon cancer. J Mater Sci Mater Med 21:2691–2699. https://doi.org/10.1007/s10856-010-4109-2
45. Zhou HY, Jiang LJ, Cao PP, Li JB, Chen XG (2015) Glycerophosphate-based chitosan thermosensitive hydrogels and their biomedical applications. Carbohydr Polym 117:524–536. https://doi.org/10.1016/J.CARBPOL.2014.09.094
46. Deng A, Kang X, Zhang J, Yang Y, Yang S (2017) Enhanced gelation of chitosan/β-sodium glycerophosphate thermosensitive hydrogel with sodium bicarbonate and biocompatibility evaluated. Mater Sci Eng C 78:1147–1154. https://doi.org/10.1016/j.msec.2017.04.109
47. Siripatrawan U, Vitchayakitti W (2016) Improving functional properties of chitosan films as active food packaging by incorporating with propolis. Food Hydrocoll 61:695–702. https://doi.org/10.1016/j.foodhyd.2016.06.001
48. Chenite A, Buschmann M, Wang D, Chaput C, Kandani N (2001) Rheological characterisation of thermogelling chitosan/glycerol-phosphate solutions. Carbohydr Polym 46:39–47. https://doi.org/10.1016/S0144-8617(00)00281-2
49. Augustine R, Dan P, Schlachet I, Rouxel D, Menu P, Sosnik A (2019) Chitosan ascorbate hydrogel improves water uptake capacity and cell adhesion of electrospun poly(epsilon-caprolactone) membranes. Int J Pharm 559:420–426. https://doi.org/10.1016/j.ijpharm.2019.01.063
50. Hossain KS, Miyanaga K, Maeda H, Nemoto N (2001) Sol-gel transition behavior of pure ι-carrageenan in both salt-free and added salt states. Biomacromolecules 2:442–449. https://doi.org/10.1021/bm000117f

51. Respiratorio S, Crítico P, García-Fernández J, Castro L (1980) I. Soporte Respiratorio en el Paciente Crítico pediátrico. 1–10. https://doi.org/10.1016/0022-2836(80)90291-0
52. Pourjavadi A, Sadeghi M, Hosseinzadeh H (2004) Modified carrageenan. Preparation, swelling behavior, salt- and pH-sensitivity of partially hydrolyzed crosslinked carrageenan-graft-polymethacrylamide superabsorbent hydrogel. Polym Adv Technol 15:645–653. https://doi.org/10.1002/pat.524
53. Watanabe T, Ohtsuka A, Murase N, Barth P, Gersonde K (1996) NMR studies on water and polymer diffusion in dextran gels. Influence of potassium ions on microstructure formation and gelation mechanism. Magn Reson Med. https://doi.org/10.1002/mrm.1910350511
54. Ahmed S, Ikram S (2016) Chitosan based scaffolds and their applications in wound healing. Achiev Life Sci 10:27–37. https://doi.org/10.1016/j.als.2016.04.001
55. Augustine R, Hasan A, Yadu Nath VK, Thomas J, Augustine A, Kalarikkal N, Al Moustafa AE, Thomas S (2018) Electrospun polyvinyl alcohol membranes incorporated with green synthesized silver nanoparticles for wound dressing applications. J Mater Sci Mater Med 29:205–212. https://doi.org/10.1007/s10856-018-6169-7
56. Guan Y, Bian J, Peng F, Zhang XM, Sun RC (2014) High strength of hemicelluloses based hydrogels by freeze/thaw technique. Carbohydr Polym 101:272–280. https://doi.org/10.1016/j.carbpol.2013.08.085
57. Kenawy ER, Kamoun EA, Mohy Eldin MS, El-Meligy MA (2014) Physically crosslinked poly(vinyl alcohol)-hydroxyethyl starch blend hydrogel membranes: synthesis and characterization for biomedical applications. Arab J Chem 7:372–380. https://doi.org/10.1016/j.arabjc.2013.05.026
58. Hassan CM, Peppas NA (2000) Structure and morphology of freeze/thawed PVA hydrogels. Macromolecules 33:2472–2479. https://doi.org/10.1021/ma9907587
59. Bai H, Li Z, Zhang S, Wang W, Dong W (2018) Interpenetrating polymer networks in polyvinyl alcohol/cellulose nanocrystals hydrogels to develop absorbent materials. Carbohydr Polym 200:468–476. https://doi.org/10.1016/j.carbpol.2018.08.041
60. Yan EK, Cao HL, Zhang CY, Lu QQ, Ye YJ, He J, Huang LJ, Yin DC (2015) Cross-linked protein crystals by glutaraldehyde and their applications. RSC Adv 5:26163–26174
61. Peppas NA, Scott JE (1992) Controlled release from poly(vinyl alcohol) gels prepared by freezing-thawing processes. J Control Release 18:95–100. https://doi.org/10.1016/0168-3659(92)90178-T
62. Takamura A, Ishii F, Hidaka H (1992) Drug release from poly(vinyl alcohol) gel prepared by freeze-thaw procedure. J Control Release 20:21–27. https://doi.org/10.1016/0168-3659(92)90135-E
63. Tashiro K, Kouno N, Wang H, Tsuji H (2017) Crystal structure of poly(lactic acid) stereocomplex: random packing model of PDLA and PLLA chains as studied by X-ray diffraction analysis. Macromolecules 50:8048–8065. https://doi.org/10.1021/acs.macromol.7b01468
64. Ikada Y, Jamshidi K, Tsuji H, Hyon SH (1987) Stereocomplex formation between enantiomeric poly(lactides). Macromolecules 20:904–906. https://doi.org/10.1021/ma00170a034
65. Lim DW, Park TG (2000) Stereocomplex formation between enantiomeric PLA-PEG-PLA triblock copolymers: characterization and use as protein-delivery microparticulate carriers. J Appl Polym Sci 75:1615–1623. https://doi.org/10.1002/(SICI)1097-4628(20000328)75:13%3c1615::AID-APP7%3e3.0.CO;2-L
66. Lim DW, Choi SH, Park TG (2000) A new class of biodegradable hydrogels stereocomplexed by enantiomeric oligo(lactide) side chains of poly(HEMA-g-OLA)s. Macromol Rapid Commun 21:464–471. https://doi.org/10.1002/(SICI)1521-3927(20000501)21:8%3c464::AID-MARC464%3e3.0.CO;2-#
67. Khan S, Ullah A, Ullah K, Rehman NU (2016) Insight into hydrogels. Des Monomers Polym 19:456–478. https://doi.org/10.1080/15685551.2016.1169380
68. Förster S, Antonietti M (1998) Amphiphilic block copolymers in structure-controlled nanomaterial hybrids. Adv Mater 10:195–217. https://doi.org/10.1002/(SICI)1521-4095(199802)10:3%3c195::AID-ADMA195%3e3.0.CO;2-V

69. Klouda L, Mikos AG (2008) Thermoresponsive hydrogels in biomedical applications. Eur J Pharm Biopharm 68:34–45
70. Jeong B, Bae YH, Kim SW (1999) Thermoreversible gelation of PEG–PLGA–PEG triblock copolymer aqueous solutions. Macromolecules 32:7064–7069. https://doi.org/10.1021/ma9908999
71. Lin HH, Cheng YL (2001) In-situ thermoreversible gelation of block and star copolymers of poly(ethylene glycol) and poly(n-isopropylacrylamide) of varying architectures. Macromolecules 34:3710–3715. https://doi.org/10.1021/ma001852m
72. Cai L, Dewi RE, Heilshorn SC (2015) Injectable hydrogels with in situ double network formation enhance retention of transplanted stem cells. Adv Funct Mater 25:1344–1351. https://doi.org/10.1002/adfm.201403631
73. Lee DS, Jeong B, Bae YH, Kim SW (1996) New thermoreversible and biodegradable block copolymer hydrogels. Proc Control Release Soc 22:228–229
74. Jeong B, Lee DS, Shon JI, Bae YH, Kim SW (1999) Thermoreversible gelation of poly(ethylene oxide) biodegradable polyester block copolymers. J Polym Sci Part A Polym Chem 37:751–760. https://doi.org/10.1002/(SICI)1099-0518(19990315)37:6%3c751::AID-POLA10%3e3.0.CO;2-0
75. Huh KM, Bae YH (1999) Synthesis and characterization of poly(ethylene glycol)/poly(L-lactic acid) alternating multiblock copolymers. Polymer (Guildf) 40:6147–6155. https://doi.org/10.1016/S0032-3861(98)00822-2
76. Bae YH, Huh KM, Kim Y, Park KH (2000) Biodegradable amphiphilic multiblock copolymers and their implications for biomedical applications. J Control Release 64:3–13. https://doi.org/10.1016/S0168-3659(99)00126-1
77. Bezemer JM, Grijpma DW, Dijkstra PJ, Van Blitterswijk CA, Feijen J (1999) A controlled release system for proteins based on poly(ether ester) block-copolymers: polymer network characterization. J Control Release 62:393–405. https://doi.org/10.1016/S0168-3659(99)00170-4
78. Bezemer JM, Radersma R, Grijpma DW, Dijkstra PJ, Feijen J, Van Blitterswijk CA (2000) Zero-order release of lysozyme from poly(ethylene glycol)/poly(butylene terephthalate) matrices. J Control Release 64:179–192. https://doi.org/10.1016/S0168-3659(99)00127-3
79. Bezemer JM, Grijpma DW, Dijkstra PJ, Van Blitterswijk CA, Feijen J (2000) Control of protein delivery from amphiphilic poly(ether ester) multiblock copolymers by varying their water content using emulsification techniques. J Control Release 66:307–320. https://doi.org/10.1016/S0168-3659(99)00287-4
80. Bezemer JM, Radersma R, Grijpma DW, Dijkstra PJ, Van Blitterswijk CA, Feijen J (2000a) Microspheres for protein delivery prepared from amphiphilic multiblock copolymers. 1. Influence of preparation techniques on particle characteristics and protein delivery. J Control Release 67:233–248. https://doi.org/10.1016/S0168-3659(00)00213-3
81. Bezemer JM, Radersma R, Grijpma DW, Dijkstra PJ, Van Blitterswijk CA, Feijen J (2000b) Microspheres for protein delivery prepared from amphiphilic multiblock copolymers. 2. Modulation of release rate. J Control Release 67:233–248. https://doi.org/10.1016/S0168-3659(00)00212-1
82. Van Dijkhuizen-Radersma R, Péters FLAMA, Stienstra NA, Grijpma DW, Feijen J, De Groot K, Bezemer JM (2002) Control of vitamin B12 release from poly(ethylene glycol)/poly(butylene terephthalate) multiblock copolymers. Biomaterials 23:1527–1536. https://doi.org/10.1016/S0142-9612(01)00286-1
83. Deschamps AA, Grijpma DW, Feijen J (2001) Poly(ethylene oxide)/poly(butylene terephthalate) segmented block copolymers: the effect of copolymer composition on physical properties and degradation behavior. Polymer (Guildf) 42:9335–9345. https://doi.org/10.1016/S0032-3861(01)00453-0
84. Akiyoshi K, Deguchi S, Moriguchi N, Yamaguchi S, Sunamoto J (1993) Self-aggregates of hydrophobized polysaccharides in water. Formation and characteristics of nanoparticles. Macromolecules 26:3062–3068. https://doi.org/10.1021/ma00064a011

85. Akiyoshi K, Deguchi S, Tajima H, Nishikawa T, Sunamoto J (1997) Microscopic structure and thermoresponsiveness of a hydrogel nanoparticle by self-assembly of a hydrophobized polysaccharide. Macromolecules 30:857–861. https://doi.org/10.1021/ma960786e
86. Akiyoshi K, Taniguchi I, Fukui H, Sunamoto J (1996) Hydrogel nanoparticle formed by self-assembly of hydrophobized polysaccharide. Stabilization of adriamycin by complexation. Eur J Pharm Biopharm 42:286–290
87. Akiyoshi K, Kobayashi S, Shichibe S, Mix D, Baudys M, Wan Kim S, Sunamoto J (1998) Self-assembled hydrogel nanoparticle of cholesterol-bearing pullulan as a carrier of protein drugs: complexation and stabilization of insulin. J Control Release 54:313–320. https://doi.org/10.1016/S0168-3659(98)00017-0
88. Taniguchi I, Akiyoshi K, Sunamoto J (1999) Self-aggregate nanoparticles of cholesteryl and galactoside groups-substituted pullulan and their specific binding to galactose specific lectin, RCA120. Macromol Chem Phys 200:1554–1560. https://doi.org/10.1002/(SICI)1521-3935(19990601)200:6%3c1554::AID-MACP1554%3e3.0.CO;2-V
89. Akiyoshi K, Kang EC, Kurumada S, Sunamoto J, Principi T, Winnik FM (2000) Controlled association of amphiphilic polymers in water: thermosensitive nanoparticles formed by self-assembly of hydrophobically modified pullulans and poly(N-isopropylacrylamides). Macromolecules 33:3244–3249. https://doi.org/10.1021/ma991798d
90. Molinaro G, Leroux JC, Damas J, Adam A (2002) Biocompatibility of thermosensitive chitosan-based hydrogels: an in vivo experimental approach to injectable biomaterials. Biomaterials 23:2717–2722. https://doi.org/10.1016/S0142-9612(02)00004-2
91. Yoo HS, Lee JE, Chung H, Kwon IC, Jeong SY (2005) Self-assembled nanoparticles containing hydrophobically modified glycol chitosan for gene delivery. J Control Release 103:235–243. https://doi.org/10.1016/j.jconrel.2004.11.033
92. Uchegbu IF, Schätzlein AG, Tetley L, Gray AI, Sludden J, Siddique S, Mosha E (1998) Polymeric chitosan-based vesicles for drug delivery. J Pharm Pharmacol 50:453–458. https://doi.org/10.1111/j.2042-7158.1998.tb06185.x
93. Sludden J, Uchegbu IF, Schätzlein AG (2000) The encapsulation of bleomycin within chitosan based polymeric vesicles does not alter its biodistribution. J Pharm Pharmacol 52:377–382. https://doi.org/10.1211/0022357001774110
94. Noble L, Gray AI, Sadiq L, Uchegbu IF (1999) A non-covalently cross-linked chitosan based hydrogel. Int J Pharm 192:173–182. https://doi.org/10.1016/S0378-5173(99)00306-3
95. Qu X, Wirsén A, Albertsson AC (2000) Novel pH-sensitive chitosan hydrogels: swelling behavior and states of water. Polymer (Guildf) 41:4589–4598. https://doi.org/10.1016/S0032-3861(99)00685-0
96. Yazdani-Pedram M, Retuert J, Quijada R (2000) Hydrogels based on modified chitosan, 1. Synthesis and swelling behavior of poly(acrylic acid) grafted chitosan. Macromol Chem Phys 201:923–930. https://doi.org/10.1002/1521-3935(20000601)201:9%3c923::AID-MACP923%3e3.0.CO;2-W
97. Kim SY, Cho SM, Lee YM, Kim SJ (2000) Thermo- and pH-responsive behaviors of graft copolymer and blend based on chitosan and N-isopropylacrylamide. J Appl Polym Sci 78:1381–1391. https://doi.org/10.1002/1097-4628(20001114)78:7%3c1381::AID-APP90%3e3.0.CO;2-M
98. Matyjaszewski K, Beers KL, Kern A, Gaynor SG (1998) Hydrogels by atom transfer radical polymerization. I. Poly(N-vinylpyrrolidinone-g-styrene) via the macromonomer method. J Polym Sci Part A Polym Chem 36:823–830. https://doi.org/10.1002/(SICI)1099-0518(19980415)36:5%3c823::AID-POLA15%3e3.0.CO;2-I
99. Ming W, Zhao Y, Cui J, Fu S, Jones FN (1999) Formation of irreversible nearly transparent physical polymeric hydrogels during a modified microemulsion polymerization. Macromolecules 32:528–530. https://doi.org/10.1021/ma9813486
100. Eagland D, Crowther NJ, Butler CJ (1994) Complexation between polyoxyethylene and polymethacrylic acid—the importance of the molar mass of polyoxyethylene. Eur Polym J 30:767–773. https://doi.org/10.1016/0014-3057(94)90003-5

101. Bell CL, Peppas NA (1996) Modulation of drug permeation through interpolymer complexed hydrogels for drug delivery applications. J Control Release 39:201–207. https://doi.org/10.1016/0168-3659(95)00154-9
102. Mathur AM, Hammonds KF, Klier J, Scranton AB (1998) Equilibrium swelling of poly(methacrylic acid-g-ethylene glycol) hydrogels. Effect of swelling medium and synthesis conditions. J Control Release 54:177–184. https://doi.org/10.1016/S0168-3659(97)00186-7
103. Nagahara S, Matsuda T (1996) Hydrogel formation via hybridization of oligonucleotides derivatized in water-soluble vinyl polymers. Polym Gels Netw 4:111–127. https://doi.org/10.1016/0966-7822(96)00001-9
104. Xue S, Wu Y, Guo M, Liu D, Zhang T, Lei W (2018) Fabrication of poly(acrylic acid)/boron nitride composite hydrogels with excellent mechanical properties and rapid self-healing through hierarchically physical interactions. Nanoscale Res Lett 13:393. https://doi.org/10.1186/s11671-018-2800-2
105. Bavaresco VP, Zavaglia CAC, Reis MC, Gomes JR (2008) Study on the tribological properties of pHEMA hydrogels for use in artificial articular cartilage. Wear 265:269–277. https://doi.org/10.1016/j.wear.2007.10.009
106. Giammona G, Pitarresi G, Cavallaro G, Spadaro G (1999) New biodegradable hydrogels based on an acryloylated polyaspartamide cross-linked by gamma irradiation. J Biomater Sci Polym Ed 10:969–987. https://doi.org/10.1163/156856299X00568
107. Çiçek H, Tuncel A (1998) Immobilization of α-chymotrypsin in thermally reversible isopropylacrylamide-hydroxyethylmethacrylate copolymer gel. J Polym Sci Part A Polym Chem 36:543–552. https://doi.org/10.1002/(SICI)1099-0518(199803)36:4%3c543::AID-POLA4%3e3.0.CO;2-Q
108. Jin Y, Yamanaka J, Sato S, Miyata I, Yomota C, Yonese M (2001) Recyclable characteristics of hyaluronate-polyhydroxyethyl acrylate blend hydrogel for controlled releases. J Control Release 73:173–181. https://doi.org/10.1016/S0168-3659(01)00234-6
109. Wichterle O, Lím D (1960) Hydrophilic gels for biological use. Nature 185:117. https://doi.org/10.1038/185117a0
110. Franssen O, Van Ooijen RD, De Boer D, Maes RAA, Herron JN, Hennink WE (1997) Enzymatic degradation of methacrylated dextrans. Macromolecules 30:7408–7413. https://doi.org/10.1021/ma970887s
111. Stubbe B, Maris B, Van den Mooter G, De Smedt SC, Demeester J (2001) The in vitro evaluation of "azo containing polysaccharide gels" for colon delivery. J Control Release 75:103–114. https://doi.org/10.1016/S0168-3659(01)00367-4
112. Ferreira L, Vidal MM, Geraldes CFGC, Gil MH (2000) Preparation and characterization of gels based on sucrose modified with glycidyl methacrylate. Carbohydr Polym 41:15–24. https://doi.org/10.1016/S0144-8617(99)00064-8
113. Hennink WE, Talsma H, Borchert JCH, De Smedt SC, Demeester J (1996) Controlled release of proteins from dextran hydrogels. J Control Release 39:47–55. https://doi.org/10.1016/0168-3659(95)00132-8
114. Van Dijk-Wolthuis WNE, Van Steenbergen MJ, Underberg WJM, Hennink WE (1997) Degradation kinetics of methacrylated dextrans in aqueous solution. J Pharm Sci 86:413–417. https://doi.org/10.1021/js9604220
115. Patil NS, Dordick JS, Rethwisch DG (1996) Macroporous poly(sucrose acrylate) hydrogel for controlled release of macromolecules. Biomaterials 17:2343–2350. https://doi.org/10.1016/S0142-9612(96)00089-0
116. Martin BD, Linhardt RJ, Dordick JS (1998) Highly swelling hydrogels from ordered galactose-based polyacrylates. Biomaterials 19:69–76. https://doi.org/10.1016/S0142-9612(97)00184-1
117. Patil NS, Li Y, Rethwisch DG, Dordick JS (1997) Sucrose diacrylate: a unique chemically and biologically degradable crosslinker for polymeric hydrogels. J Polym Sci Part A Polym Chem 35:2221–2229. https://doi.org/10.1002/(SICI)1099-0518(199708)35:11%3c2221::AID-POLA12%3e3.0.CO;2-G

118. Kim SH, Chu CC (2000) Synthesis and characterization of dextran-methacrylate hydrogels and structural study by SEM. J Biomed Mater Res 49:517–527. https://doi.org/10.1002/(SICI)1097-4636(20000315)49:4%3c517::AID-JBM10%3e3.0.CO;2-8
119. Marsano E, Gagliardi S, Ghioni F, Bianchi E (2000) Behaviour of gels based on (hydroxypropyl) cellulose methacrylate. Polymer (Guildf) 41:7691–7698. https://doi.org/10.1016/S0032-3861(00)00142-7
120. Lo CW, Jiang H (2010) Photopatterning and degradation study of dextran-glycidyl methacrylate hydrogels. Polym Eng Sci 50:232–239. https://doi.org/10.1002/pen.21531
121. McDowall DJ, Gupta BS, Stannett VT (1984) Grafting of vinyl monomers to cellulose by ceric ion initiation. Prog Polym Sci 10:1–50. https://doi.org/10.1016/0079-6700(84)90005-4
122. Lagos A, Yazdani-Pedram M, Reyes J, Campos N (1992) Ceric ion-initiated grafting of poly (methyl acrylate) onto chitin. J Macromol Sci Part A 29:1007–1015. https://doi.org/10.1080/10601329208054137
123. Gaborieau M, De Bruyn H, Mange S, Castignolles P, Brockmeyer A, Gilbert RG (2009) Synthesis and characterization of synthetic polymer colloids colloidally stabilized by cationized starch oligomers. J Polym Sci Part A Polym Chem 47:1836–1852. https://doi.org/10.1002/pola.23287
124. Singh DK, Ray AR (1994) Graft copolymerization of 2-hydroxyethylmethacrylate onto chitosan films and their blood compatibility. J Appl Polym Sci 53:1115–1121. https://doi.org/10.1002/app.1994.070530814
125. Lagos A, Reyes J (1988) Grafting onto chitosan. I. Graft copolymerization of methyl methacrylate onto chitosan with Fenton's reagent ($Fe^{2+}-H_2O_2$) as a redox initiator. J Polym Sci Part A Polym Chem 26:985–991. https://doi.org/10.1002/pola.1988.080260403
126. Matyjaszewski K, Shipp DA, Wang JL, Grimaud T, Patten TE (1998) Utilizing halide exchange to improve control of atom transfer radical polymerization. Macromolecules 31:6836–6840. https://doi.org/10.1021/ma980476r
127. Fairbanks BD, Schwartz MP, Bowman CN, Anseth KS (2009) Photoinitiated polymerization of PEG-diacrylate with lithium phenyl-2,4,6-trimethylbenzoylphosphinate: polymerization rate and cytocompatibility. Biomaterials 30:6702–6707. https://doi.org/10.1016/j.biomaterials.2009.08.055
128. Nichol JW, Koshy ST, Bae H, Hwang CM, Yamanlar S, Khademhosseini A (2010) Cell-laden microengineered gelatin methacrylate hydrogels. Biomaterials 31:5536–5544. https://doi.org/10.1016/j.biomaterials.2010.03.064
129. Benton JA, DeForest CA, Vivekanandan V, Anseth KS (2009) Photocrosslinking of gelatin macromers to synthesize porous hydrogels that promote valvular interstitial cell function. Tissue Eng Part A 15:3221–3230. https://doi.org/10.1089/ten.tea.2008.0545
130. Paul A, Manoharan V, Krafft D, Assmann A, Uquillas JA, Shin SR, Hasan A, Hussain MA, Memic A, Gaharwar AK (2016) Nanoengineered biomimetic hydrogels for guiding human stem cell osteogenesis in three dimensional microenvironments. J Mater Chem B 4:3544–3554
131. Shin H, Olsen BD, Khademhosseini A (2012) The mechanical properties and cytotoxicity of cell-laden double-network hydrogels based on photocrosslinkable gelatin and gellan gum biomacromolecules. Biomaterials 33:3143–3152. https://doi.org/10.1016/j.biomaterials.2011.12.050
132. Chou AI, Akintoye SO, Nicoll SB (2009) Photo-crosslinked alginate hydrogels support enhanced matrix accumulation by nucleus pulposus cells in vivo. Osteoarthr Cartil 17:1377–1384. https://doi.org/10.1016/j.joca.2009.04.012
133. Bryant SJ, Durand KL, Anseth KS (2003) Manipulations in hydrogel chemistry control photoencapsulated chondrocyte behavior and their extracellular matrix production. J Biomed Mater Res Part A 67:1430–1436. https://doi.org/10.1002/jbm.a.20003
134. Loessner D, Meinert C, Kaemmerer E, Martine LC, Yue K, Levett PA, Klein TJ, Melchels FPW, Khademhosseini A, Hutmacher DW (2016) Functionalization, preparation and use of cell-laden gelatin methacryloyl-based hydrogels as modular tissue culture platforms. Nat Protoc 11:727. https://doi.org/10.1038/nprot.2016.037

135. Matyjaszewski K, Wang JL, Grimaud T, Shipp DA (1998) Controlled/"living" atom transfer radical polymerization of methyl methacrylate using various initiation systems. Macromolecules 31:1527–1534. https://doi.org/10.1021/ma971298p
136. Matyjaszewski K, Hongchen D, Jakubowski W, Pietrasik J, Kusumo A (2007) Grafting from surfaces for "everyone": ARGET ATRP in the presence of air. Langmuir 23:4528–4531. https://doi.org/10.1021/la063402e
137. Sanson N, Rieger J (2010) Synthesis of nanogels/microgels by conventional and controlled radical crosslinking copolymerization. Polym Chem 1:965–977. https://doi.org/10.1039/c0py00010h
138. Draye JP, Delaey B, Van De Voorde A, Van Den Bulcke A, Bogdanov B, Schacht E (1998) In vitro release characteristics of bioactive molecules from dextran dialdehyde cross-linked gelatin hydrogel films. Biomaterials 19:99–107. https://doi.org/10.1016/S0142-9612(97)00164-6
139. Draye JP, Delaey B, Van De Voorde A, Van Den Bulcke A, De Reu B, Schacht E (1998) In vitro and in vivo biocompatibility of dextran dialdehyde cross-linked gelatin hydrogel films. Biomaterials 19:1677–1687. https://doi.org/10.1016/S0142-9612(98)00049-0
140. Lee KY, Bouhadir KH, Mooney DJ (2000) Degradation behavior of covalently cross-linked poly(aldehyde guluronate) hydrogels. Macromolecules 33:97–101. https://doi.org/10.1021/ma991286z
141. Bouhadir KH, Kruger GM, Lee KY, Mooney DJ (2000) Sustained and controlled release of daunomycin from cross-linked poly(aldehyde guluronate) hydrogels. J Pharm Sci 89:910–919. https://doi.org/10.1002/1520-6017(200007)89:7%3c910::AID-JPS8%3e3.0.CO;2-#
142. Luo Y, Kirker KR, Prestwich GD (2000) Cross-linked hyaluronic acid hydrogel films: new biomaterials for drug delivery. J Control Release 69:169–184. https://doi.org/10.1016/S0168-3659(00)00300-X
143. Wang H, Zhu D, Paul A, Cai L, Enejder A, Yang F, Heilshorn SC (2017) Covalently adaptable elastin-like protein-hyaluronic acid (ELP–HA) hybrid hydrogels with secondary thermoresponsive crosslinking for injectable stem cell delivery. Adv Funct Mater 27:1605609. https://doi.org/10.1002/adfm.201605609
144. Simonsen L, Hovgaard L, Mortensen PB, Brøndsted H (1995) Dextran hydrogels for colon-specific drug delivery. V. Degradation in human intestinal incubation models. Eur J Pharm Sci 3:329–337. https://doi.org/10.1016/0928-0987(95)00023-6
145. Gehrke SH, Uhden LH, McBride JF (1998) Enhanced loading and activity retention of bioactive proteins in hydrogel delivery systems. J Control Release 55:21–33. https://doi.org/10.1016/S0168-3659(98)00019-4
146. Alhaique F, Murtas E, Carafa M, Desideri P, Dentini M, Coviello T, Riccieri FM, Rambone G (2002) A novel co-crosslinked polysaccharide: studies for a controlled delivery matrix. J Control Release 55:57–66. https://doi.org/10.1016/s0168-3659(98)00028-5
147. Kuijpers AJ, Van Wachem PB, Van Luyn MJA, Engbers GHM, Krijgsveld J, Zaat SAJ, Dankert J, Feijen J (2000) In vivo and in vitro release of lysozyme from cross-linked gelatin hydrogels: a model system for the delivery of antibacterial proteins from prosthetic heart valves. J Control Release 67:323–336. https://doi.org/10.1016/S0168-3659(00)00221-2
148. Ohan MP, Weadock KS, Dunn MG (2002) Synergistic effects of glucose and ultraviolet irradiation on the physical properties of collagen. J Biomed Mater Res 60:384–391
149. Kuijpers AJ, Engbers GHM, Meyvis TKL, De Smedt SSC, Demeester J, Krijgsveld J, Zaat SAJ, Dankert J, Feijen J (2000) Combined gelatin-chondroitin sulfate hydrogels for controlled release of cationic antibacterial proteins. Macromolecules 33:3705–3713. https://doi.org/10.1021/ma9917702
150. Eiselt P, Lee KY, Mooney DJ (1999) Rigidity of two-component hydrogels prepared from alginate and poly(ethylene glycol)-diamines. Macromolecules 32:5561–5566. https://doi.org/10.1021/ma990514m
151. Ichi T, Watanabe J, Ooya T, Yui N (2001) Controllable erosion time and profile in poly(ethylene glycol) hydrogels by supramolecular structure of hydrolyzable polyrotaxane. Biomacromolecules 2:204–210. https://doi.org/10.1021/bm005617n

152. Ooya T, Ichi T, Furubayashi T, Katoh M, Yui N (2007) Cationic hydrogels of PEG crosslinked by a hydrolyzable polyrotaxane for cartilage regeneration. React Funct Polym 67:1408–1417
153. Peppas NA, Merrill EW (1977) Crosslinked poly(vinyl alcohol) hydrogels as swollen elastic networks. J Appl Polym Sci 21:1763–1770. https://doi.org/10.1002/app.1977.070210704
154. Jabbari E, Nozari S (2000) Swelling behavior of acrylic acid hydrogels prepared by γ-radiation crosslinking of polyacrylic acid in aqueous solution. Eur Polym J 36:2685–2692. https://doi.org/10.1016/S0014-3057(00)00044-6
155. Kofinas P, Athanassiou V, Merrill EW (1996) Hydrogels prepared by electron irradiation of poly(ethylene oxide) in water solution: unexpected dependence of cross-link density and protein diffusion coefficients on initial PEO molecular weight. Biomaterials 17:1547–1550. https://doi.org/10.1016/0142-9612(96)89781-X
156. Merrill EW, Dennison KA, Sung C (1993) Partitioning and diffusion of solutes in hydrogels of poly(ethylene oxide). Biomaterials 14:1117–1126. https://doi.org/10.1016/0142-9612(93)90154-T
157. Stringer JL, Peppas NA (1996) Diffusion of small molecular weight drugs in radiation-crosslinked poly(ethylene oxide) hydrogels. J Control Release 42:195–202. https://doi.org/10.1016/0168-3659(96)01457-5
158. Lee J, Macosko CW, Urry DW (2001) Swelling behavior of γ-irradiation cross-linked elastomeric polypentapeptide-based hydrogels. Macromolecules 34:4114–4123. https://doi.org/10.1021/ma0015673
159. Moreira Teixeira LS, Feijen J, van Blitterswijk CA, Dijkstra PJ, Karperien M (2012) Enzyme-catalyzed crosslinkable hydrogels: emerging strategies for tissue engineering. Biomaterials 33:1281–1290. https://doi.org/10.1016/j.biomaterials.2011.10.067
160. Tatsukawa H, Kojima S (2010) Recent advances in understanding the roles of transglutaminase 2 in alcoholic steatohepatitis. Cell Biol Int 34:325–334. https://doi.org/10.1042/CBI20090130
161. Mero A, Spolaore B, Veronese FM, Fontana A (2009) Transglutaminase-mediated PEGylation of proteins: direct identification of the sites of protein modification by mass spectrometry using a novel monodisperse PEG. Bioconjug Chem 20:384–389. https://doi.org/10.1021/bc800427n
162. McHale MK, Setton LA, Chilkoti A (2005) Synthesis and in vitro evaluation of enzymatically cross-linked elastin-like polypeptide gels for cartilaginous tissue repair. Tissue Eng 11:1768–1779. https://doi.org/10.1089/ten.2005.11.1768
163. Cai X, Hu S, Yu B, Cai Y, Yang J, Li F, Zheng Y, Shi X (2018) Transglutaminase-catalyzed preparation of crosslinked carboxymethyl chitosan/carboxymethyl cellulose/collagen composite membrane for postsurgical peritoneal adhesion prevention. Carbohydr Polym 201:201–210. https://doi.org/10.1016/j.carbpol.2018.08.065
164. Westhaus E, Messersmith PB (2001) Triggered release of calcium from lipid vesicles: a bioinspired strategy for rapid gelation of polysaccharide and protein hydrogels. Biomaterials 22:453–462. https://doi.org/10.1016/S0142-9612(00)00200-3
165. Sperinde JJ, Griffith LG (2000) Control and prediction of gelation kinetics in enzymatically cross-linked poly(ethylene glycol) hydrogels. Macromolecules 33:5476–5480. https://doi.org/10.1021/ma000459d
166. Yu F, Cao X, Li Y, Zeng L, Yuan B, Chen X (2014) An injectable hyaluronic acid/PEG hydrogel for cartilage tissue engineering formed by integrating enzymatic crosslinking and Diels–Alder "click chemistry." Polym Chem 5:1082–1090. https://doi.org/10.1039/c3py00869j
167. Partlow BP, Applegate MB, Omenetto FG, Kaplan DL (2016) Dityrosine cross-linking in designing biomaterials. ACS Biomater Sci Eng 2:2108–2121. https://doi.org/10.1021/acsbiomaterials.6b00454
168. Raia NR, Partlow BP, McGill M, Kimmerling EP, Ghezzi CE, Kaplan DL (2017) Enzymatically crosslinked silk-hyaluronic acid hydrogels. Biomaterials 131:58–67. https://doi.org/10.1016/j.biomaterials.2017.03.046
169. Yang G, Xiao Z, Long H, Ma K, Zhang J, Ren X, Zhang J (2018) Assessment of the characteristics and biocompatibility of gelatin sponge scaffolds prepared by various crosslinking methods. Sci Rep 8:1616 (1–13). https://doi.org/10.1038/s41598-018-20006-y

170. Valero C, Amaveda H, Mora M, García-Aznar JM (2018) Combined experimental and computational characterization of crosslinked collagen-based hydrogels. PLoS One 13:e0195820 (1–16). https://doi.org/10.1371/journal.pone.0195820
171. Ren K, Cui H, Xu Q, He C, Li G, Chen X (2016) Injectable polypeptide hydrogels with tunable microenvironment for 3D spreading and chondrogenic differentiation of bone-marrow-derived mesenchymal stem cells. Biomacromolecules 17:3862–3871. https://doi.org/10.1021/acs.biomac.6b00884
172. Hasan A, Khattab A, Islam MA, Hweij KA, Zeitouny J, Waters R, Sayegh M, Hossain MM, Paul A (2015) Injectable hydrogels for cardiac tissue repair after myocardial infarction. Adv Sci 2:1500122 (1–18). https://doi.org/10.1002/advs.201500122
173. Cheng Y-H, Chen Y-C, Yang S-H, Yang K-C, Wu S-C, Su W-Y, Cheng WT-K, Lin F-H (2010) Thermosensitive chitosan–gelatin–glycerol phosphate hydrogels as a cell carrier for nucleus pulposus. Tissue Eng Part A 16:695–703
174. Ghasemi Tahrir F, Ganji F, Mani AR, Khodaverdi E (2016) In vitro and in vivo evaluation of thermosensitive chitosan hydrogel for sustained release of insulin. Drug Deliv 23:1038–1046. https://doi.org/10.3109/10717544.2014.932861
175. Duarte BPM, Moura MJ, Gil MH, Figueiredo MM (2017) Modeling the drug release from ionic and covalent co-cross-linked chitosan hydrogels. Comput Aided Chem Eng 40:1021–1026. https://doi.org/10.1016/B978-0-444-63965-3.50172-0
176. Yegappan R, Selvaprithiviraj V, Amirthalingam S, Jayakumar R (2018) Carrageenan based hydrogels for drug delivery, tissue engineering and wound healing. Carbohydr Polym 198:385–400. https://doi.org/10.1016/j.carbpol.2018.06.086
177. Ahmadi R, De Bruijn JD (2008) Biocompatibility and gelation of chitosan-glycerol phosphate hydrogels. J Biomed Mater Res Part A 86:824–832. https://doi.org/10.1002/jbm.a.31676
178. Martins EAN, Baccarin RYA, Moraes APL, Mantovani CF, Machado TSL, Hagen SCF (2015) Evaluation of chitosan-glycerol phosphate in experimental osteochondral joint defects in horses. J Mol Genet Med s4:1747–1862. https://doi.org/10.4172/1747-0862.S4-002
179. Wu LQ, Bentley WE, Payne GF (2011) Biofabrication with biopolymers and enzymes: potential for constructing scaffolds from soft matter. Int J Artif Organs 34:215–224. https://doi.org/10.5301/IJAO.2011.6406
180. Yamamoto H, Kuno S, Nagai A, Nishida A, Yamauchi S, Ikeda K (1990) Insolubilizing and adhesive studies of water-soluble synthetic model proteins. Int J Biol Macromol 12:305–310. https://doi.org/10.1016/0141-8130(90)90019-7
181. Chen T, Embree HD, Brown EM, Taylor MM, Payne GF (2003) Enzyme-catalyzed gel formation of gelatin and chitosan: potential for in situ applications. Biomaterials 24:2831–2841. https://doi.org/10.1016/S0142-9612(03)00096-6
182. Le Thi P, Lee Y, Nguyen DH, Park KD (2017) In situ forming gelatin hydrogels by dual-enzymatic cross-linking for enhanced tissue adhesiveness. J Mater Chem B 5:757–764. https://doi.org/10.1039/c6tb02179d
183. Han B, Jaurequi J, Tang BW, Nimni ME (2003) Proanthocyanidin: a natural crosslinking reagent for stabilizing collagen matrices. J Biomed Mater Res Part A 65:118–124. https://doi.org/10.1002/jbm.a.10460
184. Butler MF, Ng YF, Pudney PDA (2003) Mechanism and kinetics of the crosslinking reaction between biopolymers containing primary amine groups and genipin. J Polym Sci Part A Polym Chem 41:3941–3953. https://doi.org/10.1002/pola.10960
185. Moura MJ, Figueiredo MM, Gil MH (2007) Rheological study of genipin cross-linked chitosan hydrogels. Biomacromolecules 8:3823–3829. https://doi.org/10.1021/bm700762w
186. Liu BS (2008) Fabrication and evaluation of a biodegradable proanthocyanidin-crosslinked gelatin conduit in peripheral nerve repair. J Biomed Mater Res Part A 87:1092–1102. https://doi.org/10.1002/jbm.a.31916
187. Huang CH, Chi CY, Chen YS, Chen KY, Chen PL, Yao CH (2012) Evaluation of proanthocyanidin-crosslinked electrospun gelatin nanofibers for drug delivering system. Mater Sci Eng C 32:2476–2483. https://doi.org/10.1016/j.msec.2012.07.029

188. Chen KY, Shyu PC, Dong GC, Chen YS, Kuo WW, Yao CH (2009) Reconstruction of calvarial defect using a tricalcium phosphate-oligomeric proanthocyanidins cross-linked gelatin composite. Biomaterials 30:1682–1688. https://doi.org/10.1016/j.biomaterials.2008.12.024
189. Migneault I, Dartiguenave C, Bertrand MJ, Waldron KC (2004) Glutaraldehyde: behavior in aqueous solution, reaction with proteins, and application to enzyme crosslinking. Biotechniques 37:790–802. https://doi.org/10.2144/04375RV01
190. Augustine R (2018) Skin bioprinting: a novel approach for creating artificial skin from synthetic and natural building blocks. Prog Biomater 7:77–92. https://doi.org/10.1007/s40204-018-0087-0

Chapter 3
Emerging Trends in the Synthesis, Properties and Applications of Nanogels Derived from Pullulan, Collagen and Gelatin

Sarojini Balladka Kunhanna, Niveditha Nagappa Bailore, and Pushparekha

Abstract Biopolymers, namely polysaccharide pullulan and the two polyamides collagen and gelatin, offer themselves as versatile materials in modern drug delivery systems by forming nanogel networks. Pullulan is highly water soluble which on conjugation with cholesterol forms CHP with increased hydrophobicity and offers itself as a matrix for nanogel formation. Self-assembly of these hybrid materials is a well-established strategy to synthesize the nanogels. Another method to make these materials is physical and chemical grafting copolymerization technique. These nanogels are usually sensitive towards environmental conditions. The thermoresponsive CHP-PNIPAM nanogels exhibit quick deswelling and reswelling behaviour at stipulated temperatures. The uronic acid-grafted pullulan derivatives exhibit pH-responsive behaviour in drug delivery. Collagen and gelatin nanohydrogels prepared through physical and chemical cross-linking as well as irradiation techniques are mainly used for drug delivery, especially in wound healing. This chapter describes the synthesis of tailor-made functional nanogels for customized use as drug carriers as well as environmental sensors.

Keywords Nanogel · Pullulan · Collagen · Gelatin · Synthesis · Drug delivery · Stimuli response

S. Balladka Kunhanna (✉)
Department of Industrial Chemistry, Mangalore University, Mangalaganothri, Karnataka 574199, India
e-mail: bksaroj35@gmail.com

N. N. Bailore
Biochemistry Section, Department of Chemistry, Mangalore University, Mangalagangothri, Karnataka 574199, India

Pushparekha
Department of Chemistry, Mangalore University, Mangalagangothri, Karnataka 574199, India

J. Jose et al. (eds.), *Nano Hydrogels*, Gels Horizons: From Science to Smart Materials,
https://doi.org/10.1007/978-981-15-7138-1_3

1 Introduction

Nanotechnology is the branch of technology which deals with the study of manipulating matter on an atomic scale. Hydrogels are a unique class of macromolecular/nanomolecular arrangements. It is a cross-linked network of hydrophilic polymers. Polymeric hydrogels can be classified into three groups based on their particle sizes; they are macrogels, microgels and nanogels. Nanogels are hydrogel networks at a nanoscale range between 1 and 100 nm [1].

Nanogels are defined as the nanosized particles synthesized through chemically or physically cross-linked hydrophilic polymer networks, which are capable of improving the swelling in the aqueous media [2]. One of the important advantages of nanogels is the faster swelling–deswelling properties. Due to its smaller size, it exhibits excellent permeation abilities and is also capable of improving the solubilization of many hydrophobic drugs and diagnostic substances [3]. Nanogels form different complexes with different drugs, proteins, peptides and DNA materials. Nanogels have great variety of applications in the field of drug delivery.

2 Classification of Nanogels

Nanogels are mainly classified as two major classes:

- Firstly on the basis of environment-responsive nature
- Secondly on the basis of type of cross-linking technology applied.

On the basis of responsive nature, nanogels can be categorized as stimuli-responsive or stimuli-nonresponsive gels [3]. Stimuli-responsive gels swell up due to environmental changes through electric and magnetic fields, pH and temperature. Nonresponsive gels just swell up when placed in an aqueous media.

Based on the second classification type, nanogels are classified as two types: chemical cross-linked gels and physical cross-linked gels [4].

Natural polymers such as polysaccharides (chitosan, hyaluronic acid (HA), heparin, chondroitin sulphate, agarose and alginate) and proteins (collagen, albumin and fibrin) are widely used for the preparation nanohydrogels. This is because of the attractive properties of natural polymers like biocompatibility, biodegradability and its lower cost [5, 6].

Polysaccharides from the natural source are most used materials in the form of food, cloth and other engineering materials since human civilization. Of late, they offer themselves as excellent materials for the preparation of hydrogel formulations [7]. The polysaccharide-based hydrogels either prepared by physical or chemical means offer versatility as materials of choice to use in medicinal fields as target drug transporters and in tissue engineering. Most of the personal care products and cosmetics preparations contain polysaccharide-based hydrogels as water replenishing agents in most of the cases [8]. They are used as water purifying agents with superabsorbent nature [9] and used for controlled release of fertilizers and herbicides as well, along with paint removal in paper and textile industries [10–12]. The structure-specific properties of polysaccharides could be related to their primary structures and masses. The reactive pendent groups present on the monomeric units make these macromolecules available to various chemical and physical modifications. Hence, customized properties could be achieved [13].

A large number of polysaccharides form hydrogel under adequate conditions. Alginate, pectins and gellan are the typical polymers that form gels by ion complexation on interaction between carboxylic groups and divalent ions; locust bean gum and xanthan on mutual interfacing form gels [14, 15].

The hydrogels of consistency could be synthesized by the treatment of borax with some polysaccharides on reacting with hydroxyl groups [16]. Cross-linking reagents possessing multifunctional reaction sites are used to chemically cross-link the functional groups present in polysaccharides to form hydrogels [17, 18]. Sometimes, the hydrogels prepared from natural polysaccharides do not meet the properties needed for specific type of applications and also there are instances that they fail to form hydrogels itself. So, semi-interpenetrating polymeric networks (semi-IPNs) and interpenetrating polymeric networks (IPNs) are synthesized to have superior properties [19]. The IPNs exhibit different physical and chemical properties than the polymers from which they are derived. According to the customized demand, these materials could be synthesized [20].

There are different methods developed to fabricate hydrogels; the number techniques are being developed to tailor the size of hydrogels. The bulk hydrogels are being used in many fields for specific applications, while the nanohydrogels are promising size-modified hydrogels which are looked upon for use in medical and engineering fields. Nanohydrogels can be generally synthesized by the polymerization of a monomer in homo- or nanoheterogeneous environment, chemical cross-linking lithography, template-assisted nanofabrication and self-assembly of polymers.

The most commonly used polysaccharides for hydrogel formation are hyaluronic acid, chitosan, gellan, scleroglucan, mannans which are prepared by varied techniques. But in this chapter, the focus will be on pullulan [PULN]–collagen-based nanohydrogels, their properties and applications.

3 Pullulan-Based Nanohydrogels

The polysaccharide-based nanohydrogels are usually prepared by the macromolecular self-assembly which result in nanostructured networks. Hence, hydrophobic and hydrophilic polymer chains are cross-linked carefully to use in drug delivery systems which is depicted in Fig. 1.

A nanohydrogel is 'an aqueous dispersion of hydrogel particles formed by physically or chemically cross-linked polymer networks of nanoscale size' as defined by

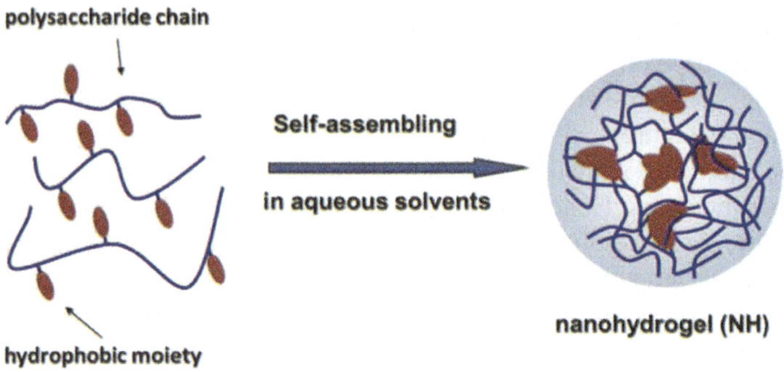

Fig. 1 Self-assembly technique for the preparation of nanogels, Ref. [13]

Kabanov and Vinogradov [21]. Sometimes during self-assembly, these nanostructured materials arrange themselves as self-assembled micelles and could be called as nanoparticles. The hydrophobized PULN was used for gelation; usually, it was identified as nanoparticles.

4 Synthesis of Nanohydrogels of Pullulan

4.1 Cholesterol-Modified Pullulan Nanohydrogels (CHP)

An exciting article by Whitesides et al. published in Science opened a new avenue to synthesize nanostructured materials by self-assembly (Fig. 2). The cholesterol-modified pullulan (CHP) was synthesized to coat liposomes [22]. The formation of polymer aggregates depended on degree of hydrophobicity. Hence, cholesterol-bearing pullulan could bind effectively on lipophilic guest molecules resulting in higher stability of colloids. In brief, first aminoethyl-carboxymethyl derivative of the polysaccharide was condensed with cholesteryl chloroformate to obtain CHP but later in an improved procedure cholesteryl *N*-(6-isocyanatohexyl) carbamate was synthesized and condensed with PULN which yielded stable nanogels [23]. The self-aggregated nanoparticles of CHP were obtained by sonication in water, but they were also prepared in water on dilution with DMSO [24].

4.2 Synthesis from Pullulan Acetates

The use of pullulan in drug delivery accounts for its film-forming capacity and high water solubility. So, PULN lipophilicity was increased by converting it into

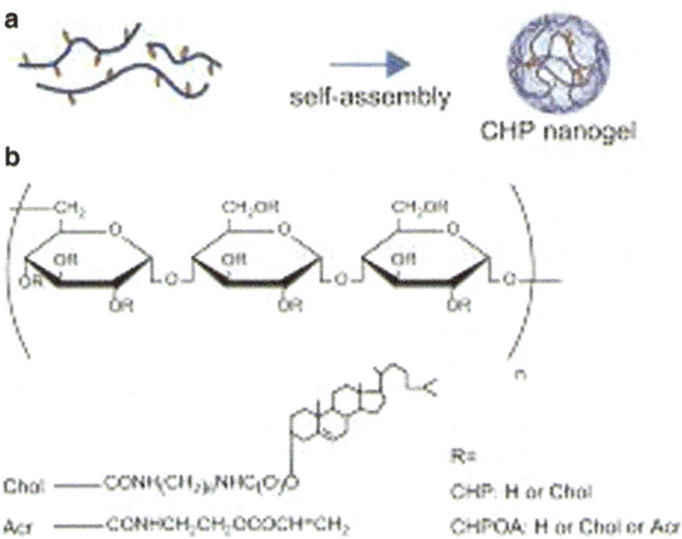

Fig. 2 Preparation of CHP, Ref. [25]

acetate which spontaneously aggregated into nanospherical particles [26]. A modified method accepted was to couple hydrophobized PULN with carboxymethylated poly(ethylene glycol). The incorporation of PEG increased craftiness of the nanoparticles for loading drugs [27].

4.3 Synthesis via Copolymerization to Hybrid Pullulan Nanogels

The hydrophobized PUL was mixed with modified poly(*N*-isopropylacrylamide) (HM-PNIPAM) to yield monodispersed nanogels via association of their hydrophobic groups which above 32 °C (i.e., the lower critical solution temperature of PNIPAM-C18Py) increased their diameter from 47 to 160 nm [28, 29]. The graft copolymerization of PNIPAM onto methacryloyl-substituted CHP nanogels in the presence of 2,2°-azobis[2-(2-imidazolin-2-yl)propane] as initiator resulted in different radii nanoparticles for customized use.

4.4 Pullulan Poly(Lactide) Nanogels

In a typical one-pot procedure, pure pullulan was dissolved in DMSO in N2 atmosphere, to this solution *L*-lactide was added slowly up to 10% (w/v) and stirring continued at 70–75 °C for another 2 h. To this mixture, triethyl amine (TEA, 1.67 w/v) was added slowly to obtain nanogel [30].

5 Properties and Applications of Pullulan Nanogels

5.1 Physical Property of CHP Nanogels

The physical properties of CHPs self-assembled structures was determined by Dynamic Light Scattering (DLS) measurements. It showed spherical shape of the particles with average diameter of 25nm. The spherical shape of the particles indicated with negative stained electron microscopic observations. On keeping this hydrogel under different environmental conditions at room temperature, the properties of nanogel was unaltered indicating its stability. The tailor-made property for these nanogels could be obtained by appropriate changes in hydrophobicity, self-assembly and association of nanoparticles.

The complexation of protease enzyme chymotrypsin with CHP hydrogel resulted in stable nanoparticles. These conjugates exhibited increased thermal stability for structure and activity on bovine serine albumin (BSA). The chymotrypsin was found to be located deep inside nanogel network which was identified by the treatment of pullulanase enzyme [25].

Insulin loading in this nanohydrogel was the most investigated mechanism, as a supramolecular assembly was formed by just mixing of the two components. The assembly was very stable, and activity of the insulin was maintained without enzymatic degradations and aggregations. The insulin loaded in gel was active even after i.v. injection [31, 32]. Similarly, enzyme lipase was also mixed instantaneously into CHP nanogel, which increased its thermal stability. The enzyme was encapsulated in the nanogel matrix by lipophilic interactions [33] (Fig. 3).

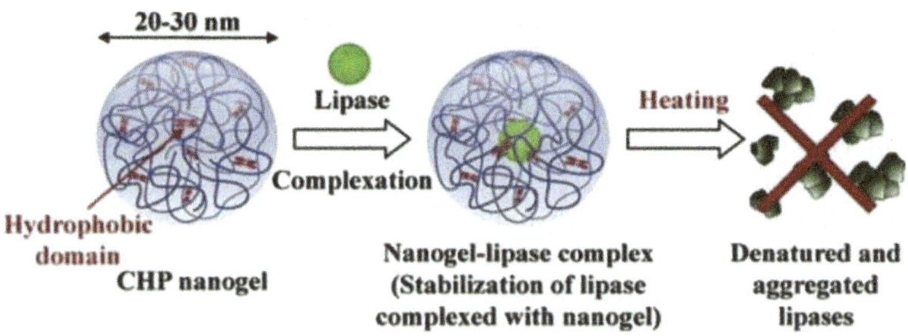

Fig. 3 Enzyme (lipase) thermal stabilization by loading within the CHP nanogel which holds the protein in the segregated nanomatrix by hydrophobic interaction (from Ref. [33] with permission)

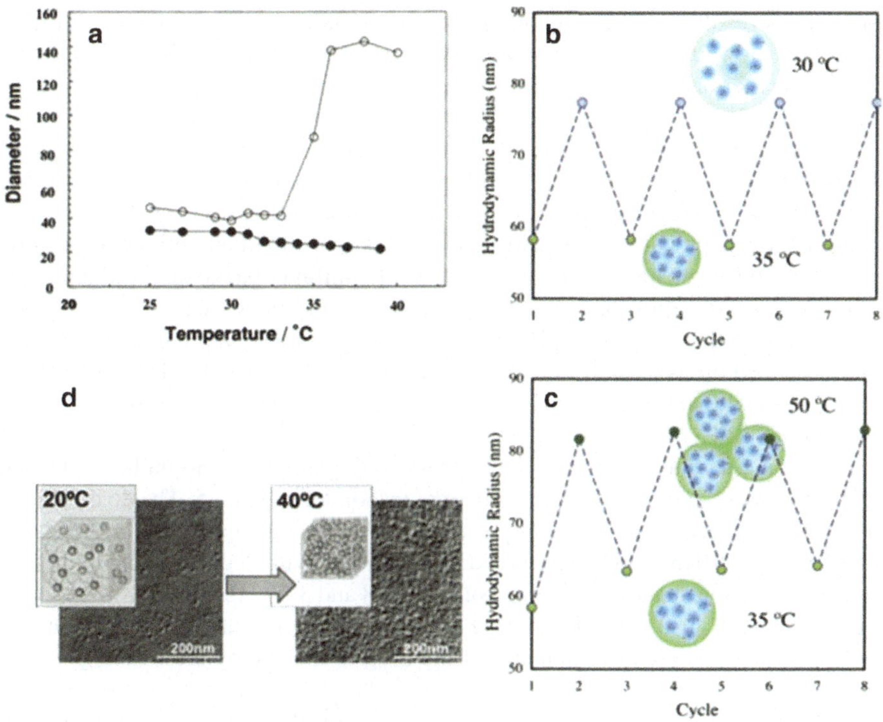

Fig. 4 Environmental-sensitive PUL nanogels. **a** Plot of the changes, as a function of temperature, of the average diameters of CHP nanogels in water (full circle) and of mixed CHP/PNIPAM-C18Py nanogels in water (open circle). **b** Changes in hydrodynamic radius of CHP nanogels with PNIPAM upon repeated changes in temperature from 35 to 30 °C and **c** from 35 to 50 °C with permission. **d** TEM image of the thermoresponsive hydrogel described in Ref. [13]

The CHP nanogels efficiently detained the inactivation of proteins and enzymes usually caused by heat, guanidinium chloride and urea. Upon addition of β-cyclodextrins, the CHP nanogel networks rapidly unfolded releasing enzymes by hydrophobic interactions. This quality makes CHP gels suitable for targeted drug delivery in hydrophobic environments, Fig. 4. The CHP application in therapeutic use was studied by using mouse embryos, which were fed with growth factor receptor FGFR2 with S252W through nanogel to treat Apert syndrome a congential disorder [34].

5.2 *Temperature- and pH-Responsive Properties*

The graft copolymerized nanogels prepared from hydrophobized pullulan and PNIPAM and NIPAM showed thermosensitive properties. The different ratios of two components resulted in different architectures of nanogels. The high concentration of NIPAM showed two-step temperature variances: one between 35–30 °C and 35–50 °C. This thermal response was attributed to the particular grape-like morphology of nanogel [35].

The nanogels prepared by cross-linking PNIPAM and cholesterol/methacryloyl PULN exhibited quick deswelling and reswelling behaviour at 20–40 °C, which could find use in releasing lipophilic and protein molecules [36] (Fig. 4).

The nanogels prepared from acid-labile cholesterol-modified pullulan with vinyl ether cholesterol substituents grafted on 100 kD pullulan backbone. The nanogels obtained showed radius 26.5 $\pm$ 5.1 nm at pH 7.0 and increased by ~135% upon acidification of the solution to pH 4.0. It was found that keeping the gel for 24 h at pH 4 degraded up to 80%. But acid-stable CHP remained undegraded at pH 4.0 as it is the case with acL-CHP at pH 4. So, these nanogels can release protein cargo at required pH [37].

The uronic acid and cholesteryl succinate conjugate grafted to pullulan showed a pH-sensitive response. These gel networks responded at pH 6.5. The doxorubicin, an antitumour drug, was physically loaded to UCPA nanogels, and drug release behaviour at a different pH was studied. The nanogel with degree of substitution of urocanyl and cholesterol in the composition of 6.8 and 3.5%, respectively, was found to be effective in vitro pH-induced drug release. The MTT assay and flow cytometry assay indicated the effective delivery of the drug to the site by these nanogels [38] (Fig. 5).

The above review has given a bird's eye view on the synthesis and their environmentally sensitive properties of pullulan-based nanogels. Pullulan offers as base material to engineer-customized nanohydrogels which respond to temperature and pH with high sensitivity. This property makes pullulan-based nanohydrogels to use in targeted drug delivery and functional-based applications.

6 Preparation of Protein-Based Gels from Collagen and Gelatin

Collagen is the principle protein of animal connective tissue and composed of approximately 30% of the total protein content of animal body [39]. The word 'collagen' is derived from the Greek words 'kolla' and 'genos' meaning glue and formation, respectively [40]. There are at least 29 different types of collagen so far identified; however, Types I to IV constitute 90% of them [41].

Collagen molecule is composed of three helical strands intertwined into one super-helix. Normally, collagen contains all essential amino acids except tryptophan. Glycine, proline and hydroxyproline are the major amino acids present in collagen at 10–20 folds the concentration found in other proteins. The most common

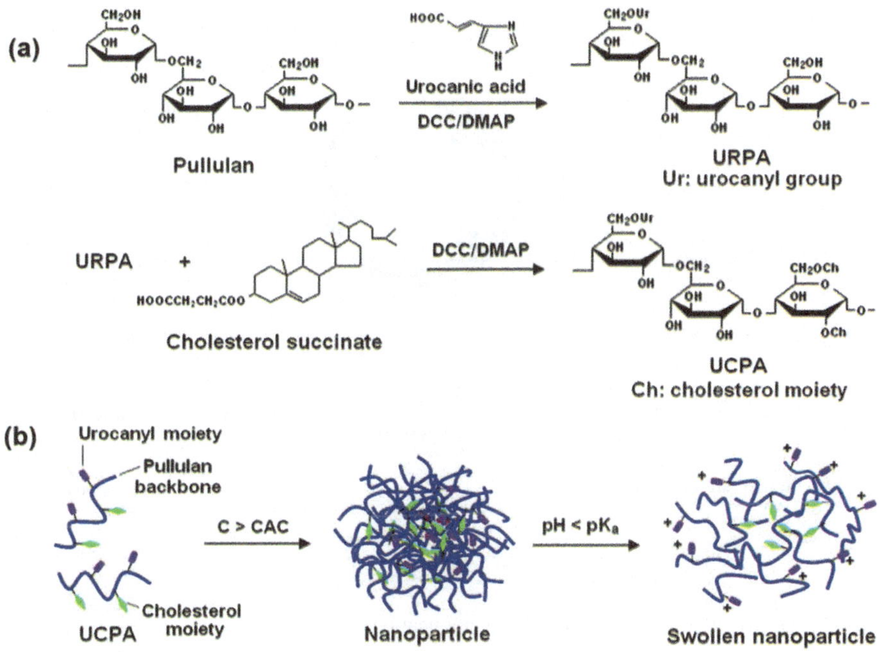

Fig. 5 pH-responsive urocanic acid-substituted nanogel, Ref. [37]

motifs in the amino acid sequence of collagen are glycine-proline-X and glycine-X-hydroxyproline, where X is any amino acid other than glycine, proline or hydroxyproline [42]. These three amino acids are very important for the formation of the specific triple helical structure and stabilization of collagen molecule [42, 43]. The hydroxyproline content is lower in fish collagen due to labile cross-links as compared to mammals [44, 45].

Collagen has widespread applications in numerous fields such as pharmaceutical, medical, biomedical, food industry and cosmetics (Fig. 6).

Soluble collagen is the starting materials used in collagen research. It can be extracted by acid-soluble collagen or pepsin-soluble collagen. In pepsin-soluble collagen, the enzyme pepsin is used to cleave the telopeptide region of collagen [47].

6.1 Properties of Collagen Nanogel

Physically formed collagen gels are thermo-reversible in nature which exhibits poor physical and chemical properties when compared to the covalently cross-linked collagen gels. The pH and temperature are the important factors involved in the gel formation. At lower temperature, collagen gels are formed which exhibits larger

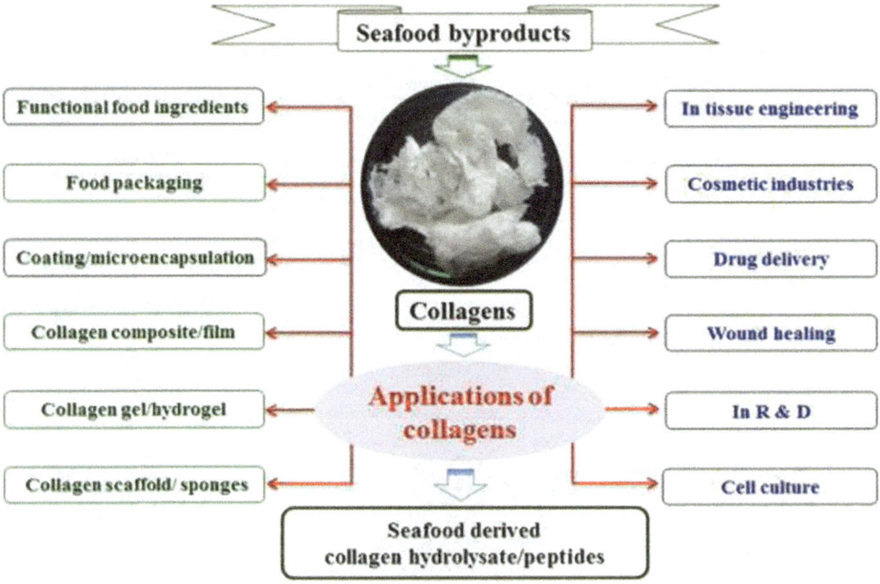

Fig. 6 Schematic representation of collagen applications [46]

pore size with enhanced cellular response [48]. On the contrary, higher temperature and higher pH accelerate fibrillogenesis but result in the formation of the gels with small diameter fibre and pore sizes [47].

For reducing the biodegradation rate of protein, numerous chemical cross-linking techniques were developed. The individual protein chains are linked with a cross-linker by covalent bond, thereby stabilizing the protein.

6.2 Preparation of Collagen Nanogels

6.2.1 Preparation of Collagen Gel with Gold Nanoparticle via EDC

The skin elasticity decreases during the ageing process, by 3-way connection through pyridinoline crosslinking of three side groups of collagen. Collagen gel was prepared by using 'multiple-way' linker as gold nanoparticles which is chemically cross-linking via 1-ethyl-3-(3-dimethyl aminopropyl) carbodiimide (EDC). The surface of gold nanoparticles contains multiple carboxyl groups; these are capable of forming multiple cross-links with the collagen. For improving properties like porosity, it used new types of cross-linking agent called as tiopronin (*N*-(2-mercaptopropionyl) glycine) which modified gold nanoparticles and form multiple cross-links with collagen molecules via EDC. There was a formation of eight bonds between each nanoparticle and the collagen molecules resulting in the reduction of the pore size, depending on the concentration of nanoclusters. This prepared new material has potential for the delivery of small molecule drugs as well as Au nanoparticles for photothermal therapies, imaging and cell targeting [49].

6.2.2 Preparation of Curcumin-Loaded Fish Scale Collagen (FSC)–Hydroxypropyl Methyl Cellulose (HPMC K100) Nanogel (CNG)

Nanoemulsion was prepared by aqueous titration method by using curcumin, oleic acid, Tween 80 and ethanol. Prepared curcumin nanoemulsion was loaded with hydroxypropyl methyl cellulose (HPMC K100) and fish scale collagen isolated from Catla fish. The prepared nanogel was evaluated for ex vivo permeation, and in vivo skin irritation and stability study. Ex vivo permeation study demonstrated that CNG prolonged release and exhibited higher per cent contraction value of wound compared to other formulations. In vivo study of CNG demonstrated higher wound contraction value compared to other formulations. Skin irritation study revealed that prepared nanogel was safe for dermatological (wound healing) applications [50].

7 Preparation of Gelatin-Based Nanogels

Gelatin is a biopolymer of animal origin (i.e., the skin and bones of bovine, porcine and fish sources) that is derived from the heat-induced hydrolytic degradation of collagen. Gelatin shows excellent biocompatibility, biodegradability, nontoxicity and high hydrophilicity in nature, and its multiple functionality (with –COOH and $–NH_2$ groups) is easily accessible for modification; due to this reason, it has been used for nanogel preparation for different applications. Gelatin nanogels can penetrate through the pores of the endothelial junctions found in tumour cells. Gelatin formed gels that are thermo-reversible in nature, and its gel-to-sol transition takes place at 30–35 °C [51–53].

Gelatin-based nanogels have been obtained via several methods as precipitation polymerization [54] and inverse miniemulsion polymerization [55].

Gelatin-based nanogels prepared without cross-linking were found to be unstable and tended to aggregate upon ageing [56, 57]. Therefore, a number of cross-linkers used are aldehydes, genipin, carbodiimide/*N*-hydroxysuccinimide, $CaCl_2$ [58] or enzymatic cross-linker as transglutaminase [59].

7.1 UV-Cross-Linked Gelatin Nanogel

Thermoresponsive behaviours of gelatin nanogel were investigated by using the preparation of UV-cross-linked gelatin nanogel without using any chemical cross-linking agents. The particle size of the nanogels decreased on heating, which is attributed to the helix-to-coil transition of gelatin [60].

7.2 Gelatin Nanogel by Desolvation Method

Gelatin nanogels were prepared via a one-step desolvation method to study the thermoresponsive property. Desolvating agents such as sodium sulphate or acetone were added to the gelatin solution. It leads to the coacervation of gelatin chains. When reaching the critical level of coacervation, the coacervate was redissolved by the addition of isopropanol. Glutaraldehyde was added to initiate the cross-links. Gelatin nanogel was prepared at various cross-linking conditions such as time, temperature and cross-linker concentration to optimize the helical structure of gelatin over the course of preparation. Thermoresponsive study showed a volume transition at 32 °C. This study shows how the temperature changes affect the particle size, the molecular configuration and factors influencing the thermoresponsive properties. It was studied by using dynamic light scattering (DLS), transmission electron microscopy (TEM) and polarimetry [61].

7.3 Stimuli-Responsive Gelatin Nanogel by Quantum Ray (60 Co Gamma) Irradiation

Akiyama et al. have studied to control the particle diameter and volume phase transition point of stimuli-responsive gelatin nanogel by quantum ray (^{60}Co gamma) irradiation at room temperature [62]. They succeeded to control the particle diameter in the range of 20–70 nm. Irradiated gelatin nanogel showed pH- and temperature-dependent response. They reversibly swelled and shrunk by stimuli of pH and temperature change. The changes in the volume phase transition point and swelling ratio are depending on the absorbed dose and the concentration of gelatin.

7.4 Polyethyleneimine-Based Core–Shell Nanogels

The core–shell nanogels were synthesized by two-stage reaction. The preparation of gelatin nanogel involves conjugation of polyethyleneimine (PEI) to the gelatin nanoparticles by desolvation and drying of the gelatin–PEI nanogels in ethanol/water mixture. The resulting nanogels show a well-defined nanostructure that contains a gelatin core and a PEI shell. They have an average diameter of 200 ± 40 nm with high uniformity. The nanogel particles possess positive zeta potential values of up to +40 mV at neutral pH, indicating that they are highly positive and very stable in aqueous media. The gelatin–PEI nanogels were able to completely condense siRNA and effectively protected siRNA against enzymatic degradation. The study shows nanogels were four times less toxic than native PEI. Due to less toxicity, the nanogels were able to effectively deliver siRNA into HeLa cells. It was studied by using confocal laser scanning microscope. This concluded that the gelatin nanogel protects siRNA against enzymatic degradation with lower toxicity and enhances cellular uptake up to 84% [63].

7.5 Preparation of Gelatin Nanogel by Gamma Ray Irradiation

Gelatin nanogels were prepared from aqueous gelatin solution by gamma ray irradiation generated from 60 °C source at room temperature around 20 °C without using any chemicals at a dose rate of 10 kGy/h.

The hydrodynamic radius of prepared nanoparticles was studied by using static and dynamic light scattering, and it was found to be 10 nm. The size of the nanoparticle could be controlled by adjusting the preparation condition of irradiation dose and concentration of gelatin. The ordered conformation of the original gelatin could be replaced by random conformation in the nanogel revealed by CD measurements. It was found to be the highly and randomly packed structure given a very high stability against the temperature change to the nanogel [64].

7.6 Curcumin-Loaded Alignate Aldehyde Gelatin Nanogels by Miniemulsion Technique

Gum arabic (GA) was oxidized to gum arabic aldehyde, and then it was cross-linked with gelatin to obtain nanogels. Physiochemical properties were studied by dynamic light scattering, NMR spectroscopy and scanning electron microscopy. Hemocompatibility and cytocompatibility of the nanogels evaluated the anticancer activity towards MCF-7 cells studied by using confocal laser scanning microscopy [65] (Fig. 7).

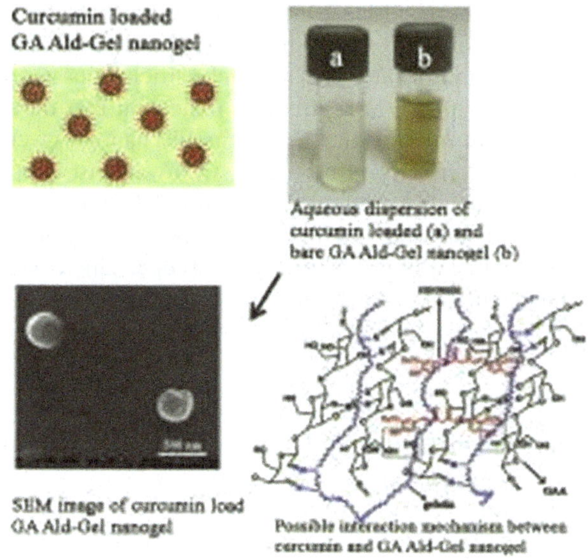

Fig. 7 Curcumin-loaded alignate aldehyde gelatin nanogels by miniemulsion technique [66]

7.7 *Gelatin Methacryloyl Nanogels by Inverse Emulsion Method*

Generally, polymeric nanoparticles have been developed mainly to deliver hydrophobic drugs to the dermis layer researchers such as Kim et al. [66] who have studied the suitability of gelatin methacryloyl (GelMA) nanogels for transdermal delivery of macromolecules and established the potency of the nanogels as a transdermal delivery carrier for hydrophilic macromolecules [51, 66]. This method involved the labelling of fluorescein isothiocyanate to bovine serum albumin (FITC-BSA) which further loaded to GelMA nanogels (FGNs) by water-in-oil emulsion droplets. The nanogel was formed by photo polymerization of methacryloyl substituents. Both GNs and FGNs existed as fine particles in aqueous condition (pH 7.4) for 7 days. High percentage of cell viability is studied by the MTT assay. The skin penetration study results showed that FGNs permeated across the epidermis and into the dermis of a porcine model when compared to the FITC-BSA dissolved in PBS. Possible penetration routes of FITC-BSA through the stratum corneum (SC) were illustrated by visualizing the SC structure with fluorescent signals of FITC-BSA. The penetration mechanism of FGNs across the SC layer was successfully demonstrated by intercellular, follicular and transcellular route. This results suggested that GNs have a potential as a transdermal delivery carrier for hydrophilic macromolecules.

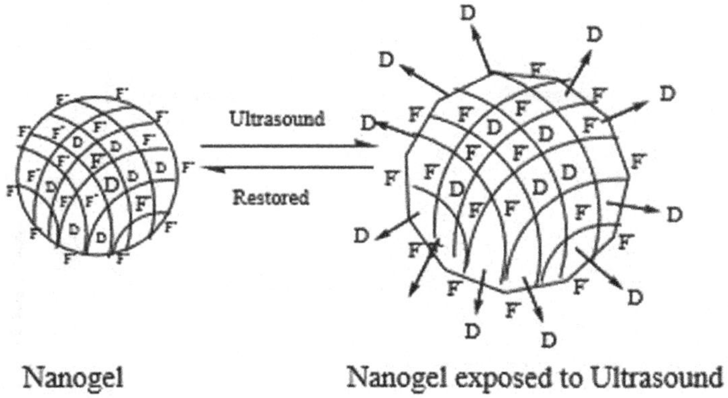

Fig. 8 Drug release of nanogel by ultrasound, Ref. [54]

7.8 Adriamycin Gelatin Nanogel Modified with Fluoride Anion (ADM-GNMF)

Gelatin nanogel was prepared by a modified co-precipitation method with fluoride anion and sodium sulphate for ultrasound-triggered drug release. Cross-linked gelatin solution was prepared by using ox-dextran. Adriamycin was introduced to cross-linked gelatin solution with Tween 20 and span 80. The size and shape of ADM-GNMF were determined by electron microscopy and photo-correlation spectroscopy. The ADM-GNMF was stable in solution with an average diameter found to be 46 ± 12 nm. This prepared nanogel releases the drug in response to ultrasound and is used as promising controlled drug release system for targeted therapy for cancer or other diseases [54] (Fig. 8).

7.9 Gelatin Nanogel by Inverse Miniemulsion Technique

Interpenetrating polymer network (IPN) nanogels composed of poly(acrylic acid) and gelatin were synthesized by one-pot inverse miniemulsion (IME) technique. Acrylic acid (AA) monomer stabilized around the gelatin macromolecules in each droplet was polymerized using ammonium persulfate (APS) and tetramethyl ethylene diamine (TEMED) and cross-linked with *N*,*N*-methylenebisacrylamide (BIS) to form semi-IPN (sIPN) nanogels, which were sequentially cross-linked by using glutaraldehyde (Glu) to form IPNs. Dynamic light scattering (DLS) and scanning electron microscopy (SEM) studies of purified nanogels showed small, spherical IPN nanogels. Interpenetration of the two networks was confirmed by FTIR, SEM, DLS, X-ray, XPS (photoelectron spectroscopy) and zeta potential studies. These nanogels have showed tailoring properties in order to use them as high-potential drug delivery vehicles for cancer targeting [67].

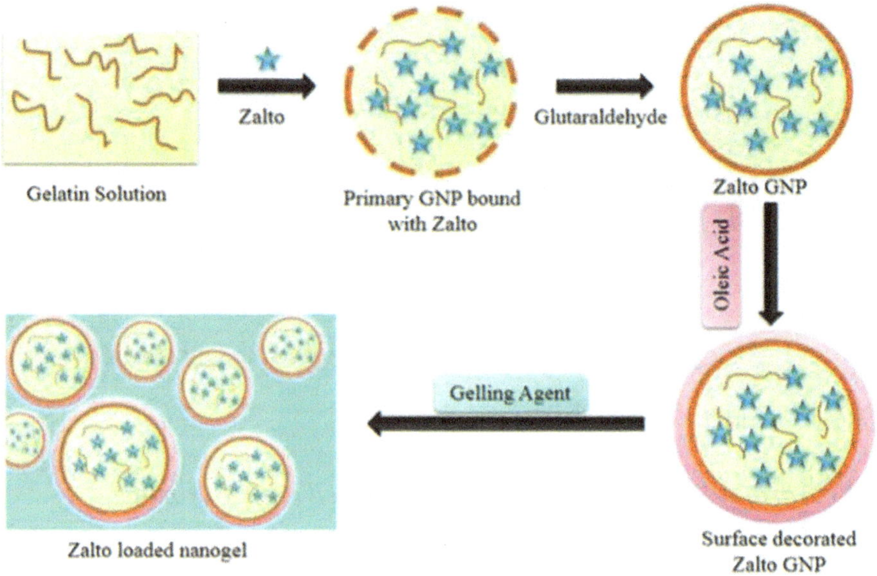

Fig. 9 Surface modification on zaltoprofen-loaded gelatin nanoparticles, Ref. [68]

7.10 Oleic Acid-Coated Gelatin Nanoparticle Impregnated Gel

Gelatin nanoparticles were first prepared by two-step desolvation method by using desolvating agent as ethanol to precipitate high molecular weight (HMW) gelatin. The supernatant was discarded, and the HMW gelatin was redissolved by adding distilled water containing zalto–cyclodextrin complex containing zaltoprofen as a result of formation of gelatin nanoparticle by the drop-wise addition of ethanol. Glutaraldehyde was added to cross-link the nanoparticles. The surface modification was done on zaltoprofen-loaded gelatin nanoparticles by adding oleic acid for preparing nanoparticulate suspension and for topical drug delivery. The smooth and spherical shape of GNP was confirmed by SEM. In vitro and ex vivo drug release showed that there was 69.47 and 78.59% drug released within 48 h. The good texture properties of nanogel were observed from texture analysis graphs. Stability data revealed stability of nanogel formulation up to 3 months [68] (Fig. 9).

7.11 Gelatin Nanogels by Sol–gel Technique

Enoxaparin-immobilized gelatin/poly(ε-caprolactone) (PCL) or Eudragit RS230D nanogels were prepared in the presence of tetraethyl orthosilicate (TEOS) that acts as polycondensation reagent by sol–gel technique for drug delivery ability. The sol–gel process was carried out under a dry nitrogen atmosphere with HCl as catalyst. For cross-linking of the organic matrix, the drug-loaded nanogel samples were exposed to ultraviolet (UV) light (150 W, XBO xenon lamp, light spectrum 200–1100 nm) for 15 min. Sol–gel formation was conducted based on hydrolysis and condensation mechanisms. Eudragit was used as model drug at different concentrations. The prepared nanogel was analysed by thermal analysis (DSC and TGA), Fourier transform infrared spectroscopy (FTIR), X-ray diffraction (XRD), and scanning and transmitting electron microscopes (SEM and TEM). The particle size, zeta potential and in vitro release profiles were investigated. The prepared nanogels exhibited amorphous nature with stable colloidal particles (9.3 nm) and high surface charge density (negative zeta potential). The immobilization of enoxaparin into the gel network led to the formation of stable nanogels with ionic functional groups, which enable the efficient loading and sustainable release [69].

8 Conclusion

Biopolymers, namely polysaccharide pullulan and the two polyamides collagen and gelatin, offer themselves as versatile materials in modern drug delivery systems by forming nanogel networks. Pullulan is highly water soluble which on conjugation with cholesterol forms CHP with increased hydrophobicity and offers itself as a matrix for nanogel formation. Self-assembly of these hybrid materials is a well-established strategy to synthesize the nanogels. Another method to make these materials is physical and chemical grafting copolymerization techniques. These nanogels are usually sensitive towards environmental conditions. The thermoresponsive CHP-PNIPAM nanogels exhibit quick deswelling and reswelling behaviour at stipulated temperatures. The uronic acid-grafted derivatives exhibit pH-responsive behaviour in drug delivery. Collagen and gelatin nanohydrogels prepared through physical and chemical cross-linking as well as irradiation techniques are mainly used for drug delivery, especially in wound healing. This chapter describes the synthesis of tailor-made functional nanogels for customized use as drug carriers as well as environmental sensors.

References

1. Jiang Y, Chen J, Deng C, Suuronen EJ, Zhong Z (2014) Click hydrogels, microgels and nanogels: emerging platforms for drug delivery and tissue engineering. Biomaterials 35(18):4969–4985
2. Kuroda K, Fujimoto K, Sunamoto J, Akiyoshi K (2002) Hierarchical self-assembly of hydrophobically modified pullulan in water: gelation by networks of nanoparticles. Langmuir 18(10):3780–3786

3. Soni KS, Desale SS, Bronich TK (2016) Nanogels: An overview of properties, biomedical applications and obstacles to clinical translation. J Control Release 240:109–126
4. Choudhary B, Paul SR, Nayak SK, Qureshi D, Pal K (2018) Synthesis and biomedical applications of filled hydrogels. In: Polymeric Gels, pp 283–302
5. Hoare TR, Kohane DS (2008) Hydrogels in drug delivery: progress and challenges. Polymer 49:1993–2007
6. Ahmed EM (2015) Hydrogel: preparation, characterization, and applications: a review. J Adv Res 6:105–121
7. Coviello T, Matricardi P, Marianecci C, Alhaique F (2007) Polysaccharide hydrogels for modified release formulations. J Control Release 119(1):5–24
8. Lautenschläger H (2009) Saccharides in cosmetic products—from alginate to Xanthan Gum. Kosmetische Praxis 4:12–15
9. Bello K, Sarojini BK, Narayana B, Rao A, Byrappa K (2018) A study on adsorption behavior of newly synthesized banana pseudo-stem derived superabsorbent hydrogels for cationic and anionic dye removal from effluents. Carbohyd Polym 181:605–615
10. Campos EVS, De Olivera JL, Fraceto LF, Sing B (2014) Polysaccharides as saferrelease systems for agrochemicals. Agron Sustain Dev 35:47–66
11. Carretti E, Bonini M, Dei L, Berrie BH, Angelova LV, Baglioni P, Weiss RG (2010) New frontiers in materials science for art conservation: responsive gels and beyond. Acc Chem Res 43:751–760
12. Mazzuca C, Micheli L, Cervelli E, Basoli F, Cencetti C, Coviello T, Palleschi A (2014) Cleaning of paper artworks: development of an efficient gel-based material able to remove starch paste. ACS Appl Mater Interfaces 6(19):16519–16528
13. Alhaique F, Matricardi P, Di Meo C, Coviello T, Montanari E (2015) Polysaccharide-based self-assembling nanohydrogels: an overview on 25-years research on pullulan. J Drug Deliv Sci Technol 30:300–309
14. Zhan DF, Ridout MJ, Brownsey G, Morris VJ (1993) Xanthan-locust bean gum interactions and gelation. Carbohyd Polym 21(1):53–58
15. Sandolo C, Bulone D, Mangione MR, Margheritelli S, Di Meo C, Alhaique F, Matricardi A (2010) Synergistic interaction of Locust Bean Gum and Xanthan investigated by rheology and light scattering. Carbohyd Polym 82:733–741
16. Coviello T, Grassi M, Lapasin R, Marino A, Alhaique F (2003) Sclero glucan/borax: characterization of a novel hydrogel system suitable for drug delivery. Biomaterials 24:2789–2798
17. Park K, Shalaby WSW, Park H (1993) Biodegradable hydrogels for drug delivery. Technomic Publishing Co., Lancaster, pp 67–98
18. Hennink WE, van Nostrum CF (2012) Novel crosslinking methods to design hydrogels. Adv Drug Deliv Rev 64:223–236
19. Jenkins AD, Kratochvíl P, Stepto RFT, Suter UW (1996) Glossary of basic terms in polymer science (IUPAC recommendations 1996). Pure Appl Chem 68(12):2287–2311
20. Matricardi P, Di Meo C, Coviello T, Alhaique F, Hennink W (2013) Interpenetrating polymer networks polysaccharide hydrogels for drug delivery and tissue engineering. Adv Drug Deliv Rev 65:1172–1187
21. Kabanov AV, Vinogradov SV (2009) Nanogels as pharmaceutical carriers: finite networks of infinite capabilities. Angew Chem Int Ed 48(30):5418–5429
22. Whitesides GM, Mathias JP, Seto CT (1991) Molecular self-assembly and nanochemistry: a chemical strategy for the synthesis of nanostructures. Science 254(5036):1312–1319
23. Akiyoshi K, Yamaguchi S, Sunamoto J (1991) Self-aggregates of hydrophobic polysaccharide derivatives. Chem Lett 20:1263–1266
24. Akiyoshi K, Nagai K, Nishikawa T, Sunamoto J (1992) Self-aggregates of hydrophobized polysaccharide as a host for macromolecular guests. Chem Lett 21(9):1727–1730
25. Nishikawa T, Akiyoshi K, Sunamoto J (1994) Supramolecular assembly between nanoparticles of hydrophobized polysaccharide and soluble protein complexation between the self-aggregate of cholesterol-bearing pullulan and .alpha.-chymotrypsin. Macromolecules, 27(26):7654–7659

26. Jeong YI, Nah JW, Na HK, Na K, Kim IS, Cho CS, Kim SH (1999) Self-assembling nano spheres of hydrophobized pullulans in water. Drug Dev Ind Pharm 25(8):917–927
27. Jung SW, Jeong YII, Kim YH, Kim SH (2004) Self-assembled polymeric nanoparticles of poly(ethylene glycol) grafted pullulan acetate as a novel drug carrier. Arch Pharm Res 27:562–569
28. Ringsdorf H, Venzmer J, Winnik FM (1991) Fluorescence studies of hydrophobically modified poly (*N*-isopropylacrylamides). Macromolecules 24(7):1678–1686
29. Akiyoshi K, Kang ES, Kurumada S, Sunamoto J, Principi T, Winnik FM (2000) Controlled association of amphiphilic polymers in water: thermo sensitive nano particles formed by self-assembly of hydrophobically modified pullulansand poly (*N*-isopropylacrylamides). Macromolecules 33:3244–3249
30. Cho JK, Park W, Na K (2009) Self-organized nanogels from pullulan-*g*-poly (*L*-lactide) synthesized by one-pot method: physicochemical characterization and in vitro doxorubicin release. J Appl Polym Sci 113(4):2209–2216
31. Akiyoshi K, Nishikawa T, Shichibe S, Sunamoto J (1995) Stabilization of insulin upon supramolecular complexation with hydrophobized polysaccharide nanoparticle. Chem Lett 24(8):707–708
32. Akiyoshi K, Kobayashi S, Shichibe S, Mix D, Baudys M, Kim SW, Sunamoto J (1998) Self-assembled hydrogel nanoparticle of cholesterol-bearing pullulan as a carrier of protein drugs: complexation and stabilization of insulin. J Control Release 54(3):313–320
33. Sawada SI, Akiyoshi K (2010) Nano-encapsulation of lipase by self-assembled nanogels: induction of high enzyme activity and thermal stabilization. Macromol Biosci 10(4):353–358
34. Yokota M, Kobayashi Y, Morita J, Suzuki H, Hashimoto Y, Sasaki Y, Moriyama K (2014) Therapeutic effect of nanogel-based delivery of soluble FGFR2 with S252W mutation on cranio synostosis. PLoS ONE 9(7):101693
35. Morimoto N, Winnik FM, Akiyoshi K (2007) Botryoidal assembly of cholesteryl-pullulan/poly(*N*-isopropylacrylamide) nanogels. Langmuir 23(1):217–223
36. Morimoto N, Ohki T, Kurita K, Akiyoshi K (2008) Thermo-responsive hydrogels with nanodomains: rapid shrinking of a nanogel crosslinking hydrogel of poly (*N*-isopropyl acrylamide). Macromol Rapid Commun 29(8):672–676
37. Wang Y, Chen H, Liu Y, Wu J, Zhou P, Wang Y, Zhang N (2013) pH-sensitive pullulan-based nanoparticle carrier of methotrexate and combretastatin A4 for the combination therapy against hepatocellular carcinoma. Biomaterials 34(29):7181–7190
38. Shiku H, Wang L, Ikuta Y, Okugawa T, Schmitt M, Gu X, Akiyoshi K, Sunamoto J, Nakamura H (2000) Development of a cancer vaccine: peptides, proteins and DNA. Cancer Chemother Pharm 46(1):S77
39. Aberoumand A (2011) Isolation of collagen from some fishes skins in Iran. J Agric Technol 7(3):783–788
40. Muralidharan N, Shakila RJ, Sukumar D, Jeyasekaran G (2013) Skin, bone and muscle collagen extraction from the trash fish, leather jacket (*Odonus niger*) and their characterization. J Food Sci Technol 50(6):1106–1113
41. Bailey AJ, Paul RG, Knott L (1998) Mechanisms of maturation and ageing of collagen. Mech Ageing Dev 106(1):1–56
42. Szpak P (2011) Fish bone chemistry and ultrastructure: implications for taphonomy and stable isotope analysis. J Archaeolog Sci 38(12):3358–3372
43. Muyonga JH, Cole CGB, Duodu KG (2004) Characterisation of acid soluble collagen from skins of young and adult Nile perch (*Lates niloticus*). Food Chem 85(1):81–89
44. Hickman D, Sims TJ, Miles CA, Bailey AJ, De Mari M, Koopmans M (2000) Isinglass/collagen: denaturation and functionality. J Biotechnol 79(3):245–257
45. Saito M, Takenouchi Y, Kunisaki N, Kimura S (2001) Complete primary structure of rainbow trout type I collagen consisting of $\alpha 1$ (I) $\alpha 2$ (I) $\alpha 3$ (I) heterotrimers. Eur J Biochem 268(10):2817–2827
46. Pal GK, Suresh PV (2016) Sustainable valorisation of seafood by-products: recovery of collagen and development of collagen-based novel functional food ingredients. Innov Food Sci Emerg Technol 37:201–215

47. Antoine EE, Vlachos PP, Rylander MN (2014) Review of collagen I hydrogels for bioengineered tissue microenvironments: characterization of mechanics, structure, and transport. Tissue Eng Part B Rev 20(6):683–696
48. Yang YL, Motte S, Kaufman LJ (2010) Pore size variable type I collagen gels and their interaction with glioma cells. Biomaterials 31(21):5678–5688
49. Castaneda L, Valle J, Yang N, Pluskat S, Slowinska K (2008) Collagen cross-linking with Au nanoparticles. Biomacromol 9(12):3383–3388
50. Pathan IB, Munde SJ, Shelke S, Ambekar W, Mallikarjuna Setty C (2018) Curcumin loaded fish scale collagen-HPMC nanogel for wound healing application: ex-vivo and in-vivo evaluation. Int J Polym Mater Polym Biomater, 1–10
51. Thakur G, Rodrigues FC, Dathathri E, Nayak SK, Pal K (2018) Protein-based gels: preparation, characterizations, applications in drug delivery, and tissue engineering. In: Polymeric Gels, pp 31–54
52. Pamfil D, Vasile C (2018) Nanogels of natural polymers. Polymer gels. Springer, Singapore, pp 71–110
53. Dalwadi C, Patel G (2015) Application of nanohydrogels in drug delivery systems: recent patents review. Recent Pat Nanotechnol 9(1):17–25
54. Wu D, Wan M (2008) A novel fluoride anion modified gelatin nanogel system for ultrasound-triggered drug release. J Pharm Pharmaceut Sci 11(4):32–45
55. Sarika PR, James NR (2015) Preparation and characterisation of gelatin–gum arabic aldehyde nanogels via inverse miniemulsion technique. Int J Biol Macromol 76:181–187
56. Bode F, da Silva MA, Drake AF, Ross-Murphy SB, Dreiss CA (2011) Enzymatically cross-linked tilapia gelatin hydrogels: physical, chemical, and hybrid networks. Biomacromol 12:3741–3752
57. Elzoghby AO, Samy WM, Elgindy NA (2012) Protein-based nanocarriers as promising drug and gene delivery systems. J Control Release 161:38–49
58. Narayanan D, Geena MG, Lakshmi H, Koyakutty M, Nair S, Menon D (2013) Poly-(ethylene glycol) modified gelatin nanoparticles for sustained delivery of the anti-inflammatory drug ibuprofen-sodium: an in vitro and in vivo analysis. Nanomedicine 9:818–828
59. Fuchs S, Kutscher M, Hertel T, Winter G, Pietzsch M, Coester C (2010) Transglutaminase: new insights into gelatin nanoparticle crosslinking. J Microencapsul 27:747–754
60. Maki Y, Saito W, Dobashi T (2018) Preparation and thermoresponsive behaviors of UV-crosslinked gelatin nanogels. J Biorheol 32(1):15–19
61. Gandhi SS, Yan H, Kim C (2014) Thermoresponsive gelatin nanogels. ACS Macro Lett 3:1210–1214
62. Akiyama Y, Fujiwara T, Takeda SI, Izumi Y, Nishijima S (2007) Preparation of stimuli-responsive protein nanogel by quantum-ray irradiation. Colloid Polym Sci 285(7):801–807
63. Mimi H, Ho KM, Siu YS (2012) Polyethyleneimine-based core-shell nanogels: A promising siRNA carrier for argininosuccinate synthetase mRNA knockdown in HeLa cells. J Control J Control Release l Rel 158:123–130
64. Furusawa K, Terao K, Nagasawa N, Yoshii F, Kubota K, Dobashi T (2004) Nanometer-sized gelatin particles prepared by means of gamma-ray irradiation. Colloid Polym Sci 283(2):229–233
65. Sarika PR, James NR, Raj DK (2016) Preparation, characterization and biological evaluation of curcumin loaded alginate aldehyde–gelatin nanogels. Mater Sci Eng C 68:251–257
66. Kim J, Gauvin R, Yoon HJ, Kim JH, Kwon SM, Park HJ, Bae H (2016) Skin penetration-inducing gelatin methacryloyl nanogels for transdermal macromolecule delivery. Macromol Res 24(12):1115–1125
67. Koul V, Mohamed R, Kuckling D, Adler HJP, Choudhary V (2011) Interpenetrating polymer network (IPN) nanogels based on gelatin and poly (acrylic acid) by inverse miniemulsion technique: Synthesis and characterization. Colloids Surf B 83(2):204–213
68. Pawar S, Pande V (2015) Oleic acid coated gelatin nanoparticles impregnated gel for sustained delivery of zaltoprofen: formulation and textural characterization. Adv Pharm Bull 5(4):537

69. Haroun AA, El Nahrawy AM, Maincent P (2014) Enoxaparin-immobilized poly (ε-caprolactone)-based nanogels for sustained drug delivery systems. Pure Appl Chem 86(5):691–700

Chapter 4
Nanobased Biodegradable Hydrogel for Biomedical Application

P. K. Sandhya, M. S. Sreekala, and Sabu Thomas

Abstract Recently, the design of hydrogels using bio-based materials has been increasingly developed for application in pharmaceutical technology. The incorporation of nanoscale structures is useful for tuning the cell behaviour and responses through optimization of mechanical properties or an enhancement in the stability of hydrogels. A considerable progress can be observed in the synthesis and technology of biodegradable nanocomposites hydrogel in the design of controlled and sustained drug delivery systems. The great interest of researchers to produce biodegradable hydrogels is due to the rich resources and huge potential to reduce the fabrication costs. Nowadays, some of the nanoparticles that are used for the preparation of the hydrogels are synthesized by green methods. The current chapter gives an idea about the preparation, characterization, various nanofillers used for the preparation of nanocomposite hydrogels and the application of biodegradable hydrogels in different fields.

1 Introduction

Nanotechnology is an interdisciplinary field which bridges the recent advances in the chemical, physical, and biological fields combined with the rising needs in the pharmaceutical and biomedical sectors. This upcoming technology has led to new developments in nanocomposite hydrogels for many applications in drug delivery, sensors, regenerative medicine, stem cell engineering, and other biomedical devices. In fact, owing to small size, drug loading capacity, surface functionality, and stability, the nanoparticles have gained increased attention for potential applications in biomedical fields [1]. Nanoparticles exist in different shapes like

P. K. Sandhya (✉) · S. Thomas
School of Chemical Sciences, Mahatma Gandhi University, Kottayam 686560, Kerala, India
e-mail: sandhyapk1@gmail.com

M. S. Sreekala
Post Graduate Research, Department of Chemistry, Sree Sankara College, Kalady 683574, Kerala, India

J. Jose et al. (eds.), *Nano Hydrogels*, Gels Horizons: From Science to Smart Materials,
https://doi.org/10.1007/978-981-15-7138-1_4

spherical, cubical, triangular, rodshaped, ellipsoidal, and so on. Some of the examples of nanomaterials are carbon-based nanomaterials (carbon nanotubes, graphene, nanodiamonds), metal/metal oxide nanoparticles (iron oxide, silver, and gold), polymeric nanoparticles (dendrimers and hyper-branched polymers) and inorganic or ceramic nanoparticles (silicates, calcium phosphate, and hydroxyapatite) [2]. On the basis of dimension, the nanoparticles are classified as one dimensional (clay), two dimensional (graphene, nanotubes), and three dimensional (metallic nanoparticles) [3].

Hydrogels are three-dimensional, highly hydrated porous networks of interconnected natural or synthetic polymer chains to produce a hydrophilic material with macro-molecular structure of a gel [4]. Due to the high water content, permeability, controllable porosity, structural similarity to extracellular matrix and tunable physical, chemical, and biological properties make hydrogels as a promising material for biological applications [1, 5]. In addition to these features, the hydrogels possess some short comings such as low strain, low thermal stability, and poor mechanical strength. Hydrogels have many applications, especially in immunomodulation, stem cell engineering, wound dressing, drug delivery systems, cancer research, cellular, contact lenses, orthodontic applications, and molecular therapies because of its biocompatibility [6, 7]. Multiple functionalities of the hydrogel network and dynamic interactions between the surrounding matrices and cells are the important demand of these applications [8]. In order to meet the requirements, a range of innovations in biomolecular engineering, polymer chemistry, micro- and nanofabrication technologies were introduced for better functionalization [8]. Recently, an increasing trend is observed in the development of nanocomposite hydrogels for different biomedical application.

The low mechanical strength is one of the disadvantages of hydrogels, and it makes them difficult to handle and load in various parts of the body, especially when used as tissue engineering scaffolds [9]. Now, various approaches are introduced in the field of optimization of mechanical and chemical properties of hydrogels for specific biomedical purposes. The limitations of hydrogels can be reduced by the addition of nanoparticles, where these nanostructures undergo physical or covalent interaction with the polymeric chains to create the novel properties in hydrogels [10]. The properties of nanoparticles such as a high surface area-to-volume and aspect ratio made them a suitable candidate for use in the network of polymeric materials [11]. For example, the surface area-to-volume ratio increases the bioavailability, surface reactivity, mechanical properties, and release of loaded bioactive agents. Moreover, the nanoparticles can penetrate tissues via capillaries and epithelial lining, and they can influence the transport properties which ultimately lead to an effective delivery of therapeutic agents to target the cells [12–14].

Nanocomposite hydrogels are also known as hybrid hydrogels, and they are crosslinked three-dimensional water-swollen networks in the presence of nanoparticles. The physical and chemical interactions of polymeric chains with nanoparticles lead to the formation of network with new exclusive properties [6]. The inclusion of the nanoparticles provides unique properties like thermal behaviour, optical activity, barrier resistance, mechanical resistance etc. [15]. The limitations of conventional

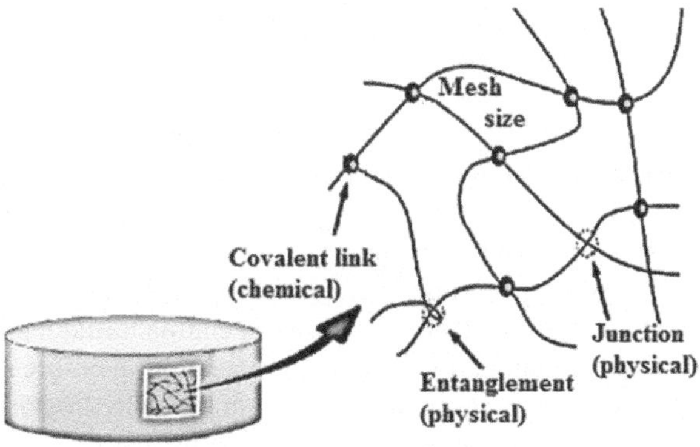

Fig. 1 Structural chemistry of a hydrogel [21]

hydrogels can be overcome by extraordinary features of nanocomposite hydrogels. For instance, in order to make the hydrogels mechanically stronger than conventional hydrogels, clays are used as catalyst, absorbents, metal chelating agents as well as polymer nanocomposites [16]. For wound dressing, the water absorption is controlled with the inclusion of clay nanofillers [17]. The nanofillers such as graphene and carbon nanotubes are used in hydrogels for tissue engineering, drug delivery, and coating the electrodes in solar cell operated medical devices [18, 19]. While considering the increased requirements of nanocomposite hydrogels for biomedical use, various strategies have been explored to conquer its drawbacks but at the same time maintain the advantages of nanoparticles and hydrogels [20].

A three-dimensional network of crosslinked polymer chains constitutes the solid portion of the hydrogel and is usually referred to as a mesh with the spaces filled up with a fluid like water. The fluid present in the meshes exerts an elastic force that leads to the expansion and contraction of the hydrogel [21]. These processes are responsible for the solidity of the hydrogel. Ionisable groups bound onto the polymer chains, and a number of mobile ions are present in the ionic phase of hydrogels. The mobile ions include counter-ions and co-ions due to the presence of the electrolytic solvent, which surrounds the hydrogel. Figure 1 represents the structural chemistry of the hydrogel.

2 Preparation of Biodegradable Hydrogels

The nanocomposite hydrogels prepared from natural polymers are biodegradable, possess good mechanical strength, and highly hydrophilic. The natural polymers commonly used to fabricate nanocomposite hydrogels are starch, cellulose, chitin, alginate, gelatin, and carrageenan. The stiffness and water absorbing capacity of the nanocomposite hydrogels can be increased by the presence of alcohols, amides, and carboxylic acid as hydrophilic moieties in the structure of nanocomposite hydrogels. Under extreme conditions of pressure, temperature, and pH, the stability of nanocomposite hydrogels can be increased by the addition of cross-linker during their synthesis [15].

The naocomposite hydrogels can be made through the combination of nanoparticles and hydrogels by various mechanisms. The simplest and widely used method for the preparation of a variety of nanocomposite hydrogels containing various nanoparticles is the gelation of a suspension of pre-ready nanoparticles in a solution of hydrogel forming monomer. For example, Sershen et al. [22] prepared gold nanoparticle hydrogel composites by adding nanoshell gold particles into a solution of monomers followed by addition of gelation initiator and an accelerator. The aggregation of the nanoparticles in monomer solution before and during the gelation process and the leaching of nanoparticles out of the hydrogel matrix if the cross-link density is low limits the wide application of this method of preparation [23, 24]. The other method used for the preparation of nancomposite hydrogels is the physical introduction of nanoparticles into a hydrogel networks after gelation. This method is suitable for hydrogels that can highly swell in water but dramatically shrink in aprotic solvent acetone. Repeated swelling–shrinking process is employed for the introduction of naoparticles into this kind of hydrogels [25, 26]. Pardo-Yissar et al. [25] incorporated gold nanoparticles into polyacrylamide gel after the electropolymerization formation of the hydrogel. The next method of preparation of nanocomposite hydrogels involves the loading of nanoparticle precursors into a gel [27]. Marcelo et al. [28] used redox active catechol side chain in acrylamide-N-isopropylacrylamide (NIPAAm) to form nanoparticle hydrogel composite from gold precursor, and great reinforcement of mechanical property was observed for the resulting hydrogel. The use of crosslinker groups on the outer surface of nanoparticles is an interesting method for the preparation of nanocomposite hydrogels. Further developments in the field of using nanoparticles as cross-linking agent were introduced by Rose et al. [29] for adhesion between two hydrogels. This method depends on certain factors such as the ability of the nanoparticles to adsorb onto the polymer gels, to act as a connector between the polymer chains and the ability of the polymer chains to recognize, and dissipate energy under stress when adsorbed onto the nanoparticles. By using the interactions among the nanoparticles, polymers, and distinct gelator molecules, nanocomposite hydrogels can also be prepared [30]. For instance, Wu et al. [30] has reported the incorporation of silicon (Si) nanoparticles into a conducting polymer hydrogel for Si-based anodes. These different approaches for the preparation of nanocomposite hydrogels have introduced new chances in manufacturing advanced biomaterials for various applications in the field of biotechnology and biomedicine. Figure 2 illustrates the schematic representation of formation of nanocomposite hydrogels in different ways.

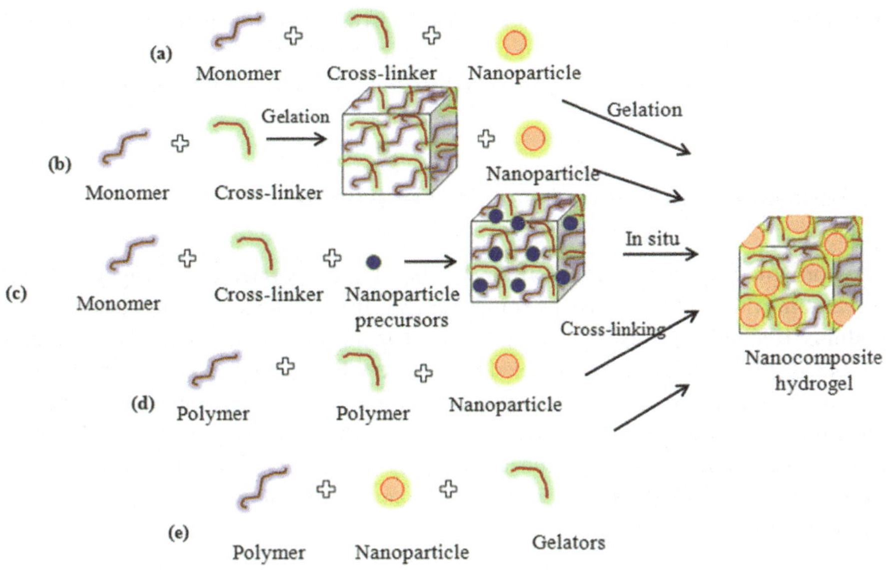

Fig. 2 Schematic representation of formation of nanocomposite hydrogels by different methods **a** gelation of a suspension of pre-ready nanoparticles in a solution of hydrogel forming monomer **b** physical introduction of nanoparticles into a hydrogel networks after gelation **c** loading of nanoparticle precursors into a gel **d** use of crosslinker groups on the outer surface of nanoparticles **e** using the interactions among the nanoparticles, polymers, and distinct gelator molecules

3 Characterization Techniques

Physicochemical properties of these materials depend on the type of compound used for a hydrogel matrix preparation. The most commonly used characterization techniques for studying the morphology of the nanocomposite hydrogels are scanning electron microscopy (SEM), transmission electron microscopy (TEM), and atomic force microscopy (AFM) [31, 32]. UV–visible spectroscopy and Fourier transform infrared spectroscopy are used to determine the chemical composition of the nanocomposite hydrogels [31]. Light scattering provides information about the structure and molecular dynamics of nanoparticles as well as their size distribution [33]. This technique is essential for the characterization of soft material. Viscosimetry technique involves the preparation of dilute solutions of nanogels to determine viscosity. If the intrinsic viscosity of the solution is known, the average molecular weight can be determined and can be used for monitoring the size changes of the nanogels during their synthesis. Gel permeation chromatography (GPC) determines the molecular weight of the nanogel particles [31]. Differential scanning calorimetry (DSC) is used for determining the heat absorbed or released by a substance. It measures the melting, phase transition, crystallization, and glass transition temperatures of the polymers constituting the nanogels. It also finds the degree of swelling of the nanogels by analysing the presence of associated and non-associated water in the nanogels.

Depending on the applications and nature of the hydrogels, the other characterization techniques used are the response of nanoparticles to the changes in temperature and pH, biocompatibility studies and in vitro dissolution and release of drugs [34].

4 Nanofillers in Nanocomposite Hydrogels

Many organic and inorganic nanofillers are being incorporated in hydrogel matrices to overcome the drawbacks like poor mechanical strength, tensile strength, and elastic modulus. Recently, the researchers are focused on the incorporation of many nanoparticulate systems such as carbon-based nanomaterials (graphene, carbon nanotubes), ceramic nanoparticles, metal/metal oxide nanopatrticles, and polymeric nanoparticles into the hydrogels for preparing nanocomposite hydrogels. The addition of these nanoparticles may reinforce the starting hydrogels and result in nanocomposite hydrogels with responsiveness to mechanical, magnetic, electric, and thermal stimuli [35].

4.1 Graphene-Based Nanocomposite Hydrogels

Graphene is a two-dimensional carbon atom monolayer with excellent electrical, mechanical, and thermal properties which makes it as a suitable candidate for improvement of many properties of composite materials [36–38]. It is easy to introduce hydroxyl, carboxylic acid, and epoxide groups in the plane of graphene, and it can be converted into graphene oxide (GO) and reduced graphene oxide (RGO). These graphene derivatives possess a combination of hydrophilic as well as hydrophobic (π–π interactions) which provides them dipole interactions, hydrogen bonding, colloidal stability, pH-dependent surface charges, and other surface reactions along with non-covalent functionalization. Graphene derivatives shows high drug entrapment ability with particular sensitivity for hydrophobic drug molecules due to their amphiphilic nature and ability to be functionalize [18]. In hydrogels, graphene acts as a gelator to self-assemble into the hydrogels and also as a filler to blend with small molecules and macromolecules for the preparation of multifunctional hydrogels [39, 40]. Graphene-based hydrogels attracted great attention in the field of tissue engineering because the water-rich graphene-based hydrogels is similar to natural soft tissues, in addition to high conductivity, biocompatibility, good mechanical strength, and non-covalent bonds between graphene derivatives and polymers (chitosan, poly(N,N′-dimethylacrylamide etc.).

Ligorio et al. [41] used GO as a nanofiller for the design of hybrid peptide hydrogel for the delivery of nucleus pulposus (NP) cells. There is a strong interaction between peptide and GO, promoting high cell viability and metabolic activity, mimicking the mechanical properties of the NP tissue. Liu and colleagues [42] developed a highly efficient near-infrared (NIR) and pH-responsive carboxymethyl chitosan functionalized reduced graphene oxide/aldehyde functionalized polyethylene glycogel which shows excellent delivery performance of antitumor drug, doxorubicin hydrochloride (DOX).

Rasoulzadehzali and Namazi [43] prepared novel pH-sensitive bio-nanocomposite hydrogel beads based on chitosn and graphene oxide–silver nanohybrid particles for controlled release of anti-cancer drugs. Jing et al. [44] prepared chitosan/graphene oxide composite hydrogels by the incorporation of the mussel-inspired protein polydopamine (PDA) with self-adhesive and self-healing properties. The hydrogen bonds, covalent bonds, π–π stacking, and supramolecular interactions allow the nanocomposite hydrogels strong mechanical behaviour, good adhesiveness, high stability, fast recovery ability, and self-healing properties. These hydrogels found application in the field of electroactive tissue engineering. Shin et al. [45] incorporated reduced graphene oxide in gelatine methacryloyl hydrogel matrix to improve the mechanical and electrical properties of the hydrogel which leads to a more natural microenvironment for the cardiomyocytes and improving the cardiac tissue morphogenesis and beating behaviour. The graphene/Ag composite hydrogel prepared by cross-linking reaction of graphene with acrylic acid and methylene bisacrylamide exhibited good biocompatibility and high swelling ratio, and it accelerates healing in the treatment of artificial wounds in rats [46].

4.1.1 Carbon Nanotube-Reinforced Nanocomposite Hydrogels

Carbon nanotubes (CNTs) are cylindrical nanostructure with hexagonal arrangement of sp^2 hybridized carbon atom. CNTs are formed by rolling the graphene sheets, and the wall of CNT discriminates it as single-walled carbon nanotubes (SWCNT) or multi-walled carbon nanotubes (MWCNT) [47]. SWCNTs show perfect quality control as drug carrier whereas MWCNTs occurred with defects in the nanostructure which are quite unstable and can be modified easily [48]. CNTs consist of carbon only, and they have superior biocompatibility, immunogenicity, and low toxicity which made them suitable for biomedical applications.

The properties of carbon nanotubes (CNTs) such as high tensile strength, chemical stability, electrical conductivity, and thermal stability encouraged the usage of CNT as a reinforcing agent in tissue engineering and drug delivery systems [49–52]. Kouser et al. [53] prepared biocompatible nanocomposite hydrogels through solution blending method using microporous multiwall carbon nanotubes (MWCNT) dispersed chitosan (CH)-acrylonitrile (AN), N,N′-methylenebisacrylamide (MBAAm) and linseed polyol. The addition of nanoparticle increases the swelling ability, biodegradability, modulus and tensile strength, and biocompatibility. By varying the concentration of MWCNT, the properties can be finely tuned, and these nanostructure hydrogel is found applications in the field of tissue engineering. Saeednia et al. [54] incorporated carbon naotubes into a thermosensitive and injectable hydrogel formed by chitosan and β-glycerophophate (β-GP), and the prepared hybrid hydrogel can be used as a potential breast cancer therapy system for controlled delivery of methotexate (MTX). Choudhary et al. [55] studied the variation in the properties of tamarind gum hydrogels by incorporating CNT, OH–CNT, and COOH–CNT. The microscopic studies of the prepared nancomposite hydrogels showed that the alteration in the microstructure is due to the alteration in the interactive forces among the polymeric chains of the hydrogel, and it tailored the electrical and mechanical properties. These hydrogels can be used in the differential drug release patterns of the model drug, tigecycline. Multi-walled carbon nanotube-alginate nanocomposite hydrogels were developed by encapsulating COOH-functionalized MWCNT as a reinforcing phase within alginate [56]. The resulted nanocomposite hydrogels showed better handling characteristics, stability, enhanced cell clustering, improved stiffness, and they can act as a new substrate for mimicking cancer progression in a dish or for cell therapy and tissue engineering.

4.1.2 Ceramic Nanoparticle-Reinforced Nanocomposite Hydrogel

By combining inorganic ceramic nanoparticles with natural or synthetic polymeric hydrogels, it is possible to fabricate several advanced nanocomposite hydrogels. Synthetic silicate nanoparticles, silica, glass ceramic, hydroxyapatite (HAP), bioactive glass, b-wollastonite and calcium phosphate are examples of bioactive nanoparticles [35]. Ceramic nanoparticles are characterized by high mechanical and thermal stability, excellent biocompatibility, easy functionalization, and facile surface modification. Moreover, most of these silicon-based nanoparticles are already present in the body and are essential for the functioning of human tissues [57]. Silicon stimulates the osteogenic differentiation in human stem cells, and it promotes the collagen type 1synthesis. Apart from that silicon is very important in skeletal development. HAP is an essential ingredient of normal bone and teeth, and it is used as biomaterial for bone regeneration. They can promote new bone growth without causing any local or systematic toxicity, inflammation or foreign body response through osteoconduction mechanism [58, 59]. High mechanical strength and unique bioactive properties of silicon-based nanoparticles and nanoclays will be of great interest for the repair and regeneration of human tissues and body functions [60]. Nanoclays and their composites are nontoxic, and they are used for various biomedical applications such as drug delivery, wound healing, bone cement, and enzyme immobilization [61]. The effect of incorporation of clay nanoparticles on the mechanical and biological properties of photo-crosslinked triblock copolymer hydrogel PTMC-PEG-PTMC (poly (trimethylene carbonate)-poly (ethylene glycol)-poly(trimethylene carbonate)). The prepared hydrogels were enzymatically degradable by cholesterol esterase and by the action macrophages [62]. Entezam et al. [63] investigated the effect of modified nanoclay by chitosan on the physical, mechanical, and antimicrobial properties of poly (vinyl alcohol) hydrogels for wound dressing applications. Filipowska et al. [64] assed osteogenic potential of three groups of bipolymeric hydrogel-based surfaces made of plain collagen, chitosan, or collagen/chitosan modified with silica particles of two sizes. They analysed the biocompatibility and osteoinductive properties of the resulting composites in the human bone marrow-derived mesenchymal stromal cells. New porous silicon-based gelatin hydrogel composites showed property enhancements such as mechanical stiffness, higher hydrolytic stability, and swelling capability attributed to the porous silicon microparticles capacity of producing multiple bonds within the hydrogel network [65]. Lima et al. [66] successfully developed hydrogel nanocomposites based on alginate and mesoporous silica with reduced release burst and enhanced elastic moduli using prednisolone as a model drug. The synthesized nanocomposites can be used as a tool for further physiological and pathological applications like drug delivery device.

4.1.3 Metal and Metal Oxide-Based Nanocomposite Hydrogel

The unique characters of metal and metal nanoparticles that are not commonly found in polymer materials made them as reinforcing elements to prepare composite hydrogels with unique characteristic and tunable properties. Different types of metal and metal oxide nanoparticles are incorporated into the polymer hydrogels by covalent or non-covalent interactions to prepare nanocomposite hydrogels [20]. Metallic nanoparticle affects the hydrogel depend on the type of interaction, a weaker interaction improve the conductivity, stimuli responses and antimicrobial properties, but it has little effect on the mechanical properties of nanocomposite hydrogel. The improvement in swelling behaviour, localized surface plasmon resonance, sensitivity towards pH, electricity, and heat are the results obtained when there is a strong interaction between metallic nanoparticles and hydrogels. Natural polymers are good choice for the synthesis of nanocomposite hydrogel with metals because of its non-toxic and biocompatible nature.

Modification of hydrogels based on chitosan by inserting gold nanoparticles was done by Tyliszczak et al. [67], and the hydrogels act as an interesting material that affects the development in the fields of nanotechnology and polymer technology as well as they are the potential components for the preparation of modern wound dressing. The use of a covalent click chemistry strategy to cross-link chitosan hydrogels using functionalized gold nanoparticles (Au NPs) as multifunctional cross-linkers and the prepared nanocomposite hydrogels open a new avenue to bioengineering of pH-responsive surfaces or novel drug delivery systems [68]. Thermo-switchable electronic properties, enhanced electrochemical properties are the characteristics of gold nanoparticle based hydrogels and used as a light-responsive hydrogel for drug delivery, catalysts, tissue engineering, cancer therapy, and sensors [47]. A novel chitosan-Ag nanoparticle-reinforced hydrogels were successfully produced by a green and simple method with homogeneous porous network structures, better mechanical properties, and proper water-retention capacity [69]. The synthesized nanohydrogels found application in the field of wound dressing materials. Jing et al. [70] prepared stretchable gelatine/silver nanowires (GE-AgNWs) composite hydrogel with enhanced electrical conductivity, and mechanical properties has been developed through chemical grafting and physical cross-linking. The prepared nanocomposite hydrogels were biocompatible and can be used as a strain sensor to detect multiple human motions. These hydrogels found application in the field of biosensors, electric skins, and health monitoring applications. It is found that the addition of silver nanoparticles into the hydrogels enhanced the antibacterial, antifungal, and electronic properties of the hydrogels [47]. Starch/CuO nanocomposite hydrogels were successfully prepared by in situ formation of CuO nanoparticles in the oxidized starch hydrogel matrix [71]. With increase in CuO nanoparticle content, an increase in sustained and controlled drug release was observed. Zhai et al. [72] fabricated porous keratin–chitosan/n-ZnO nanocomposite bandages by the inclusion of nano-ZnO into the keratin–chitosan hydrogel. The prepared nanocomposite hydrogels exhibit biological application due to its excellent mechanical, bactericidal, swelling, and bactericidal properties.

4.1.4 Polymer-Based Nanocomposite Hydrogels

A wide range of polymers like homo- and copolymers, branched polymers, cross-linked polymers, block copolymers, graft copolymers, and blends of two or more biopolymers are used as polymer matrix for the preparation of nanocomposite hydrogels [73–75]. Hydrogels can be divided into natural and synthetic polymer-based hydrogels on the basis of source of the polymer. Natural polymer-based hydrogels consists of natural hydrophilic polymers like gelatin, chitosan, cellulose, alginate, hyaluronic acid, peptides, agar–agar, and some of their derivatives [76–78]. Synthetic polymer-based hydrogels include poly(vinyl alcohol) (PVA), poly(ethylene glycol) (PEG), poly(acrylic acid) (PAA), polyacrylamide (PAAm), and poly(*N*-isopropylacrylamide) (PNIPAAm), and their copolymers [79–82]. The natural polymer-based hydrogels are drawing great attention in various fields like wound dressing, healthcare monitoring, biomedical daily care, and human–machine interfaces due to its biocompatibility, biodegradability and tissue mimicking consistency characteristics [83–87].

4.1.5 Cellulose-Based Nanocomposite Hydrogel

Cellulose is a natural polymer composed of β-(1–4) linked D-glucose units, and it is widely used for the synthesis of biocompatible hydrogels due to its properties like hydrophilicity, biodegradability, low-cost, biocompatibility, and non-toxicity [88]. The back bone of cellulose and its derivatives consists of large number of hydrophilic functional groups such as carboxyl, hydroxyl, and aldehyde groups which make them suitable candidate for the preparation of hydrogels for various biomedical applications. The specific applications of cellulose-based hydrogels include wound dressing, tissue engineering, drug delivery, bioimaging, and wearable epidermal sensors [88]. Using glutaraldehyde (GA) as a cross-linker cellulose nanocrystal (CNC)-reinforced poly(vinyl alcohol) (PVA) hydrogels were prepared with water content of ~92%. The prepared nanocomposite hydrogels can be used in the fields of biomedical and tissue engineering [89]. Javanbakht and Namazi [90] designed a novel hydrogel nanocomposite film by the incorporation of graphene quantum dot as a nanoparticle into carboxymethyl cellulose hydrogel using doxorubicin as the drug model. The synthesized biodegradable nanocomposite hydrogel films act as a novel anticancer drug carrier. A green smart cellulose/black phosphorous nanosheet nanocomposite hydrogels were developed by a facile, green chemical cross-linking reaction in alkaline solutions [91]. Black phosphororus has recently emerged as an intriguing photothermal agent against cancer due to its biocompatibility, biodegradability, and high photothermal efficiency. Functional inorganic nanoparticle-reinforced cellulose hydrogels shows considerable potential in biomedical applications. A total biocompatibility within tissues, cells, and other components of the living body is shown by cellulose hydrogels with considerable amounts of water. With the addition of nanoparticles into cellulose hydrogel, it improves mechanical property, photoluminescence, conductivity, magnetic, catalytic, and mechanical properties [92]. For the preparation of cellulose-based hydrogels poly(vinyl alcohol) is a good candidate for the preparation of hydrogels which can be cross-linked by several methods such as irradiation, electron beam, chemical agents, and chemical thermal cycling. In the case biomedical applications, physical cross-linking is the most suitable method for the preparation of hydrogels than chemical or irradiation techniques because it avoids the residual amounts of toxic chemical cross-linker [93]. Freezing–thawing technique via physical cross-linking is the usual method used for the preparation of novel PVA/cellulose hydrogels [94].

Chitosan-Based Nanocomposite Hydrogel

Chitosan is a potential candidate for the applications in the field of biochemical and biomedical fields due to the presence of numerous functional groups with peculiar properties like biodegradability and biocompatibility, high water absorption capacity, mechanical strength, long life, easy availability, and non-toxicity. Chitosan is a polysaccharide which mainly consists of β(1, 4)-linked 2-deoxy-2-amino-D-glucopyranose units and is obtained from alkaline hydrolysis of chitin [95–99]. Chitosan chain consists of a large number of amine groups (-NH_2), and hydroxyl groups (–OH) can be used as cross-linking agents for in situ chemical cross-linking [100]. In addition to that below pH 6.3, the amine groups can be easily converted into ammonium groups, which make them as a suitable candidate for the preparation of pH-responsive hydrogels. Moreover, non-toxic oligosaccharides are the products obtained from the degradation of chitosan and can be excreted or incorporated to glycosoaminoglycans and glycoproteins. By increasing the pH or by dissolving in a solvent, chitosan undergoes self-crosslinking. Song et al. [101] developed a complex physical hydrogel of cordycepin and chytosan through a one-step freezethaw operation, and the prepared complex gel exhibited outstanding antimicrobial properties and wound-recovering ability without side effects. These hydrogels displayed a quicker re-epithelization of skin wounds and

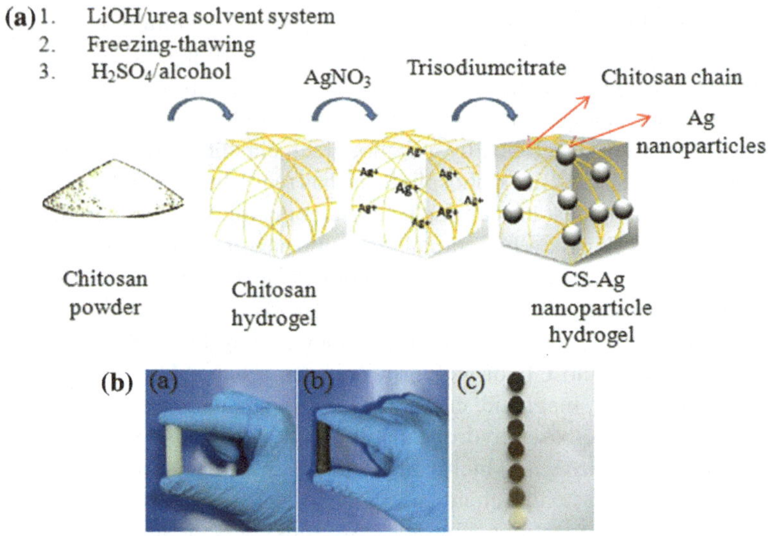

Fig. 3 **A** Schematically represents the formation of Ag nanoparticles in the chitosan hydrogel network. **B a** Chitosan hydrogels, **b** chitosan-Ag nanoparticles hydrogels, **c** hydrogels with different Ag content [69]

promoted collagen deposition. Santos et al. [102] reported the preparation and characterization of nanocomposite hydrogels with chitosan-embedded poly(lactic-co-glycolic acid) (PLGA) employed for the encapsulation of an enriched flavaniod fraction of Cecropia glaziovii Senthl. New photo-crosslinkable thermogels were prepared by photo-crosslinking of glycidyl methacrylate-modified hydroxypropyl chitin (GM-HPCH) under physiological conditions and in the presence of photoinitiator [103]. The synthesized hydrogels found applications in the field of tissue engineering. Smart polymeric hydrogels of chitosan and modified amino acid (acryloyl-phenylalanine)-based hydrogels were synthesized by in situ polymerization using ammonium persulfate as a redox intiator, and the synthesized hydrogels showed good intrinsic self-healing property [104]. Xie et al. [69] prepared chitosan hydrogels reinforced by silver nanoparticles with ultrahigh mechanical and high antibacterial properties for accelerating wound healing and Fig. 3A represents the steps involved in the formation of chitosan–silver nanocomposite hydrogel and 3B shows the photographic images of chitosan and chistosan-Ag nanoparticle hydrogels.

Carrageenan-Based Nanocomposite Hydrogel

Carrageenan (crg) is a naturally occurring anionic sulphated polysaccharide obtained from the red seaweeds of Rhodophyceae class, which consists of galactose and anhydrogalactose linked through glycosidic bonds [105]. The anionic nature of crg is due to the long linear chains of D-galactose and D-anhydrogalactose with ester sulphates [106]. They exist in three types, kappa-crg-1 sulphate group, iota-crg-2 sulphate groups, and lamda-crg-3 sulphate groups, based on the number of sulphate groups per disaccharide. Crg is widely used in the fields of drug delivery, tissue engineering, and wound healing in addition to food, cosmetic, and pharmaceutical industries [107]. Thermoreversible gelation, ionic crosslinking, and ionic modification of Crg backbone with photo-crosslinking methacrylate moieties are the different methods employed for the formation of Crg hydrogels [108]. First study introducing a photo-crosslinked kappa-carrageenan with controllable elastic moduli, pore size distribution, and swelling ratios were conducted by Mihalia et al. [109]. In this study, methacrylated kappa-carrageenan was synthesized by reacting kappa-carrageenan with various amount of methacrylic anhydride. Bio-nanocomposite hydrogel beads based on kappa-carrageenan as hydrogel matrix and bio-synthesized silver nanoparticles as an antimicrobial agent were prepared and studied the swelling behaviour, cytotoxicity, and antibacterial activity [110]. This trend acts as a motivation for researchers in developing nanocomposite hydrogels with strong antimicrobial activity using green synthesized nanoparticles in hydrogels. Mahdaviniaet al. [111] developed ionically crosslinked and magnetic kappa-carrageenan/chitosan for in vitro release of the methotrexate drug using a facile and green route. They selected an in situ method of preparation for the synthesis of magnetic Fe_3O_4 nanoparticles in the presence of kappa-carrageenan and then crosslinked using the polycation chitosan biopolymer. Yegappan and colleagues [108] developed an injectable carrageenan nanocomposite hydrogel incorporated with whitlockite nanoparticles and an angiogenic drug, dimethyloxallylglycine with enhanced mechanical strength, physiological stability, thereby achieving sustained drug release and enhanced protein adsorption. Feng and co-workers [112] synthesized collagen–hydroxyapatite/k-crg composite material which can be used as a substitute for bone tissue. Gonzalez and Ossa [113] studied the injectability of bone graft substitutes based on carrageenan and hydroxyapatite nanorods. Pourjavadi et al. [114] developed an injectable hydrogel from biocompatible polysaccharides and poly-*N*-isopropyl acryl amide enriched with gold nanoparticles. The studies showed that the gels modified with gold nanoparticles showed significant enhancement in cell proliferation and adhesion and these hydrogels found application in tissue engineering.

Gelatin Based Nanocomposite Hydrogel

Gelatin is derived from collagen and it is abundantly available, low cost, biodegradable, biocompatible and low antigenicity. Due to these properties it is widely used in the field of tissue engineering. Gelatine contains peptide sequences for the recognition of integrin receptors in the cells which is very essential for the cell adhesion in wound dressing materials [115]. Moreover, the nanofiber formation ability of gelatin can be used for skin generation. Pristine gelatin is seldom used for skin regeneration so that chemical modification or physical blending has been adopted for improving the gelling condition of gelatin. Grafting and crosslinking of gelatine and poly(ethylene glycol) diglycidyl ether in the presence of chitosan and hydroxyethyl cellulose lead to reproducible and mechanically robust hybrid hydrogels showed superb performance for human foreskin fibroblasts cell line [116]. These biodegradable/resorbable hydrogel can promote cell growth, viability and proliferation. El-Feky et al. [117] prepared chitosan gelatine hydrogel loaded with timolol maleate (TM) for intraocular pressure (IOP) lowering was successfully developed by utilizing the semisynthetic biocompatible oxidized sucrose as crosslinker. A facile approach without chemical modification to construct injectable gelatin-based hydrogels with excellent shear-thinning as well as self-recovering for wound healing was introduced by Zheng et al. [115] The addition of gelatin and bioactive glass to chitosan hydrogels produce enhanced properties can be used as injectable systems for biomedical applications [118]. Song et al. [119] introduced a muco-adhesive ophthalmic drug delivery system, developed using chitosan–gelatin that crosslinked with β-glycerophosphate disodium salt hydrate (β-GD) and genipin. A new method to photopolymerize gelatine methacryloyl (GelMA) using a visible light curing unit with parameters similar to those used in the dental office were developed and can be directly established in regenerative procedures in dental care [120]. Bacterial cellulose and gelatine-based composite hydrogels were successfully prepared with glutaraldehyde as a crosslinking agent and they are considered as good candidates for drug delivery systems [121]. Maharana and co-workers [122] reported a study on the fabrication of filled hydrogels using gelatin, tamarid gum and carbon nanotubes for various biomedical applications such as tissue engineering, wound healing and drug delivery. The prepared hydrogels showed cytocompatibility with human keratinocytes. Glycerol phosphate crosslinked to chitosan–gelatin hydrogel base ocular drug delivery systems are reported and these hydrogels exhibited low cytotoxicity, prolonged precorneal retention time, high drug loading capacity [123, 124]. Bakravi et al. [125] prepared a series of gelatin-based hydrogel nanocomposites containing CuO nanoparticles by immersion of gelatin hydrogel in $CuCl_2$ solution with different concentrations and the prepared nanocomposite hydrogels were used as drug delivery agent.

Starch-Based Nanocomposite Hydrogel

Starch is widely used for the purpose of wound dressing because it is biodegradable, biocompatible, cheap, possess ease of physical and chemical modification and good physical properties. The poor mechanical properties of starch can be reduced by starch blends or composites with polymers like PVA. The PVA/starch hydrogels found application in the field of wound dressing because of its excellent mechanical, hydrophilic, biocompatible and non-toxic properties [126, 127]. Batool et al. [128] synthesized silver nanoparticles from fruit extract and used for the preparation of starch-based nanocomposite hydrogel and investigated their mechanical as well as antimicrobial activity. Successful preparation of a new drug delivery approach for the preparation of starch/CuO nanocomposite hydrogels was reported and the drug release studies revealed that CuO nanoparticles extend the release of drugs from the oxidized starch hydrogels [71]. New oxidized starch/ZnO nanocomposites hydrogels were effectively synthesized by in situ oxidation of Zn^{2+} ions in the oxidized starch hydrogel medium and find applications in biomedical field [129].

5 Biomedical Applications of Biodegradable Nanocomposite Hydrogels

Nanocomposite gels combine the advantages of both hydrogel and nano-fillers. With the addition of nano-fillers with its properties such as mechanical, electrical, magnetic, and optical would endow the nanocomposite gel with extraordinary functionalities made them great potential in biomedical practice.

5.1 Drug Delivery

The process of transferring a drug into the body over a period of time at a specific rate with the desired drug concentration is called drug delivery. Nanocomposite hydrogels have many attractive physical properties like diffusion coefficient, swelling ratio, and mesh size, swelling ration) can be modified and tuned to improve performance of nanocomposite hydrogels of both water-soluble and insoluble drugs for drug delivery applications. The particular properties of hydrogels made them to be used as ideal drug delivery systems because they are similar to body's tissues, rubbery consistency, and high water content. Hydrogels are capable of handling both dry and swollen networks for drug loading and releasing. Physical entrapment method is generally used for the incorporation of drugs into hydrogels [125].

The incorporation of metal oxides like ZnO and CuO nanoparticles into the polymeric matrix improved the drug loading and drug release profiles of nanocomposite hydrogels. Gelatin/copper oxide hydrogel nanocomposites, a physical interaction between cephalexin and gelatine exists and carboxylic acid and amine groups in cephalexin are converted to carboxylate and ammonium group [125]. Starch/CuO nanocomposite hydrogels were used for drug delivery, a sustained and controlled drug releases were observed with increases in CuO nanoparticle content [71]. The hybrid hydrogel composites can discharge the drugs from polymer matrices in measured and more persistent manner. The particular characteristics of these materials are they can accurately and precisely control the duration, drug delivery timings, and the amount of drug to be delivered. The delivery of atenolol drug using gum dammar crosslinked polyacrylamide and zirconium-based biodegradable hydrogel composites are reported elsewhere [130]. Hydrogels based on carboxymethyl chitosan-poly (vinyl alcohol) containing Ag nanoparticles showed sustained and controlled drug releases that increased with increase in Ag nanoparticles content which can lead to prolong the release of the drug [131].

Graphene quantum dots possess large surface area with delocalized electrons, solubility in the variety of solvents, high fundamental fluorescence, chemical inertness, ability of drug loading by π–π interactions and easy variability of size and shape, local functional groups at the edges made them applied for cellular imaging and drug delivery. Easy functionalization through the oxygen groups or through π–π interactions provides graphene quantum dots as a drug delivery platform. In chemotherapy, a typical anticancer drug used is doxorubicin (DOX), which kills cells by incorporating with DNA. Moreover, it prevents the cell division and the DNA replication process [132, 133]. So it is necessary to prepare a drug carrier which is capable of releasing anticancer drugs effectively in the location of cancer cells and direct delivery of drugs into the cancer cells. Carboxymethyl cellulose/graphene quantum dot nanocomposite hydrogel films loaded with DOX were prepared and nanparticles could efficiently conjunct with DOX then deliver it to the cancer tissues and dramatically enhance cytotoxicity of DOX [90]. An antibacterial chitosan/graphene oxide-Ag bio-nanocomposite (CH/GO-Ag) hydrogel beads were used for controlled release of doxorubicin [43] and the Fig. 4 shows the drug release behaviour of the DOX-loaded CH/GO-Ag nanocomposite beads containing various amount of GO-Ag nanohybrid particles in the different pHs of 1.2 and 6.8. The release time of doxorubicin from DOX-loaded CH/GO-Ag nanocomposite beads were prolonged by increase in the GO-Ag nanohybrid content. This is due to the existence of GO-Ag nanohybrid particles into prepared nanocomposite beads make a longer path for the

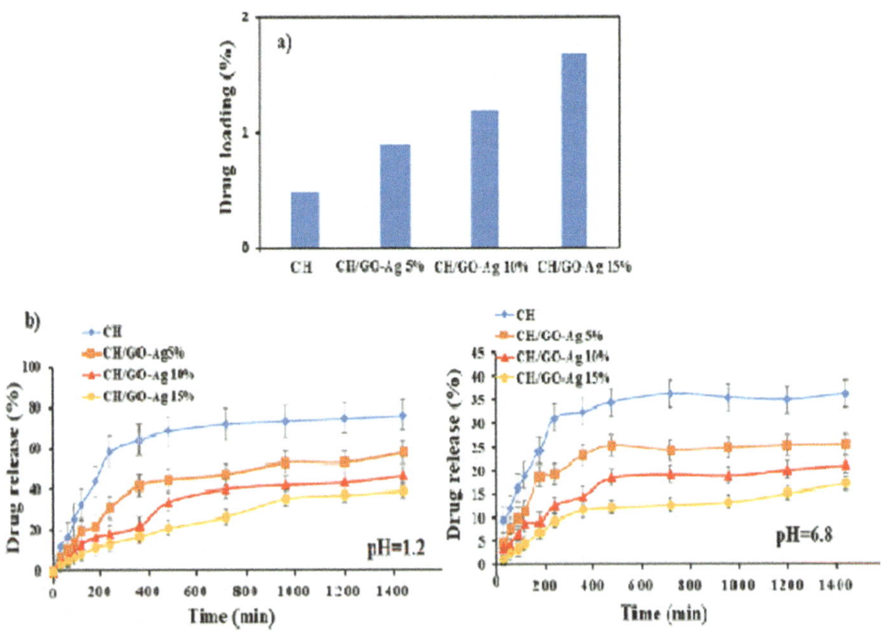

Fig. 4 Percentage of DOX loaded into **a** and released from b CH and CH/GO-Ag (5, 10 and 15%) nanocomposite hydrogel beads [43]

migration of doxorubicin from nanocomposite beads into the release medium and hydrogen bonding and electrostatic attraction interactions between doxorubicin and GO-Ag nanohybrid particles reduce the initial burst release of doxorubicin.

Addition of nanoparticles to nanocomposite hydrogels provides stability of drug as well as slower and continuous drug release, and reduces burst release effect [15]. Changes in temperature, magnetic field, pH, and electric field help to release drug from nanocomposite matrix. Nanocomposite hydrogels can act as reservoir of drug molecules with interaction between drug molecule and nanofiller is necessary for the delivery of drugs [134]. The electro-stimulated drug release behaviour is observed with PVA/CNT-based hydrogel using tetracycline as a model drug [135]. Fe_3O_4 nanoparticles reinforced with kappa-carrageenan, starch and cellulose base hydrogels were used for drug delivery applications reported elsewhere [20].

5.2 Tissue Engineering

For the regeneration or replacement of damaged tissues, tissue engineering is considered as a developing field. An appropriate scaffold that supports the recruitment, adhesion, proliferation, and differentiation of cells is necessary. Recently, hydrogels play the role of replacing defective tissues, but they have limited mechanical strength. To improve their properties, nanomaterials such as organic/polymeric and inorganic (hydroxyapatite, clay, graphene, and metallic nanoparticles) are embedded into the hydrogel's matrix. Those nanocomposites improve the properties of hydrogels and make them suitable in cartilage regeneration practices. The major challenges faced by the use of hydrogels for tissue engineering is the highly hydrated condition and poor mechanical properties in vitro and in vivo. The insertion of nanomaterials in the hydrogel's matrix during the crosslinking of scaffold, resulted in more homogeneous distribution and availability of much more particles for the same equivalent weight of carriers. In cell growth as well as tissue regeneration, the biomimetic properties of nanomaterials are important. . The direct interactions of nanostructured extracellular matrix with natural tissues and organs have nanometer dimensions [136].

In the case of thermally responsive hydrogels, the gelation and swelling behaviour can be triggered by temperature change, and they attracted great interest in the field of tissue engineering [137]. Other excellent materials for tissue engineering are chitin and chitosan due to their properties, such as high biocompatibility, biodegradability, nonantigenicity, antibacterial activity, and high adsorption [138]. PVA hydrogel shows high potential for cartilage tissue engineering due to its structure and material properties similarities with natural cartilage. Alginate is a biomaterial that has some properties like excellent biocompatibility, low immunological motivation, degradability, and flexibility and forms hydrogels tissue engineering [139].

The primary focus in the area of bone tissue engineering is the development of scaffolds and bone substitutes that provide structural and functional support in treating the bone defect. When incorporated with functional bioactive cues, carrageenan (crg) has the ability to allow apatite layer formation. The incorporation of kappa-carrageenan into collagen–hydroxyapatite composite gel increased the compressive strength and improvement in mechanical property which justifies crg an efficient bone repair material [112]. Nano-hydroxyapatite (nHAP)-based bone substitutes have been widely used for their effective ion exchange, bioactivity, and biocompatibility [140].

The mechanical properties of silk fibroin (SF) can be improved by various strategies like combining SF with other biopolymers has a double network, showing an enhanced mechanical and biological property. Carboxymethyl chitosan (CMCS) is a biopolymer having the properties such as water-soluble, non-toxic, antibacterial and good degradability. The multiple functional chemical groups in CMCS effectively promote osteoblasts adhesion and proliferation. One of the essential features of bone repairing scaffold is osteoinductivity. SF has intrinsic abilities to regenerate bone, but it is insufficient to repair large areas of bone defects so that several bioactive ceramics like hydroxyapatite (HAp) have been used to make bone repair scaffolds by combing with SF [141, 142]. Strontium (Sr) can accelerate the regeneration and maturation of bone by promoting the differentiation of osteoblasts [143, 144]. Silk fibroin/carboxymethyl chitosan/strontium-substituted hydroxyapatite/cellulose nanocrystal composite scaffolds which can be used for bone tissue engineering [145].

5.3 Wound Dressing

One of the most attractive areas of research is the development of nanocomposite hydrogel in the field of tissue engineering and as wound dressings. The bacterial infections of wounds can be minimized with the help of wound dressings with antimicrobial effects. The difficulty of infection control in wound healing process is one of most serious challenges in wound care. The epidermal damages are common in our daily life so that dressing these damages could be useful for wound healing. The important characteristics of wound dressings are protecting the wounds from side infection, maintaining a moist environment for skin wound healing, penetration of microorganisms, and bacterial invasion [146]. Wound dressings can be used as bioactive agents and deliver to the wound sites for promoting epithelialization and treatment of severe injuries. Wound dressing in biomedical application should be fabricated into a three-dimensional (3D) architecture with a high porosity with oxygen and water vapour permeability, antibacterial properties, an appropriate pore size, high mechanical strength, and excellent biocompatibility [147, 148]. Silver, due to its polycationic nature, was used as antimicrobial agents since many centuries. Different types of wound dressings exist which depend on materials containing natural or synthetic polymers or their combinations. The microporous architecture of some natural polymers improves wound healing process by their antimicrobial activities [149]. Synthetic hydrogels composed of natural polymer collagen to obtain novel dressing materials for healing burns and wound dressing were introduced by Yannas's group [150]. The similarity of some polysaccharides (chitosan, gelatin, chitin etc.) to the human body macromolecules, they could be currently used to make different wound dressings. Chitin is one the natural polymers variety application including drug delivery, tissue engineering, wound dressing, and other biomedical applications [149]. Biodegradable silk fibroin/chitin/silver nanoparticles 3D scaffolds can be used as a bandage for antimicrobial wound dressing [149]. Figure 5A shows the cell viability data, and it revealed that both silk fibroin and chitin had viability of below 25% for 24 h of incubation which reached to 36–39% after 48 h. DAPI or 4′, 6-diamidino-2-phenylindole was used as nuclear stain of the normal fibroblast (nHFFF2) cells attached on the bandages and was confirmed by the cytocompatible nature of the bandages as shown in Fig. 5B. From the images, it is clear that higher number of cells were attached on composite bandages containing lower concentration of Ag and vice versa.

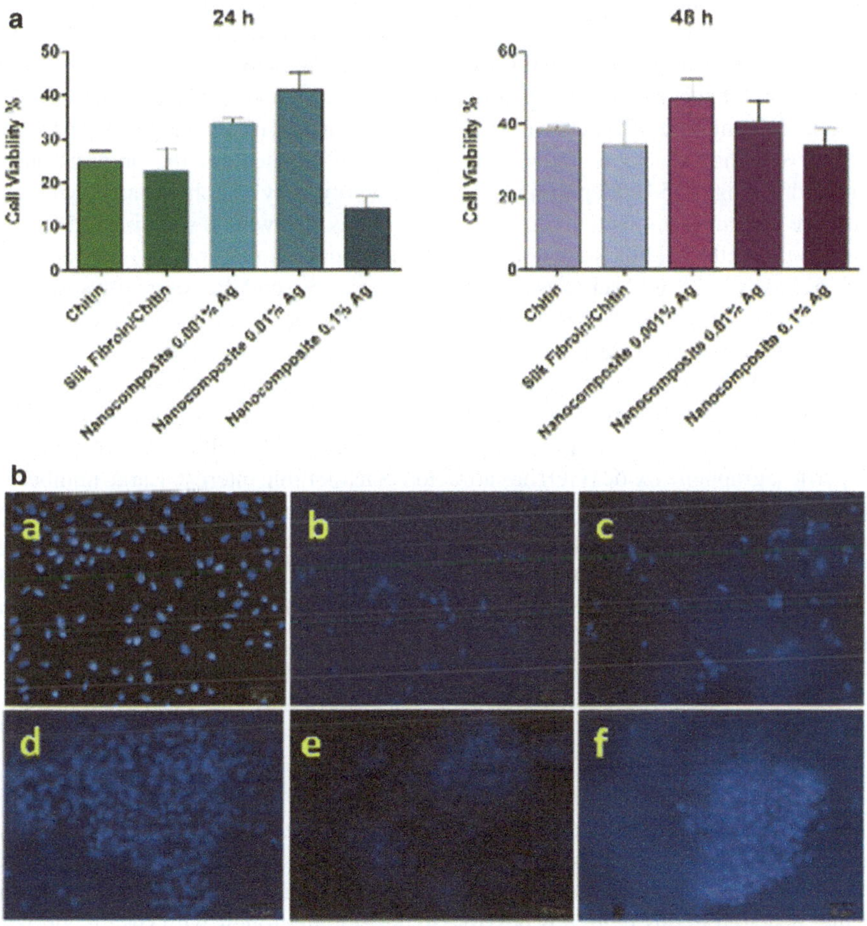

Fig. 5 **A** Proliferation and cell viability of nHFFF2 cell cultured on chitin, silk fibroin/chitin, and scaffolds with different Ag NPs contents after 24 and 48 h. **B** DAPI staining of the nHFFF2 cells attached on the chitin (**b**), silk fibroin/chitin (**c**), and nanocomposite scaffolds with 0.001% (**d**), 0.01% (**e**), and 0.1% Ag NPs (**f**). The cells with no samples used as a control (**a**) [149]

PVA is one of the most frequently used polymers and employed as wound dressings, wound management, and drug delivery systems. But the properties of PVA hydrogel such as stiff membrane, inadequate elasticity, and very incomplete hydrophilic characteristics which restrict its use alone as wound dressing polymeric membranes. Hydrogels prepared using PVA blended with some natural polysaccharides and some other synthetic ones are attractive. PVA/starch nanocomposites hydrogel membranes reinforced with silver nanoparticles demonstrate their potential to be employed for the wound dressing applications in dried as well as in the form of gel due to antimicrobial activity [128]. Sericin/poly(vinyl alcohol) hydrogel can be used as a drug delivery carrier for potential wound dressing application [151]. ZnO nanoparticles in the hydrogels are spherical and can be used in wound dressing applications. Hyaluronic acid-zinc oxide ((HA-ZnO) nanocomposite hydrogels (NCHs) was prepared by one-pot synthesis method and can be used for wound dressing [152]. Good biocompatibility and positive effects on wound healing were shown by chitosan, and it can accelerate repair of different tissues and facilitate contraction of wounds. A combination of heparinized PVA, chitosan, and nZnO was used to produce hydrogels using the freeze–thaw method which is applied for the preparation of wound dressings [153]. Heparinized nano-ZnO/poly(vinyl alcohol)/carboxymethyl cellulose bionanocomposite hydrogels are employed for wound dressing [154].

Carboxymethyl cellulose nanocomposite hydrogel containing ZnO impregnated mesoporous silica could serve as a kind of promising wound dressing with sustained drug delivery properties [155]. Carboxymethylcellulose hydrogel and mesoporous silica system can be used for wound dressing due to its water uptake properties which help in maintaining a moist environment and absorption of wound exudates, while releasing antibacterial agent preventing the wound against infections [147]. Due to the excellent biocompatibility, surface functionalizability, and mechanical properties, graphene oxide (GO) has attracted considerable interest. Large number of hydrophilic oxygenated functional groups on its surface enhances its hydrophilicity and miscibility within polymer matrices, potentially improving hydrogel swelling and mechanical property. Bacterial nanocellulose/poly(acrylic acid)/graphene oxide composite hydrogel uses two electron beam irradiation methods making them an effective wound dressing material [156].

6 Conclusion

The present chapter gives an outline of the increased usage of nanoparticle-reinforced biodegradable hydrogels for applications in various fields such as drug delivery, tissue engineering, and wound dressing with along with its advantages. By carrying out further research in this field, it is possible to develop hydrogels with specific properties by simple and cost-effective manner. In the designing of drug delivery systems as well as other biomedical applications, biodegradable hydrogels act as an alternative material of choice. Biodegradable nanocomposite hydrogels can act as a highly engineered platform for multiple biomedical applications, providing renewable and permanent solutions to life sciences. Future studies in the field of nanocomposite hydrogels will focus on new fabrication technologies, understanding the interactions between polymeric chains and nanoparticles at different length scales and fabrication of multi-component network of hydrogels.

References

1. Palmese LL et al (2019) Hybrid hydrogels for biomedical applications. Curr Opin Chem Eng
2. Rafieian S et al (2019) A review on nanocomposite hydrogels and their biomedical applications. Sci Eng Compos Mater **26**(1):154–174
3. Pal SL et al (2011) Nanoparticle: an overview of preparation and characterization. J Appl Pharm Sci **1**(6):228–234
4. Curvello R, Raghuwanshi VS, Garnier G (2019) Engineering nanocellulose hydrogels for biomedical applications. Adv Colloid Interface Sci
5. De France KJ et al (2016) Enhanced mechanical properties in cellulose nanocrystal–poly (oligoethylene glycol methacrylate) injectable nanocomposite hydrogels through control of physical and chemical cross-linking. Biomacromolecules 17(2):649–660
6. Conte R et al (2019) Hydrogel nanocomposite systems: characterization and application in drug-delivery systems. In: Nanocarriers for Drug Delivery, pp 319–349
7. Feksa LR et al (2018) Hydrogels for biomedical applications. In: Nanostructures for the engineering of cells, tissues and organs. William Andrew Publishing, pp 403–438.
8. Gaharwar AK, Peppas NA, Khademhosseini A (2014) Nanocomposite hydrogels for biomedical applications. Biotechnol Bioeng 111(3):441–453
9. Haraguchi K (2007) Nanocomposite hydrogels. Curr Opin Solid State Mater Sci 11(3–4):47–54
10. Asadi N et al (2019) Fabrication and in vitro evaluation of nanocomposite hydrogel scaffolds based on gelatin/PCL–PEG–PCL for cartilage tissue engineering. ACS Omega **4**(1):449–457 (2019)
11. Sasaki Y, Akiyoshi K (2010) Nanogel engineering for new nanobiomaterials: from chaperoning engineering to biomedical applications. Chem Rec **10**(6):366–376
12. Asghari F et al (2017) Biodegradable and biocompatible polymers for tissue engineering application: a review. Artif. Cells Nanomed Biotechnol **45**(2):185–192
13. Eftekhari H et al (2017) Assessment of polycaprolacton (PCL) nanocomposite scaffold compared with hydroxyapatite (HA) on healing of segmental femur bone defect in rabbits. Artif Cells Nanomed Biotechnol **45**(5):961–968
14. Liao JF et al (2017) Injectable alginate hydrogel cross-linked by calcium gluconate-loaded porous microspheres for cartilage tissue engineering. ACS Omega 2(2):443–454.
15. Sharma G et al (2018) Applications of nanocomposite hydrogels for biomedical engineering and environmental protection. Environ Chem Lett 16(1):113–146
16. Bullo S, Hussein MZB (2015) Inorganic nanolayers: structure, preparation, and biomedical applications. Int J Nanomed 10:5609
17. Kokabi M, Sirousazar M, Hassan ZM (2007) PVA–clay nanocomposite hydrogels for wound dressing. Eur Polym J 43(3):773–781
18. Goenka S, Sant V, Sant S (2014) Graphene-based nanomaterials for drug delivery and tissue engineering. J Control Rel 173:75–88
19. Yun J-M et al (2011) Solution-processable reduced graphene oxide as a novel alternative to PEDOT: PSS hole transport layers for highly efficient and stable polymer solar cells. Adv Mater 23(42):4923–4928
20. Zhao F et al (2015) Composites of polymer hydrogels and nanoparticulate systems for biomedical and pharmaceutical applications. Nanomaterials 5(4):2054–2130

21. Ullah F et al (2015) Classification, processing and application of hydrogels: a review. Mater Sci Eng C 57:414–433
22. Sershen SR et al (2002) Independent optically addressable nanoparticle-polymer optomechanical composites. Appl Phys Lett 80(24):4609–4611
23. Holtz JH, Asher SA (1997) Polymerized colloidal crystal hydrogel films as intelligent chemical sensing materials. Nature 389(6653):829
24. Xia Y et al (2003) One-dimensional nanostructures: synthesis, characterization, and applications. Adv Mater 15(5):353–389
25. Pardo-Yissar V et al (2001) Gold nanoparticle/hydrogel composites with solvent-switchable electronic properties. Adv Mater 13(17):1320–1323
26. Sheeney-Haj-Ichia L, Sharabi G, Willner I (2002) Control of the Electronic properties of thermosensitive poly (N-isopropylacrylamide) and au-nano-particle/poly (N-isopropylacrylamide) composite hydrogels upon phase transition. Adv Func Mater 12(1):27–32
27. Wang C, Flynn NT, Langer R (2004) Controlled structure and properties of thermoresponsive nanoparticle–hydrogel composites. Adv Mater 16(13):1074–1079
28. Marcelo G et al (2014) Poly (N-isopropylacrylamide)/gold hybrid hydrogels prepared by catechol redox chemistry. Characterization and smart tunable catalytic activity. Macromolecules **47**(17):6028–6036
29. Rose S et al (2014) Nanoparticle solutions as adhesives for gels and biological tissues. Nature 505(7483):382
30. Wu H et al (2013) Stable Li-ion battery anodes by in-situ polymerization of conducting hydrogel to conformally coat silicon nanoparticles. Nat Commun 4:1943
31. Escalona Rayo O, Quintanar Guerrero D (2014) Polymeric nanogels: a new alternative for drug delivery. Rev Mex Cienc Farm 45(3):17–38
32. Nita LE et al (2016) Multifunctional nanogels with dual temperature and pH responsiveness. Int J Pharm 515(1–2):165–175
33. Koul V et al (2011) Interpenetrating polymer network (IPN) nanogels based on gelatin and poly (acrylic acid) by inverse miniemulsion technique: synthesis and characterization. Colloids Surf B: Biointerfaces 83(2): 204–213
34. Veiga M-D et al (2018) Hydrogels: biomedical uses. In: Design and development of new nanocarriers. William Andrew Publishing, pp 509–554
35. Biondi M et al (2015) Nanoparticle-integrated hydrogels as multifunctional composite materials for biomedical applications. Gels 1(2):162–178
36. Geim AK (2009) Graphene: status and prospects. Science 324(5934):1530–1534
37. Li D et al (2008) Processable aqueous dispersions of graphene nanosheets. Nat Nanotechnol 3(2):101
38. Weiss NO et al (2012) Graphene: an emerging electronic material. Adv Mater 24(43):5782–5825
39. Wang R, Chaohe Xu, Lee J-M (2016) High performance asymmetric supercapacitors: New NiOOH nanosheet/graphene hydrogels and pure graphene hydrogels. Nano Energy 19:210–221
40. Zhao Y et al (2017) Construction of three-dimensional hemin-functionalized graphene hydrogel with high mechanical stability and adsorption capacity for enhancing photodegradation of methylene blue. ACS Appl Mater Interfaces 9(4):4006–4014
41. Ligorio C et al (2019) Graphene oxide containing self-assembling peptide hybrid hydrogels as a potential 3D injectable cell delivery platform for intervertebral disc repair applications. Acta Biomaterialia
42. Liu W et al (2019) Reduced graphene oxide (rGO) hybridized hydrogel as a near-infrared (NIR)/pH dual-responsive platform for combined chemo-photothermal therapy. J Colloid Interface Sci 536:160–170
43. Rasoulzadehzali M, Namazi H (2018) Facile preparation of antibacterial chitosan/graphene oxide-Ag bio-nanocomposite hydrogel beads for controlled release of doxorubicin. Int J Biol Macromol 116:54–63

44. Jing X et al (2017) Mussel-inspired electroactive chitosan/graphene oxide composite hydrogel with rapid self-healing and recovery behavior for tissue engineering. Carbon 125:557–570
45. Shin SR et al (2016) Reduced graphene oxide-gelMA hybrid hydrogels as scaffolds for cardiac tissue engineering. Small 12(27):3677–3689
46. Fan Z et al (2014) A novel wound dressing based on Ag/graphene polymer hydrogel: effectively kill bacteria and accelerate wound healing. Adv Funct Mater 24(25):3933–3943
47. Vashist A et al (2018) Advances in carbon nanotubes–hydrogel hybrids in nanomedicine for therapeutics. Adv Healthcare Mater 7(9):1701213
48. Foldvari M, Bagonluri M (2008) Carbon nanotubes as functional excipients for nanomedicines: I. Pharmaceutical properties. Nanomed Nanotechnol Biol Med 4(3):173–182
49. Prato M, Kostarelos K, Bianco A (2007) Functionalized carbon nanotubes in drug design and discovery. Acc Chem Res 41(1):60–68
50. Li X et al (2013) Nanostructured scaffolds for bone tissue engineering. J Biomed Mater Res Part A 101(8):2424–2435
51. Cirillo G et al (2014) Carbon nanotubes hybrid hydrogels in drug delivery: a perspective review. BioMed Res Int 2014
52. Pok S et al (2014) Biocompatible carbon nanotube–chitosan scaffold matching the electrical conductivity of the heart. ACS Nano 8(10):9822–9832
53. Kouser R et al (2018) Biocompatible and mechanically robust nanocomposite hydrogels for potential applications in tissue engineering. Mater Sci Eng C 84:168–179
54. Saeednia L et al (2019) Sustained releasing of methotrexate from injectable and thermosensitive chitosan–carbon nanotube hybrid hydrogels effectively controls tumor cell growth. ACS Omega 4(2):4040–4048
55. Choudhary B et al (2018) Understanding the effect of functionalized carbon nanotubes on the properties of tamarind gum hydrogels. Polymer Bull 75(11):4929–4945
56. Joddar B et al (2016) Development of functionalized multi-walled carbon-nanotube-based alginate hydrogels for enabling biomimetic technologies. Sci Rep 6:32456
57. Hoppe A, Güldal NS, Boccaccini AR (2011) A review of the biological response to ionic dissolution products from bioactive glasses and glass-ceramics. Biomaterials 32(11):2757–2774
58. Song W et al (2012) Poly (vinyl alcohol)/collagen/hydroxyapatite hydrogel: Properties and in vitro cellular response. J Biomed Mater Res Part A 100(11):3071–3079
59. Kokubo T, Takadama H (2006) How useful is SBF in predicting in vivo bone bioactivity? Biomaterials 27(15):2907–2915
60. Annabi N et al (2014) 25th anniversary article: rational design and applications of hydrogels in regenerative medicine. Adv Mater 26(1):85–124
61. Peña-Parás L, Sánchez-Fernández JA, Vidaltamayo R (2017) Nanoclays for biomedical applications. In: Handbook of ecomaterials, pp 1–19
62. Sharifi S et al (2012) Biodegradable nanocomposite hydrogel structures with enhanced mechanical properties prepared by photo-crosslinking solutions of poly (trimethylene carbonate)–poly (ethylene glycol)–poly (trimethylene carbonate) macromonomers and nanoclay particles. Acta Biomaterialia 8(12):4233–4243
63. Entezam M et al (2019) Physicomechanical and antimicrobial characteristics of hydrogel based on poly (vinyl alcohol): performance improvement via inclusion of chitosan-modified nanoclay. J Appl Polym Sci 136(20):47444
64. Filipowska J et al (2018) In vitro osteogenic potential of collagen/chitosan-based hydrogels-silica particles hybrids in human bone marrow-derived mesenchymal stromal cell cultures. Int J Biol Macromol 113:692–700
65. Rocha-García D et al (2018) Gelatin-based porous silicon hydrogel composites for the controlled release of tramadol. Eur Polym J 108:485–497
66. de Lima HHC et al (2018) Bionanocomposites based on mesoporous silica and alginate for enhanced drug delivery. Carbohydrate Polym 196:126–134
67. Tyliszczak B et al (2017) In vitro cytotoxicity of hydrogels based on chitosan and modified with gold nanoparticles. J Polym Res 24(10):153

68. García-Astrain C et al (2016) Click crosslinked chitosan/gold nanocomposite hydrogels. Macromol Mater Eng 301(11):1295–1300
69. Xie Y et al (2018) Novel chitosan hydrogels reinforced by silver nanoparticles with ultrahigh mechanical and high antibacterial properties for accelerating wound healing. Int J Biol Macromol 119:402–412
70. Jing X et al (2019) Stretchable gelatin/silver nanowires composite hydrogels for detecting human motion. Mater Lett 237:53–56
71. Gholamali I et al (2019) Preparation and characterization of oxidized starch/CuO nanocomposite hydrogels applicable in a drug delivery system. Starch-Stärke 71(3–4):1800118
72. Zhai M et al (2018) Keratin-chitosan/n-ZnO nanocomposite hydrogel for antimicrobial treatment of burn wound healing: characterization and biomedical application. J Photochem Photobiol B: Biol 180 (2018):253–258
73. Carvalho HWP et al (2010) Removal of metal ions from aqueous solution by chelating polymeric hydrogel. Environ Chemis Lett 8(4):343–348
74. Pathania D et al (2016) Novel guar gum/Al_2O_3 nanocomposite as an effective photocatalyst for the degradation of malachite green dye. Int J Bio Macromol 87:366–374
75. Thakur M et al (2017) Efficient photocatalytic degradation of toxic dyes from aqueous environment using gelatin-Zr (IV) phosphate nanocomposite and its antimicrobial activity. Colloids Surf B: Biointerfaces 157:456–463
76. Alvarez-Lorenzo C, Blanco-Fernandez B, Puga AM, Concheiro A (2013) Adv Drug Deliv Rev 65:1148–1171
77. De France KJ, Hoare T, Cranston ED (2017) Review of hydrogels and aerogels containing nanocellulose. Chem Mater **29**(11):4609–4631
78. Dou X-Q, Feng C-L (2017) Amino acids and peptide-based supramolecular hydrogels for three-dimensional cell culture. Adv Mater 29(16):1604062
79. Jeong B, Kim SW, Bae YH (2012) Thermosensitive sol–gel reversible hydrogels. Adv Drug Deliv Rev 64:154–162
80. Ahmed EM (2015) Hydrogel: preparation, characterization, and applications: a review. J Adv Res 6(2):105–121
81. Xu B et al (2017) A mineralized high strength and tough hydrogel for skull bone regeneration. Adv Funct Mater 27(4):1604327
82. Ge G et al (2018) Stretchable, transparent, and self-patterned hydrogel-based pressure sensor for human motions detection. Adv Funct Mater 28(32):1802576
83. Elshaarani T et al (2018) Synthesis of hydrogel-bearing phenylboronic acid moieties and their applications in glucose sensing and insulin delivery. J Mater Chem B6.23:3831–3854
84. Deligkaris K et al (2010) Hydrogel-based devices for biomedical applications. Sens Actuat B Chem 147(2):765–774
85. Ghobril C, Grinstaff MW (2015) The chemistry and engineering of polymeric hydrogel adhesives for wound closure: a tutorial. Chem Soc Rev 44(7):1820–1835
86. Li J et al (2017) Self-healable gels for use in wearable devices. Chem Mater 29(21):8932–8952
87. Lei Z et al (2017) A bioinspired mineral hydrogel as a self-healable, mechanically adaptable ionic skin for highly sensitive pressure sensing. Adv Mater 29(22):1700321
88. Fu L-H et al (2019) Multifunctional cellulose-based hydrogels for biomedical applications. J Mater Chem B7(10):1541–1562
89. Tanpichai S, Oksman K (2016) Cross-linked nanocomposite hydrogels based on cellulose nanocrystals and PVA: Mechanical properties and creep recovery. Compos A Appl Sci Manuf 88:226–233
90. Javanbakht S, Namazi H (2018) Doxorubicin loaded carboxymethyl cellulose/graphene quantum dot nanocomposite hydrogel films as a potential anticancer drug delivery system. Mater Sci Eng C 87:50–59
91. Xing C et al (2018) Conceptually novel black phosphorus/cellulose hydrogels as promising photothermal agents for effective cancer therapy. Adv Healthcare Mater 7(7):1701510
92. Chang C, Zhang L (2011) Cellulose-based hydrogels: present status and application prospects. Carbohyd Polym 84(1):40–53

93. Păduraru OM et al (2012) Synthesis and characterization of polyvinyl alcohol/cellulose cryogels and their testing as carriers for a bioactive component. Mater Sci Eng: C 32(8):2508–2515
94. Ciolacu DE, Suflet DM (2018) Cellulose-based hydrogels for medical/pharmaceutical applications. In: Biomass as renewable raw material to obtain bioproducts of high-tech value. Elsevier, pp 401–439
95. Shin SR et al (2013) Carbon-nanotube-embedded hydrogel sheets for engineering cardiac constructs and bioactuators. ACS Nano 7(3):2369–2380
96. Nair LS, Laurencin CT (2007) Biodegradable polymers as biomaterials. Prog Polym Sci 32(8–9):762–798
97. Ching KY (2014) Mechanically adjustable and degradable scaffolds for the treatment of articular cartilage defects. Dissertation. University of Southampton
98. Yang Y et al (2014) Advances in self-assembled chitosan nanomaterials for drug delivery. Biotechnol Adv 32(7):1301–1316
99. Pujana MA et al (2013) Biodegradable chitosan nanogels crosslinked with genipin. Carbohydrate Polym 94(2):836–842
100. Xiao C et al (2016) Tunable functional hydrogels formed from a versatile water-soluble chitosan. Int J Biol Macromol 85:386–390
101. Song R et al (2019) A natural cordycepin/chitosan complex hydrogel with outstanding self-healable and wound healing properties. Int J Biol Macromol 134:91–99
102. dos Santos TC et al (2018) Nanocomposite chitosan hydrogels based on PLGA nanoparticles as potential biomedical materials. Eur Polym J 99:456–463
103. Yuan M et al (2018) Thermosensitive and photocrosslinkable hydroxypropyl chitin-based hydrogels for biomedical applications. Carbohydrate Polym 192:10–18
104. Sharma S et al (2018) Development of a novel chitosan based biocompatible and self-healing hydrogel for controlled release of hydrophilic drug. Int J Biol Macromol 116:37–44
105. Sharma A et al (2013) Three-dimensional supermacroporous carrageenan-gelatin cryogel matrix for tissue engineering applications. BioMed Res Int
106. Liu J et al (2015) Review for carrageenan-based pharmaceutical biomaterials: favourable physical features versus adverse biological effects. Carbohydrate Polym 121:27–36
107. Yegappan R et al (2018) Carrageenan based hydrogels for drug delivery, tissue engineering and wound healing. Carbohydrate Polym
108. Yegappan R et al (2019) Injectable angiogenic and osteogenic carrageenan nanocomposite hydrogel for bone tissue engineering. Int J Biol Macromol 122:320–328
109. Mihaila SM et al (2013) Photocrosslinkable kappa-carrageenan hydrogels for tissue engineering applications. Adv Healthcare Materials 2(6):895–907
110. Azizi S et al (2017) Hydrogel beads bio-nanocomposite based on Kappa-Carrageenan and green synthesized silver nanoparticles for biomedical applications. Int J Biolog Macromol 104:423–431
111. Mahdavinia GR et al (2017) Magnetic-and pH-responsive κ-carrageenan/chitosan complexes for controlled release of methotrexate anticancer drug. Int J Biol Macromol 97:209–217
112. Feng W et al (2017) A novel composite of collagen-hydroxyapatite/kappa-carrageenan. J Alloys Compd 693:482–489
113. González JI, Ossa CPO (2017) Injectability evaluation of bone-graft substitutes based on carrageenan and hydroxyapatite nanorods. In: Proceedings of the 3rd Pan American Materials Congress. Springer, Cham
114. Pourjavadi A et al (2019) Injectable chitosan/κ-carrageenan hydrogel designed with au nanoparticles: a conductive scaffold for tissue engineering demands. Int J Biol Macromol 126:310–317
115. Zheng Y et al (2018) Gelatin-based hydrogels blended with gellan as an injectable wound dressing. ACS Omega 3(5):4766–4775
116. Dey K et al (2019) Preparation and properties of high performance gelatin-based hydrogels with chitosan or hydroxyethyl cellulose for tissue engineering applications. Int J Polym Mater Polym Biomater 68(4):183–192

117. El-Feky GS et al (2018) Chitosan-gelatin hydrogel crosslinked with oxidized sucrose for the ocular delivery of timolol maleate. J Pharm Sci 107(12):3098–3104
118. Moreira CDF et al (2018) Nanostructured chitosan/gelatin/bioactive glass in situ forming hydrogel composites as a potential injectable matrix for bone tissue engineering. Mater Chem Phys 218:304–316
119. Song Y et al (2018) In situ formation of injectable chitosan-gelatin hydrogels through double crosslinking for sustained intraocular drug delivery. Mater Sci Eng C 88: 1–12
120. Monteiro N et al (2018) Photopolymerization of cell-laden gelatin methacryloyl hydrogels using a dental curing light for regenerative dentistry. Dental Mater 34(3):389–399
121. Treesuppharat W et al (2017) Synthesis and characterization of bacterial cellulose and gelatin-based hydrogel composites for drug-delivery systems. Biotechnol Rep 15:84–91
122. Maharana V et al (2017) Reinforcing the inner phase of the filled hydrogels with CNTs alters drug release properties and human keratinocyte morphology: A study on the gelatin-tamarind gum filled hydrogels. J Mech Behav Biomed Mater 75:538–548
123. Cheng Y-H et al (2016) Thermosensitive chitosan-based hydrogel as a topical ocular drug delivery system of latanoprost for glaucoma treatment. Carbohydrate Polym 144:390–399
124. Chen X et al (2012) Chitosan-based thermosensitive hydrogel as a promising ocular drug delivery system: preparation, characterization, and in vivo evaluation. J Biomater Appl 27(4):391–402
125. Bakravi A et al (2015) Synthesis of gelatin-based biodegradable hydrogel nanocomposite and their application as drug delivery agent. Adv Polym Technol 37(7):2625–2635
126. Ninan N et al (2015) Natural polymer/inorganic material based hybrid scaffolds for skin wound healing. Polym Rev 55(3):453–490
127. Kamoun EA, Kenawy E-R, Chen X (2017) A review on polymeric hydrogel membranes for wound dressing applications: PVA-based hydrogel dressings. J Adv Res 8(3):217–233
128. Batool S et al (2019) Biogenic synthesis of silver nanoparticles and evaluation of physical and antimicrobial properties of Ag/PVA/starch nanocomposites hydrogel membranes for wound dressing application. J Drug Deliv Sci Technol 52:403–414
129. Namazi H, Hasani M, Yadollahi M (2019) Antibacterial oxidized starch/ZnO nanocomposite hydrogel: synthesis and evaluation of its swelling behaviours in various pHs and salt solutions. Int J Biol Macromol 126:578–584
130. Sharma P et al (2019) Sustained delivery of atenolol drug using gum dammar crosslinked polyacrylamide and zirconium based biodegradable hydrogel composites. Colloids Surf A Physicochem Eng Aspects 562:136–145
131. Gholamali I, Asnaashariisfahani M, Alipour E (2019) Silver nanoparticles incorporated in ph-sensitive nanocomposite hydrogels based on carboxymethyl chitosan-poly (vinyl alcohol) for use in a drug delivery system. Regener Eng Transl Med:1–16
132. Schroeder KL, Goreham RV, Nann T (2016) Graphene quantum dots for theranostics and bioimaging. Pharm Res 33(10):2337–2357
133. Yousef T, Hassan N (2017) Supramolecular encapsulation of doxorubicin with β-cyclodextrin dendrimer: in vitro evaluation of controlled release and cytotoxicity. J Incl Phenom Macrocycl Chem 87(1–2):105–115
134. Zhang J, Qin W, Wang A (2010) In situ generation of sodium alginate/hydroxyapatite nanocomposite beads as drug-controlled release matrices. Acta Biomaterialia 6(2):445–454
135. Choi EJ et al (2015) Synthesis of electroconductive hydrogel films by an electro-controlled click reaction and their application to drug delivery systems. Polym Chem 6(24):4473–4478
136. Zhang L, Webster TJ (2009) Nanotechnology and nanomaterials: promises for improved tissue regeneration. Nano Today 4(1):66–80
137. Klouda L (2015) Thermoresponsive hydrogels in biomedical applications: A seven-year update. Eur J Pharm Biopharm 97:338–349
138. Shabestari Khiabani S et al (2017) Magnetic nanoparticles: preparation methods, applications in cancer diagnosis and cancer therapy. Artif Cells Nanomed Biotechnol 45(1):6–17
139. Zhao W et al (2013) Degradable natural polymer hydrogels for articular cartilage tissue engineering. J Chem Technol Biotechnol 88(3):327–339

140. Morais DS et al (2013) Development and characterization of novel alginate-based hydrogels as vehicles for bone substitutes. Carbohyd Polym 95(1):134–142
141. Huang Y et al (2012) Micro-/nano-sized hydroxyapatite directs differentiation of rat bone marrow derived mesenchymal stem cells towards an osteoblast lineage. Nanoscale 4(7):2484–2490
142. Pina S, Oliveira JM, Reis RL (2015) Natural-based nanocomposites for bone tissue engineering and regenerative medicine: A review. Adv Mater 27(7):1143–1169
143. Marie PJ, Felsenberg D, Brandi ML (2011) How strontium ranelate, via opposite effects on bone resorption and formation, prevents osteoporosis. Osteoporosis Int 22(6):1659–1667
144. Sila-Asna M et al (2007) Osteoblast differentiation and bone formation gene expression in strontium-inducing bone marrow mesenchymal stem cell. Kobe J Med Sci 53(1–2):25–35
145. Zhang X et al (2019) Biocompatiable silk fibroin/carboxymethyl chitosan/strontium substituted hydroxyapatite/cellulose nanocrystal composite scaffolds for bone tissue engineering. Int J Biol Macromol
146. Lee OJ et al (2016) Fabrication and characterization of hydrocolloid dressing with silk fibroin nanoparticles for wound healing. Tissue Eng Regener Med 13(3):218–226
147. Namazi H et al (2016) Antibiotic loaded carboxymethylcellulose/MCM-41 nanocomposite hydrogel films as potential wound dressing. Int J Biol Macromol 85:327–334
148. Salehi R et al (2015) pH-Controlled multiple-drug delivery by a novel antibacterial nanocomposite for combination therapy. RSC Adv 5(128):105678–105691
149. Mehrabani MG et al (2018) Preparation of biocompatible and biodegradable silk fibroin/chitin/silver nanoparticles 3D scaffolds as a bandage for antimicrobial wound dressing. Int J Biol Macromol 114:961–971
150. Yannas IV et al (1981) Crosslinked collagen-mucopolysaccharide composite materials. U.S. Patent No. 4,280,954, 28 July 1981
151. Tao G et al (2019) Design and performance of sericin/poly (vinyl alcohol) hydrogel as a drug delivery carrier for potential wound dressing application. Mater Sci Eng C 101:341–351
152. Rao KM et al (2019) One-pot synthesis of ZnO nanobelt-like structures in hyaluronan hydrogels for wound dressing applications. Carbohydrate Polym 115124
153. Khorasani MT et al (2018) Incorporation of ZnO nanoparticles into heparinised polyvinyl alcohol/chitosan hydrogels for wound dressing application. Int J Biol Macromol 114:1203–1215
154. Jourabloo A et al (2019) Fabrication of heparinized nano ZnO/poly (vinylalcohol)/carboxymethyl cellulose bionanocomposite hydrogels using artificial neural network for wound dressing application. J Ind Eng Chem 70:253–263
155. Rakhshaei R, Namazi H (2017) A potential bioactive wound dressing based on carboxymethyl cellulose/ZnO impregnated MCM-41 nanocomposite hydrogel. Mater Sci Eng C 73:456–464
156. Halib N, Amin MCIM, Ahmad I (2010) Unique stimuli responsive characteristics of electron beam synthesized bacterial cellulose/acrylic acid composite. J Appl Polym Sci 116(5):2920–2929

Chapter 5
Stimulus-Responsive Polymers

Vincent Joseph and Jiya Jose

1 Introduction

Smart polymers or stimuli-responsive polymers are high-performance polymers that change according to the environment they are in. Such materials can be sensitive to a number of factors, such as temperature, humidity, pH, the wavelength or intensity of light or an electrical or magnetic field, and can respond in various ways, like altering colour or transparency, becoming conductive or permeable to water or changing shape (shape memory polymers). Usually, slight changes in the environment are sufficient to induce large changes in the polymer's properties [1, 2].

Smart polymers appear in highly specialized applications and everyday products alike. They are used for the production of hydrogels, biodegradable packaging, and to a great extent in biomedical engineering. One example is a polymer that undergoes conformational change in response to pH change, which can be used in drug delivery. Another is a humidity-sensitive polymer used in self-adaptive wound dressings that automatically regulate moisture balance in and around the wound. The nonlinear response of smart polymers is what makes them so unique and effective. A significant change in structure and properties can be induced by a very small stimulus. Once that change occurs, there is no further change, meaning a predictable all-or-nothing response occurs, with complete uniformity throughout the polymer. Smart polymers may change conformation, adhesiveness, or water retention properties, due to slight changes in pH, ionic strength, temperature, or other triggers.

Another factor in the effectiveness of smart polymers lies in the inherent nature of polymers in general. The strength of each molecule's response to changes in stimuli is

V. Joseph
School of Chemical Sciences, Mahatma Gandhi University, Kottayam 686560, Kerala, India

J. Jose (✉)
International and Inter University Centre for Nanoscience and Nanotechnology, Mahatma Gandhi University, PD Hills (PO), Kottayam 686560, Kerala, India
e-mail: jiyajose@gmail.com

J. Jose et al. (eds.), *Nano Hydrogels*, Gels Horizons: From Science to Smart Materials,
https://doi.org/10.1007/978-981-15-7138-1_5

the composite of changes of individual monomer units which, alone, would be weak. However, these weak responses, compounded hundreds or thousands of times, create a considerable force for driving biological processes.

In physiology, a stimulus is a detectable change in the internal or external environment. The ability of an organism or organ to respond to external stimuli is called sensitivity. Several polymer systems respond to temperature, undergoing an lower critical solution temperature phase transition. One of the better-studied such polymers is poly(*N*-isopropylacryamide), with a transition temperature of approximately 33 °C. Several homologous *N*-alkyl acrylamides also show LCST behaviour, with the transition temperature depending on the length of the hydrophobic side chain. Above their transition temperature, these polymers become insoluble in water. This behaviour is believed to be entropy drive.

The strategy underlying polymer-containing responsive systems is a dramatic physicochemical change caused by stimuli. At the macromolecular level, polymer chains can be altered in different ways, including changes in hydrophilic-to-hydrophobic balance, conformation, solubility, degradation, and bond cleavage, and these, in turn, will cause detectable behavioural changes to self-assembled structures. Many designs that vary the location of responsive moieties or functional groups are possible. Locations include, but are not limited to: side chains on one of the blocks, chain end groups, or junctions between blocks. The response may be reversible or not, depending on the strategy employed.

2 Physical Forms of Stimuli-Responsive Polymers

2.1 Dentrimers

Dentrimers are usually highly branched stared-shaped molecules with a dimension generally of nanometer range. Dentrimers are monodisperse macromolecules, unlike linear polymers. Because of their molecular architecture, dentrimers show some significantly improved physical and chemical properties when compared to traditional linear polymers. They can be used as delivery vessels, carriers of imaging agents, and therapeutically active compounds [3–5].

2.2 Micelles

Block copolymer micelles are generally formed by the spontaneous self-assembly of amphiphilic copolymer molecules in an aqueous environment. Usually, they are spherically shaped core–shell structures with sizes varying in the range of 10–100 nm. The hydrophobic block forms the micelle cores, while the hydrophilic block forms the micelle corona (shells). This can be thus very much utilized in the field of targeted drug delivery to deliver the drug to the specific point.

2.3 Vesicles

Spherical shell structures in which an aqueous compartment is enclosed by a bilayer membrane made of amphiphilic block copolymers are commonly referred to as polymer vesicles which is also called polymersomes. They have the advantages of greater toughness, greater stability, tunable membrane properties, capacity to transport both hydrophilic andhydrophobic compounds like genes, proteins, imaging agents, anticancer and anti-inflammatory drugs, and others, making them good candidates for applications including drug delivery, nano-reactors, and templates for micro- or nanostructured materials making them to be used in stimuli-responsive systems [6–8].

2.4 Smart Surfaces

New modulation systems that control the surface properties or solubility of materials in response to an external signal are designed using the stimuli-responsive polymers on a material surface or by modifying the surface with active substances that are more sensitive to a trigger. Indeed, smart surfaces that respond to specific chemical and biological species have been the basis for the fabrication of highly sensitive, reagentless, re-usable biosensors [9]. Surface-grafted polymers can be defined as long chain polymer molecules that are attached to a surface through one or a few anchor sites [10]. Two primary covalent attachment techniques, i.e. "grafting-to" and "grafting-from", have been reported to create polymer brushes. In the "grafting-to" technique, a pre-formed end-functionalised polymer in a solution reacts with a suitable substrate surface to form a tethered polymer brush. In the "grafting-from" method, also called the surface-initiated polymerization method, monomers are polymerised from surface-anchored initiators generally immobilized by the self-assembled monolayer technique (SAM) [11, 12]. SAMs offer ease of preparation and versatile surface chemistry, while polymer brushes can be produced by surface-initiated polymerization techniques with improved control of surface coverage, thickness, and composition. Stimuli-responsive polymer films can be prepared on substrate surfaces using several deposition techniques of differing complexities and applicability, such as spin coating, chemical vapour deposition, laser ablation, plasma deposition, and chemical or electrochemical reactions [13–15]. The choice of deposition methods depends on the physicochemical properties of the polymer material, the film quality requirements, and the substrate being coated.

2.5 Polymer–Protein–Drug Conjugates

Polymers conjugated with therapeutic agents have been extensively investigated over the past years. Conjugation of polymers to therapeutic molecules resulted in macromolecular systems that synergistically combined the individual properties of the components. As a result of these conjugation drug solubilization, protein efficacy and stability are increased by conjugation, while immunogenicity and toxicity are lowered.

3 Stimulus-Responsive Polymers

The condition for polymer-responsive systems depends on the type of stimuli applied to the system. The effect depends on the physiochemical changes brought about by the stimuli. These changes at the molecular levels can be in various forms such as changes in hydrophilic-to-hydrophobic nature or vice-versa, conformation, degradation, solubility, etc., which can cause a detectable change in the self-assembled structures of the polymer or to the stable conformation state of the polymer [16]. Mostly, these changes are as shift in the functional moieties which are sensitive to the applied stimuli. Depending on the nature of the stimuli, these can be reversible or non-reversible. Based on the various stimulus that are seen commonly, the stimuli can be classified broadly into three, namely physical, chemical, and biological [17, 18]. The physical stimuli usually modify the energy level of the polymer/solvent system or simply the chain dynamics, whereas the chemical stimuli are usually resulted as a result of the changes bought by the change in the molecular interactions between polymer and solvent molecules or even between polymer chains. The physical stimulus commonly includes light, temperature, ultrasound, magnetic, mechanical, and electrical. The chemical stimulus includes solvent, ionic strength, electrochemical, pH, etc. [19]. Biological stimuli which usually include enzymes and receptors which usually relate to the actual functioning of the molecules like enzymatic reactions or recognition of the molecules [20]. An additional stimuli commonly referred to as dual stimuli-responsive polymer are the ones in which the polymer responds to more than one stimuli.

3.1 Physically Dependent Stimuli

The physically dependent stimuli include temperature, electric field, light, ultrasound, magnetic fields, and mechanical deformation. The physical stimuli include the change in the properties or the structure as a function of temperature light or electric field. As mentioned, these bring about a change to the chain dynamics in the system. The major changes that are brought about by these stimuli are in the energy levels of the interacting materials, i.e. the polymer–solvent system.

3.1.1 Temperature-Responsive Polymers

The temperature-responsive polymers have attracted greater importance these days because the variation in the temperature is easily detectable and most systems show deflection in temperature in response to even a small stimulus. The greater attentions of these are seen in fields of bioengineering and biotechnology as the detection of disease is mainly characterized by change in temperature of the system [21]. It is generally observed in case of copolymers that the hydrophobic and hydrophilic interactions between the polymer chains and aqueous media change around a small range of temperature known as the critical solution temperature. Thus, a volume expansion particularly expansion or collapse in the chain occurs which is resulted from the disruption of intra- and intermolecular electrostatic and hydrophobic interactions. Polymer solutions generally possess an upper critical solution temperature (UCST) above which one polymer phase exists and below which a phase separation appears. Polymer solutions that appear as a single phase below a specific temperature and appear as biphasic above it generally possess a so-called lower critical solution temperature (LCST). Some copolymers that fall into the category of the temperature-responsive polymers include poly(*N*-isopropylacrylamide) (PNiPAAm) [22, 23], poly(*N*-vinylalkylamides), e.g. poly(*N*-vinylcaprolactam) (PNVC) [24], and copolymers such as poly(L-lactic acid)-poly(ethylene glycol)-poly(L-lactic acid) (PLLA-PEG-PLLA) triblock copolymers [25], and poly(ethylene oxide)-poly(propylene oxide)-poly(ethylene oxide) (PEO–PPO–PEO) copolymers [26].

Temperature-Responsive Dentrimers

Various temperature-responsive dentrimer systems which differ in architecture and chemical composition usually used to encapsulate and release drugs are developed. The generation and the molecular mass of the dentrimers are responsible for the temperature sensitivity of the dentrimers [27]. Common examples include star-shaped poly(e-caprolactone)-b-poly(2-(dimethylamino)ethyl methacrylate) (HPs-Star-PCL-b-PDMAEMA) [28], core–shell dendritic poly(ether-amide) (DPEA) modified with carboxyl end-capped linear poly(*N*-isopropylacrylamide) (PNIPAAm–COOH), and carboxyl end-capped methoxy polyethylene glycol (PEG–COOH) [29].

Temperature-Responsive Vesicles

Looking on to the thermo-responsiveness vesicles, some of the reported vesicles show these properties are discussed. Thermo-responsive cross-linked polymer vesicles were formed by self-assembly of the block copolymer poly(2-cinnamoylethyl methacrylate)-b-poly(*N*-isopropylacrylamide) (PCEMA-b-PNIPAM) and following photo-cross-linking of PCEMA shells and were used for temperature-(higher than 32 °C) triggered release of 4-aminopyridine [30]. Self-assembly of amphiphilichyper-branched star copolymers with a hydrophobic hyperbranchedpoly[3-ethyl-3-(hydroxymethyl)oxetane] (HBPO) core and many hydrophilic polyethylene oxide (PEO) arms also showed thermo-sensitive behaviour [31]. Thermo-responsiveness can also be obtained by using the synthetic poly(trimethylene carbonate)-b-poly(L-glutamic acid) (PTMC-b-PGA), di block copolymer [32]. Temperature-induced reversible crystallization/melting of the PTMC-b-PGA vesicles in water depended on the vesicle size (membrane thickness). The disruption of the vesicular structure occurred when the temperature was increased above the melting point of the PTMC block (34–35 °C).

Temperature-Responsive Surfaces

The most widely studied temperature-controlled films are built from PNiPAAm, a thermo-responsive polymer that has an LCST of 32 °C in aqueous solution [33]. PNiPAAm chains present a widespread hydrogen bonding network between the amide groups and water molecules. Above LCST, PNiPAAm films undergo a phase transition, from a hydrated swollen state to yield a collapsed morphology (solvent is forced out) [34–36]. The reversible volume phase transition of PNiPAAm films can be utilized to develop thermo-responsive culture media for cells [37–39]. Surface-attached stimuli-responsive polymers do not aggregate to form a separate phase, but the conformational transition from the hydrophilic-to-hydrophobic state endows the surface with regulated hydrophobicity.

Temperature-Responsive Conjugates

Consider the system protein–polymer conjugates are based on biocompatible polyethyleneglycol methacrylate (PEGMA) [40]. Hybrid polymer–protein (PEGMA–trypsin) conjugates are promising candidates for biomedical applications. The first hybrid (diblock conjugate) and the second hybrid (triblock) demonstrated behaviour depending on their architectures but also their enzymatic activities—hydrolysis of peptide and protein substrates were different for various hybrids. This is an example of polymer–protein conjugates with varied architectures, and it can be used to regulate the properties of the protein polymer hybrids in terms of stability and reactivity.

3.1.2 Electro-responsive Polymers

The presence of ions of different sizes and charge were found to change the heights of the polyelectrolyte brushes in response to the stimuli. When polymer chains bond with counter ions, it is observed that the swelling and the hydrophilic/hydrophobic properties of the polymer layer change. Due to the precise control over the magnitude of current, the duration of an electrical pulse or the interval between pulses, these are used for electrical and electrochemical-responsive stimuli applications [9, 41]. Electrochemical stimulation can produce different effects like.

1. An influx of the counter ion and solvent molecules causes an increase in the osmotic pressure in the polymer which results in a volumetric expansion.
2. Control of loading/adsorption of polyelectrolyte on to oppositely charged porous materials.
3. Formation and swelling of redox-active polyelectrolyte multilayers.

Consider a case wherein an electrochemical stimulus is applied to multilayer polyacrylamide films. The result of the stimulus is the shrinking of the film on the anode side. This happens because of the combined effects of H^+ ions migrating to the region of the cathode and the electrostatic attraction between the anode surface and the negatively charged acrylic acid groups [42, 43].

3.1.3 Photo-responsive Polymers

Light can be applied instantaneously and under specific conditions with high precision and accuracy. This is utilized by the light-responsive polymers and leads to highly advantageous applications [44]. Thus, this light can be precisely used at the polymer surface or can be delivered to distinct locations by the use of optical fibres. The near-infrared part of the spectrum is less harmful and has deeper penetration in tissues than visible light and thus can be used as biologically friendly window [45]. Most photo-responsive polymers contain light-sensitive chromophores such as azobenzene groups [46, 47], spiropyran groups [48, 49], or nitrobenzyl groups [50, 51]. A variety of azobenzene or spiropyran-containing photo-responsive polymers, as for example PAA [52, 53], PHPMAm [54, 55], and PNIPAM [56, 57], have been reported.

Photo-Responsive Dentrimers

The conversion of photo-energy into dynamic energy or in drug delivery systems led to the development of photo-responsive carbosilane dendrimers containing 4-phenylazo benzonitrile units at each terminal end [58]. It was also seen that the molecular size of the dentrimer was a factor deciding the photo-responsiveness as in case of the photo- and heat isomerization abilities of the azobenzene unit which depended on the molecular size of the dentrimer. The photo-response can also be obtained by introducing O-nitrobenzyl groups to the surface of hyperbranched polyglycerols (HPGs) for drug release [59]. The presence of a hexa(ethylene glycol) outershell instead of the hexane increased the stability of the formed host–guest complexes but resulted in lower guest release.

Photo-Responsive Micelles

The photo-switchable PSPMA core micelle upon exposure to UV light, ring-opening isomerization of spiropyran (non-polar, hydrophobic, and colourless under visible light irradiation) occurred, resulting in the coloured, polar, hydrophilic form. These micelles were used for encapsulation and controlled release and re-encapsulation of the model drug coumarin 102. Another example of the same is in the case of Spiropyran-decorated amphiphilic polypeptide-based block copolymers PLGASP-b-PEO (poly(L-glutamicacid)-b-polyethylene oxide) that form micelles, and micellar aggregates also showed conformational changes (from alpha-helix to random coil and vice versa) under UV and visible light, respectively [60]. Because the light used was a medically non-invasive, highly penetrating UV source, these photoresponsive rod-coil block polypeptides could be applied as viable model systems to study photo-induced drug release or light-controlled biomedical applications.

Photo-Responsive Surfaces

As described previously, there are mainly two types of photo-responsive molecules that may be used for a phototriggered response. Spiropyran derivatives can transform from a hydrophobic spiro conformation to a polar hydrophilic zwitterionic merocyanine conformation under UV light and can reversibly change with visible light [61, 62]. This change from the hydrophobic to the hydrophilic state upon isomerisation has been applied to demonstrate UV light-induced modification of surfaces [62]. The second type is azobenzene molecules that can change from the stable trans form to the cis state under UV light irradiation (300–400 nm) and reverse the isomerisation by irradiation with visible light [63–65]. A photo-responsive copolymer monolayer combining PNiPAAm and spiropyran chromophores has been used to tailor cell adhesion by switching light on or off [66]. Change in surface hydrophilicity was obtained by irradiation with 365 nm light and 'reset' by visible light irradiation (400–440 nm) [61].

3.2 Chemically Dependent Stimuli

The chemically dependent stimuli comprises mainly of pH, ionic strength, redox, and solvent. The physical stimuli include the change in the molecular as a function of pH, ionic strength, or solvent. As mentioned, these bring about the change in the molecular interaction of the system. The major changes in molecular interactions are observed between the polymers-solvent or polymer–polymer, or solvent–solvent systems.

3.2.1 pH-Responsive Polymers

pH is a very important environmental parameter, observed mainly in the many specific or pathological component which brings about the high potential in the field of biomedical applications. Human body is a very good example which is sensitive to the pH. As we take the different parts of the body, different pHs are observed which is set for the particular anabolic or catabolic actions of the body. Considering the pH along the gastrointestinal tract from stomach which is about 1–3 changes to 5–8 when it reaches the intestine. The chronic wounds are found to have a pH in between 7.4 and 5.4 [67]. Tumorous tissues are found to have pH acidic extracellularly [68, 69]. The key element for pH-responsive polymers is the presence of ionisable, weak acidic, or basic moieties that attach to a hydrophobic backbone, such as polyelectrolytes [16, 44, 70]. On ionization, a dramatic extension of the coiled chains occur due to the electrostatic repulsion of the charges generated upon ionizations. It can also arise due to the electrostatic effect arising from the adjacent ionized groups [71]. Another way the pH-responsive polymers works is by the protonation or deprotonation that can occur by the charge distribution over the ionisable group such as carboxyl or amino groups that are present in the molecule [72]. The phase transition occurs very abruptly in the case of pH responsible polymer of within 0.2–0.3 U of pH [73]. The commonly used pH-responsive polymers include chitosan [74], albumin [75], gelatin [76], poly(acrylic acid) (PAAc)/chitosan IPN [77], poly(methacrylic acid-g-ethylene glycol) [P(MAA-g-EG)] [78, 79], poly(ethylene imine) (PEI) [80], poly(*N*,*N*-diakylaminoethylmethacrylates) (PDAAEMA), and poly(lysine) (PL) [81, 82].

pH-Responsive Dendrimers

It could be seen that the cationic (non-acetylated) and acetylated (acetylation is a convenient strategy to neutralize the peripheral amine group) dendrimers exhibited different pH-dependent micellization, complexation, and encapsulation behaviour. The acetylated dendrimer encapsulated the Dp21 under acidic conditions (pH = 3.0), while the cationic dendrimer encapsulated the drug under both acidic (pH = 3 and pH = 5.0) and neutral conditions (pH = 7.4). In addition, pH-responsive release was different for an acetylated- and a non-acetylated dendritic matrix. Non-acetylated dendrimers showed a much slower release rate than acetylated dendrimers under conditions of lower pH, and a much faster release rate from non-acetylated dendrimer as pH values decreased. Degradable 1,3,5-triazaadamantane (TAA) dendrimers were able to be triggered by the addition of HCl [83].

pH-Responsive Micelle

The role of the pH is inevitable part when we consider the responsive materials. Miscelles which can release materials on the basis of the change in pH can be extremely useful because of the fact that the different metabolic activities of the body happens at different pH. Thus, the release of different materials in accordance with the pH can be extremely useful and can be exploited. Acid labile micelles of a model amphiphilic block copolymer, poly(hydroxyethyl acrylate)-b-poly(n-butyl acrylate) (PHEA-b-PBA) with encapsulated doxorubicin (DOX) demonstrated that hydrolysis of less than half of the cross-links in the core was sufficient to release DOX at acidic pH (5.0) faster than at neutral pH (7.4) [84].

pH-Responsive Vesicles

pH-responsive polymervesicles obtained by the aqueous self-assembly of carboxyterminated hyperbranched polyesters have the advantage of simple and the possibility of controlling vesicle size (from 200 to 10 mm) by pH changes [85]. The potential of a drug to be released as triggered by pH changes can be understood bypoly(ethylene oxide)-bpoly-(glycerolmonomethacrylate) (PEO-b-PG2MA) drug conjugates [86]. At a pH close to neutral, ester-bond linkages were stable and vesicular structures were formed. When pH was lowered to 2.0–3.5, hydrolysis of the ester bond took place and the drug was released.

pH-Responsive Surfaces

Polyelectrolyte brushes are pH-responsive materials that undergo structural changes at interfaces when their chains are charged and/or discharged because of the protonation/dissociation of acid/base groups [87]. As a result, upon an alteration in pH, polyelectrolyte brushes transform from the swollen state to a shrunken state in which the polymer chains collapse [88]. For example, surfaces grafted with an Os-complex redox unit modified poly(4-vinyl pyridine) [89]. Another type of surface was obtained from a mixed polyelectrolyte brush consisting of poly(2-vinylpyridine) and poly(acrylic acid) that had switchable permeability for both anions and cations [90].

3.2.2 Ion-Responsive Polymers

For a polymer to be ion responsive, the polymer should have ionisable groups within itself. The responsiveness to ionic strength can be can be related to the property of the polymer containing ionisable group. Such systems exhibit unusual rheological property. This rheological property arises as a result of the attractive columbic interactions between oppositely charged species that may render the polymer insoluble in deionized water but soluble in the presence of a critical concentration of added electrolytes where the attractive charge–charge interactions are shielded [91–93]. Thus, it can be concluded that the change in the ionic strength can result in the change of the polymer chain length, the polymer solubility, and the fluorescence quenching kinetics of chromophores bound to electrolytes [92, 94, 95]. In the polyphosphazene-functionalized diaminobutane poly(propyleneimine) (DAB-PN) dendrimeric system used for hydrophobic drug delivery, release was triggered by sodium chloride ions [96]. Cations such as Na^+, K^+ on polyphosphazene chains result in the swelling of the polyphosphazene external groups.

3.2.3 Redox-Responsive Polymers

The major criteria for redox-responsive polymers are the presence of liable groups in it. The redox responsiveness in polyanhydrides [97, 98], poly(lactic/glycolic acid) (PLGA) [99], and poly(b-amino esters) (PbAEs) [100] are bought about by the presence of acidic liable moieties in them. Disulfide groups are unstable in reducing environment that is being cleaved in favour of the corresponding thiol groups which in turn induces redox responsiveness [101, 102]. It is found that those polymers with disufide crosslinks degrade when exposed to reductive amino-acid-based molecules, namely cysteine or glutathione [103]. Poly(NiPAAm-co-Ru(bpy)3) generates a chemical wave by the periodic redox change of Ru(bpy)3 into an oxidized state of lighter colour [104]. This can also result in the swelling and deswelling of the polymer, caused by the change in the hydrophobic and hydrophilic properties of the chain.

Redox-Responsive Dentrimers

Redox-triggered release of dendrimer end groups can be caused by the physiological redox cofactors. Degradable polylysinedendrimers with multiple spermine groups on the surface and non-covalently bound DNA were synthesized via attachment of the spermine by a disulphide linker [105], which was cleaved by mild reducing agents such as glutathione (GSH), therefore causing the release of DNA. Chemically and electrochemically triggered release of dendrimer end groups was obtained, based on different generations of poly(propyleneimine) dendrimers with redox-labile, trimethyl-locked quinone (TLQ) end groups [106].

3.3 Biologically Dependent Stimuli

The biologically dependent stimuli comprise of analytes and biomacromolecules such as glucose, glutathione, enzymes, receptors, and over-produced metabolites in inflammation. These stimuli can bring about the changes in the polymers. The trigger of the change can be any changes mentioned above.

3.3.1 Glucose-Responsive Polymers

Oxidation-responsive vesicles from amphiphilic block copolymers based on ethylene glycol and propylene sulphide (PPS) exposed to oxidative conditions were destabilized [107]. Thioethers in the hydrophobic PPS blocks were changed into hydrophilic sulfoxides, influencing the hydrophilic–lipophilic balance of the amphiphile and inducing its solubilization. Considering self-regulated modes of insulin delivery, [17, 108], it becomes clear that precisely engineered glucose-sensitive polymers have huge potential in the quest to generate. The working of the glucose-responsive polymers can be explained as follows. The glucose oxidase is a smart, pH-sensitive polymer. This glucose oxidase oxidizes glucose to gluconic acid which causes a pH change in the environment [44]. With respect to the decrease in pH [108], the volume transition occurs. In this way, drastic changes in the polymer conformation are regulated by the body's glucose level, which, in turn, significantly affects enzyme activity and substrate access.

3.3.2 Enzyme-Responsive Polymers

In nature, bacteria located mainly in the colon produce special enzymes, including reductive enzymes (e.g. azoreductase) or hydrolytic enzymes (e.g. glycosidases) which are capable of degrading various types of polysaccharides, such as pectin, chitosan, amylase/amylopectin, cyclodextrin, and dextrin [109–111]. In most enzyme-responsive polymer systems, enzymes are used to destroy the polymer or its assemblies. The biggest advantage of enzyme-responsive polymers is that they do not require an external trigger for their decomposition, exhibit high selectivity, and work under mild conditions. For example, polymer systems based on alginate/chitosan or DEXS/chitosan microcapsules are responsive to chitosanase [112]. Andazoaromatic bonds are sensitive to azoreductase [113]. In this respect, they have great potential for in vivo biological applications. However, the main disadvantage is the difficulty of establishing a precise initial response time.

Enzyme-Responsive Dentrimers

An interesting example of an enzyme-responsive dendrimer was obtained by the synthesis of dendrimers with a hexyl ester functionality as the hydrophobic part and polyethylene glycol (PEG) as the hydrophilic part [114]. These dendrimers are found to disassembled in response to an enzymatic trigger (enzymeporcine liver esterase) due to the incorporation of enzyme-cleavable ester moieties at the hydrophobic part of the dendrimers. A similar strategy was used for the preparation of dendritic micellar containers [115], based on receptor–ligand binding interactions. PEG was chosen as the hydrophilic part and a decyl chain as the hydrophobic part. In order to disintegrate the dendritic structure, biotyn was incorporated (via click chemistry) as a ligand that bonded to a specific proteinextravidin. The disintegration of the system was caused by the biotin–extravidin interaction, which dramatically changed the hydrophilic–lipophilic balance (HLB) of the dendrimer molecule. The selectivity of this binding and release is based on molecular recognition.

Enzyme-Responsive Micelles

Some of the common examples of polymer peptide conjugates, particles of which disintegrated in response to the proteinase K signal [116], are the graft-type polymers (NIPAM–PEP and NIPAM–PEPEP; NIPAM is *N*-isopropylacrylamide; PEP and PEPEP are peptide units) containing a substrate peptide of protein kinase A (PKA). The micellization of the complex of the polymer poly(potassium acrylate) (PPA) and the surfactant cetyltrimethylammonium bromide (CTAB), using the fluorescent pyrene as a guest molecule,resulted in an enzyme-responsive system [117, 118].

3.3.3 Inflammation-Responsive Polymers

The inflammatory process is initiated by T- and B-lymphocytes, but amplified and perpetuated by polymorphonuclear (PMN) leukocytes and macrophages. Various chemical mediators in the process, including arachidonic acid metabolites, proteolytic enzymes, and oxygen metabolites, can cause tissue damage. For inflammation-responsive systems, the reactive oxygen metabolites (oxygen-free radicals) released by PMNs and macrophages during the initial phase of inflammation are the stimuli [119].

3.4 Dual Stimuli

Smart materials usually respond to more than one stimulus simultaneously. The efficiency of a stimuli-responsive polymeric system can be bought if the material responds to more than one stimulus. These usually combine of any of the three systems such as physically, chemically, or biologically responsive systems. These materials are of greater importance because the same material can be used efficiently for different triggers. Moreover, these provide an effective method for the response polymers. These dual-responsive polymers increase the efficiency of the system and thus becoming a promising material for the future smart polymers. An example of this type is explained as follows. A dual stimuli-responsive delivery system, using both pH and glutathione-responsive polymeric modules, was developed to therapeutically deliver medicinal molecules [120]. A poly(ethylene glycol)-b-poly(styrene boronic acid) (PEG-b-PSBA) system with boronic acid moieties showed both pH- and sugar-responsive behaviour [121]. Disruption of the assemblies occurred after adding 0.5 M NaOH to the vesicle solution. In addition, in the presence of 200 mM D-glucose, vesicles were also disrupted. The binding of the sugar molecules to the ionized boronic acid increased solubility of the PSBA blocks in water. The polymersomes disassembled completely in the presence of D-fructose (100 mM) in medium of pH 10.

3.4.1 Dual Stimuli-Responsive Surfaces

A smart and stable polymer brush interface based on PNiPAAm, PAA, and poly(*N*-isopropylacrylamide-coacrylic acid) was able to reversibly respond to temperature, ionic strength, and pH, independently or simultaneously [122]. The reversible change in hydrogen bonding between the two components (NIPAm and AAc) and water, and the ionization of carboxylate groups under different environmental condition resulted in the dual stimuli response. Chitosan-based PNiPAAm films possessing both thermal and pH sensitivity were prepared by blending chitosan with PNiPAAm and PEG [123]. The resulting film had an LCSTat around 32 °C, due to PNiPAAm and showed pH responsiveness due to the amino groups of chitosan component.

3.4.2 Dual-Responsive Conjugates

Dual-response conjugates are also known. A biotin-terminated poly(N-isopropylacrylamide)-b-poly(acrylic acid)(PNiPAAm)-b-(PAA) was conjugated to streptavidin (SA)via the terminal biotin on the PNiPAAm block [124]. Interestingly, the usual aggregation and phase separation of PNiPAAm-SA following the thermally triggered collapse and dehydration of PNIPAAM (the lower critical solution temperature of PNiPAAm is 32 °C in water) was prevented by the shielding of the PAA block. In addition, the aggregation properties of the [(PNiPAAm)-b-(PAA)]-SA conjugate were pH dependent. By varying temperature and pH, the sizes of these particles differed from 60 nm (pH 7.0, temperatures above the lower critical solution temperature of PNiPAAm) to 218 nm (pH 5.5 and 20 °C). This was explained by hydrogen bonding between the –COOH groups of PAA with other –COOH groups and also with the –CONH groups of PNIPAAM. The aggregation properties of the block copolymer–streptavidin conjugate differ from those of the free block copolymer.

References

1. Galaev IY, Mattiasson B (1999) Trends Biotechnol 17:335–340
2. Hoffman AS, Stayton PS, Bulmus V, Chen G, Chen J, Cheung C, Chilkoti A, Ding Z, Dong L, Fong R, Lackey CA, Long CJ, Miura M, Morris JE, Murthy N, Nabeshima Y, Park TG, Press OW, Shimoboji T, Shoemaker S, Yang HJ, Monji N, Nowinski RC, Cole CA, Priest JH, Harris JM, Nakamae K, Nishino T, Miyata T (2000) J Biomed Mater Res 52:577–586
3. Boas U, Heegaard PMH (2004) ChemSoc Rev 33:43
4. Cheng Y, Xu Z, Ma M, Xu T (2007) J Pharm Sci 97:123–143

5. Patri AK, Majoros IJ, Baker JR Jr (2002) Curr Opin Chem Biol 6:466–471
6. Discher DE, Ahmed F (2006) Annu Rev Biomed Eng 8:323–341
7. Meng F, Zhong Z (2011) J Phys Chem Lett 2:1533–1539
8. Meng F, Zhong Z, Feijen J (2009) Biomacromol 10:197–209
9. Mendes PM (2008) Chem Soc Rev 37:2512–2529
10. Milner ST (1991) Science 251:905–914
11. Jordan R (2006) Surface-initiated polymerization I. Springer, New York
12. Sakellariou G, Park M, Advincula R, Mays JW, Hadjichristidis N (2006) J Polym Sci Part A Polym Chem 44:769–782
13. Mittal KL, Lee K-W (1997) Polymer surfaces and interfaces: characterization, modification and applications. VSP, Utrecht
14. Norrman K, Ghanbari-Siahkali A, Larsen NB (2005) Annu Rep Sect C (Phys Chem) 101:174–201
15. Wise DL, Wnek GE, Trantolo DJ, Cooper TM, Gresser JD (1998) Electrical and optical polymer systems. Marcel Dekker, New York
16. Schmaljohann D (2006) Adv Drug Deliv Rev 58:1655–1670
17. Gil ES, Hudson SM (2004) Prog Polym Sci 29:1173–1222
18. Delcea M, Möhwald H, Skirtach AG (2011) Adv Drug Deliv Rev 63:730–747
19. Liechty WB, Kryscio DR, Slaughter BV, Peppas NA (2010) Annu Rev Chem Biomol Eng 1:149–173
20. Delcea M, Möhwald H, Skirtach AG (2011) Adv Drug Deliv Rev (in Press, Corrected Proof)
21. Zhang L, Xu T, Lin Z (2006) J Membr Sci 281:491–499
22. Liu Y, Meng L, Lu X, Zhang L, He Y (2008) Polym Adv Technol 19:137–143
23. Ohya S, Sonoda H, Nakayama Y, Matsuda T (2005) Biomaterials 26:655–659
24. Suwa K, Morishita K, Kishida A, Akashi M (1997) J Polym Sci Part a PolymChem 35:3087–3094
25. Na K, Lee KH, Lee DH, Bae YH (2006) Eur J Pharm Sci 27:115–122
26. Sosnik A, Cohn D (2004) Biomaterials 25:2851–2858
27. Haba Y, Harada A, Takagishi T, Kono K (2004) J Am Chem Soc 126:12760–12761
28. Zhou J, Wang L, Ma J, Wang J, Yu H, Xiao A (2010) Eur Polym J 46:1288–1298
29. Yang Z, Zhang W, Zou J, Shi W (2007) Polymer 48:931–938
30. Chen X, Ding X, Zheng Z, Peng Y (2006) New J Chem 30:577–582
31. Zhou Y, Yan D, Dong W, Tian Y (2007) J Phys Chem B 111:1262–1270
32. Sanson C, Le Meins JF, Schatz C, Soum A, Lecommandoux S (2010) Soft Matter 6:1722
33. Pelton R (2000) Adv Colloid Interface Sci 85:1–33
34. Chung JE, Yokoyama M, Okano T (2000) J Controlled Rel 65:93–103
35. Dimitrov I, Trzebicka B, Muller AHE, Dworak A, Tsvetanov CB (2007) Prog Polym Sci 32:1275–1343
36. Dreher MR, Simnick AJ, Fischer K, Smith RJ, Patel A, Schmidt M, Chilkoti A (2007) J Am Chem Soc 130:687–694
37. Okano T, Yamada N, Sakai H, Sakurai Y (1993) J Biomed Mater Res 27:1243–1251
38. Takezawa T, Mori Y, Yoshizato K (1990) Bio Technol 8:854–856
39. Yamada N, Okano T, Sakai H, Karikusa F, Sawasaki Y, Sakurai Y (1990) Die Makromolekulare Chemie Rapid Commun 11:571–576
40. Yaşayan G, Saeed AO, Fernández-Trillo F, Allen S, Davies MC, Jangher A, Paul A, Thurecht KJ, King SM, Schweins R, Griffiths PC, Magnusson JP, Alexander C (2011) Polym Chem 2:1567
41. Anal AK (2007) Recent Pat Endocr Metab Immune Drug Discov 1:83–90
42. Gong JP, Nitta T, Osada Y (1994) J Phys Chem 98:9583–9587
43. Tanaka T, Nishio I, Sun S-T, Ueno-Nishio S (1982) Science 218:467–469
44. Qiu Y, Park K (2001) Adv Drug Deliv Rev 53:321–339
45. Roggan A, Friebel M, Dörschel K, Hahn A, Müller G (1999) J Biomed Opt 4:36–46
46. Ichimura K, Oh S-K, Nakagawa M (2000) Science 288:1624–1626
47. Ichimura K, Suzuki Y, Seki T, Hosoki A, Aoki K (1988) Langmuir 4:1214–1216

48. Wang S, Song Y, Jiang L (2007) J Photochem Photobiol C Photochem Rev 8:18–29
49. Yoshida M, Lahann J (2008) ACS Nano 2:1101–1107
50. Jiang X, Lavender CA, Woodcock JW, Zhao B (2008) Macromolecules 41:2632–2643
51. Li Y, Jia X, Gao M, He H, Kuang G, Wei Y (2009) J PolymSci Part A Polym Chem 48:551–557
52. Czaun M, Hevesi L, Takafuji M, Ihara H (2008) Chem Commun 44:2124–2126
53. Szabo´ D, Szeghy G, Zrı´nyi M (1998) Macromolecules 31:6541–6548
54. Korth BD, Keng P, Shim I, Bowles SE, Tang C, Kowalewski T, Nebesny KW, Pyun J (2006) J Am Chem Soc 128:6562–6563
55. Marin A, Muniruzzaman M, Rapoport N (2001) J Controlled Rel 71:239–249
56. Norris P, Noble M, Francolini I, Vinogradov AM, Stewart PS, Ratner BD, Costerton JW, Stoodley P (2005) Antimicrob Agents Chemother 49:4272–4279
57. Rapoport NY, Christensen DA, Fain HD, Barrows L, Gao Z (2004) Ultrasonics 42:943–950
58. Koyama T, Hatano K, Matsuoka K, Esumi Y, Terunuma D (2009) Molecules 14:2226–2234
59. Burakowska E, Zimmerman SC, Haag R (2009) Small 5:2199–2204
60. Kotharangannagari VK (2011) Sa´nchez-Ferrer A, Ruokolainen J, Mezzenga R. Macromolecules 44:4569–4573
61. Edahiro J-I, Sumaru K, Tada Y, Ohi K, Takagi T, Kameda M, Shinbo T, Kanamori T, Yoshimi Y (2005) Biomacromol 6:970–974
62. Higuchi A, Hamamura A, Shindo Y, Kitamura H, Yoon BO, Mori T, Uyama T, Umezawa A (2004) Biomacromol 5:1770–1774
63. Auernheimer JR, Dahmen C, Hersel U, Bausch A, Kessler H (2005) J Am ChemSoc 127:16107–16110
64. Hayashi G, Hagihara M, Dohno C, Nakatani K (2007) J Am Chem Soc 129:8678–8679
65. Pearson D, Downard AJ, Muscroft-Taylor A, Abell AD (2007) J Am Chem Soc 129:14862–14863
66. Garcia A, Marquez M, Cai T, Rosario R, Hu Z, Gust D, Hayes M, Vail SA, Park C-D (2006) Langmuir 23:224–229
67. Dissemond J, Witthoff M, Brauns TC, Haberer D, Goos M (2003) Hautarzt 54:959–965
68. Rofstad EK, Mathiesen B, Kindem K, Galappathi K (2006) Cancer Res 66:6699–6707
69. Vaupel P, Kallinowski F, Okunieff P (1989) Cancer Res 49:6449–6465
70. Gupta P, Virmani K, Garg S (2002) Drug Discov Today 7:569–579
71. Park SY, Bae YH (1999) Macromol Rapid Commun 20:269–273
72. Lee YM, Shim JK (1997) Polymer 38:1227–1232
73. Soppimath KS, Kulkarni AR, Aminabhavi TM (2001) J Controlled Rel 75:331–345
74. Abdelaal MY, Abdel-Razik EA, Abdel-Bary EM, El-Sherbiny IM (2007) J Appl Polym Sci 103:2864–2874
75. Park H-Y, Song I-H, Kim J-H, Kim W-S (1998) Int J Pharm 175:231–236
76. Kurisawa M, Yui N (1998) Macromol Chem Phys 199:1547–1554
77. Lee JW, Kim SY, Kim SS, Lee YM, Lee KH, Kim SJ (1999) J Appl Polym Sci 73:113–120
78. Nakamura K, Murray RJ, Joseph JI, Peppas NA, Morishita M, Lowman AM (2004) J Controlled Rel 95:589–599
79. Zhang J, Peppas NA (1999) Macromolecules 33:102–107
80. Sideratou Z, Tsiourvas D, Paleos CM (2000) Langmuir 16:1766–1769
81. Burke SE, Barrett CJ (2003) Biomacromol 4:1773–1783
82. Toncheva V, Wolfert MA, Dash PR, Oupicky D, Ulbrich K, Seymour LW (1998) Biochim Biophys Acta 1380:354–368
83. Kohman RE, Zimmerman SC (2009) Chem Commun 45:794–796
84. Chan Y, Wong T, Byrne F, Kavallaris M, Bulmus V (2008) Biomacromol 9:1826–1836
85. Shi Z, Zhou Y, Yan D (2008) Macromol Rapid Commun 29:412–418
86. Giacomelli C, Schmidt V, Borsali R (2007) Macromolecules 40:2148–2157
87. Minko S (2006) J Macromol Sci Part C Polym Rev 46:397–420
88. Netz RR, Andelman D (2003) Phys Rep 380:1–95
89. Tam TK, Ornatska M, Pita M, Minko S, Katz E (2008) J Phys Chem C 112:8438–8445
90. Motornov M, Tam TK, Pita M, Tokarev I, Katz E, Minko S (2009) Nanotechnology 20:434006

91. Corpart JM, Candau F (1993) Macromolecules 26:1333–1343
92. Kathmann EEL, White LA, McCormick CL (1997) Macromolecules 30:5297–5304
93. Salamone JC, Rodriguez EL, Lin KC, Quach L, Watterson AC, Ahmed I (1985) Polymer 26:1234–1238
94. Morrison ME, Dorfman RC, Clendening WD, Kiserow DJ, Rossky PJ, Webber SE (1994) J Phys Chem 98:5534–5540
95. Szczubiałka K, Jankowska M, Nowakowska M (2003) J Mater Sci Mater Med 14:699–703
96. Cho SY, Allcock HR (2007) Macromolecules 40:3115–3121
97. Leong KW, Brott BC, Langer R (1985) J Biomed Mater Res 19:941–955
98. Mathiowitz E, Jacob JS, Jong YS, Carino GP, Chickering DE Chaturvedi P, Santos CA, Vijayaraghavan K, Montgomery S, Bassett M, Morrell C (1997) Nature 386:410–414
99. Cohen S, Yoshioka T, Lucarelli M, Hwang LH, Langer R (1991) Pharm Res 8:713–720
100. Shenoy D, Little S, Langer R, Amiji M (2005) Pharm Res 22:2107–2114
101. Cerritelli S, Velluto D, Hubbell JA (2007) Biomacromol 8:1966–1972
102. Oh JK, Siegwart DJ, Lee H-I, Sherwood G, Peteanu L, Hollinger JO, Kataoka K, Matyjaszewski K (2007) J Am Chem Soc 129:5939–5945
103. Matsumoto S, Christie RJ, Nishiyama N, Miyata K, Ishii A, Oba M, Koyama H, Yamasaki Y, Kataoka K (2008) Biomacromol 10:119–127
104. Yoshida R, Yamaguchi T, Kokufuta E (1999) J Artif Organs 2:135–140
105. Kostiainen MA, Rosilo H (2009) Chem Eur J 15:5656–5660
106. Ong W, McCarley RL (2006) Macromolecules 39:7295–7301
107. Napoli A, Boerakker MJ, Tirelli N, Nolte RJM, Sommerdijk NAJM, Hubbell JA (2004) Langmuir 20:3487–3491.
108. Chaterji S, Kwon IK, Park K (2007) Prog Polym Sci 32:1083–1122
109. Chambin O, Dupuis G, Champion D, Voilley A, Pourcelot Y (2006) Int J Pharm 321:86–93
110. Sinha VR, Kumria R (2001) Int J Pharm 224:19–38
111. Vandamme TF, Lenourry A, Charrueau C, Chaumeil JC (2002) Carbohydr Polym 48:219–231
112. Itoh Y, Matsusaki M, Kida T, Akashi M (2006) Biomacromol 7:2715–2718
113. Akala EO, Kopečková P, Kopeček J (1998) Biomaterials 19:1037–104
114. Azagarsamy MA, Sokkalingam P, Thayumanavan S (2009) J Am Chem Soc 131:14184–14185
115. Azagarsamy MA, Yesilyurt V, Thayumanavan S (2010) J Am Chem Soc 132:4550–4551
116. Katayama Y, Sonoda T, Maeda M (2001) Macromolecules 34:8569–8573
117. Gonza´lez DC, Savariar EN, Thayumanavan S (2009) J Am Chem Soc 131:7708–7716
118. Savariar EN, Ghosh S, Thayumanavan S (2008) J Am Chem Soc 130:5416–5417
119. Rao NA (1990) Trans Am Ophthalmol Soc 88:787–850
120. Miyata K, Kakizawa Y, Nishiyama N, Harada A, Yamasaki Y, Koyama H, Kataoka K (2004) J Am Chem Soc 126:2355–2361
121. Kim KT, Cornelissen JJLM, Nolte RJM, van Hest JCM (2009) Adv Mater 21:2787–2791
122. Zhou J, Wang G, Hu J, Lu X, Li J (2006) Chem Commun 42:4820–4822
123. Sun H, Liu S, Ge B, Xing L, Chen H (2007) J Membr Sci 295:2–10
124. Kulkarni S, Schilli C, Grin B, Müller AHE, Hoffman AS, Stayton PS (2006) Biomacromolecules 7:2736–2741

Chapter 6
Polymer–Water Interactions in Hydrogels

S. Snigdha, Nandakumar Kalarikkal, Sabu Thomas, and E. K. Radhakrishnan

Abstract Hydrogels are water/polymer systems that are in high demand due to their broad-spectrum applications in the industrial and bio-medical sectors. A basic hydrogel is a polymer network capable of absorbing a large quantity of water. Water–polymer interactions play a vital role in maintaining the structural integrity, physical properties and overall applicability of the hydrogel system. This chapter focuses on the various water–polymer interactions within the hydrogel matrix, techniques to analyze these interactions and the effects of these interactions on the property of the hydrogels.

keywords Hydrogels · Polymer-water network · Hydrogel matrix · Interactions · Monte Carlo models

1 Introduction

Hydrogels are finding increased applications in various fields such as industry, biotechnology, medicine and environment [1]. They act as building blocks for technological and biological industries, with properties between those of solids and liquids. All these applications exploit various properties of the hydrogel such as integrity, solubility and diffusion of substances [8]. Smart/intelligent hydrogel systems are

S. Snigdha · N. Kalarikkal · S. Thomas
International and Inter University Centre for Nanoscience and Nanotechnology, Mahatma Gandhi University, PD Hills (PO), Kottayam, Kerala 686 560, India

E. K. Radhakrishnan (✉)
School of Biosciences, Mahatma Gandhi University, PD Hills (PO), Kottayam, Kerala 686 560, India
e-mail: radhakrishnanek@mgu.ac.in

S. Thomas
School of Chemical Sciences, Mahatma Gandhi University, PD Hills (PO), Kottayam, Kerala 686 560, India

N. Kalarikkal
School of Pure and Applied Physics, Mahatma Gandhi University, PD Hills (PO), Kottayam, Kerala 686 560, India

J. Jose et al. (eds.), *Nano Hydrogels*, Gels Horizons: From Science to Smart Materials,
https://doi.org/10.1007/978-981-15-7138-1_6

designed to respond to changes in stimuli [12]. Many applications of hydrogels also make use of their unique mechanical abilities due to random alignment of polymer fibres and large percentage of water within the matrix [28, 29].

Hydrogels are crosslinked water-insoluble polymer networks that are capable of holding a vast amount of water. Depending upon the functional group of the constituent polymer side chains, the hydrogels may be neutral or ionic [23]. The water holding capacity of these three-dimensional polymeric structures is several times their weight (~100 g/g of dry polymer or higher). Integrity of the hydrogels is maintained due to its insolubility in water. Various types of natural macromolecules and synthetic polymers are crosslinked to in order to achieve a stable and water-insoluble network. The crosslinking may be of physical or chemical nature [23]. Some of the natural macromolecules used in preparing hydrogels include alginates, agar, polypeptides and their derivatives. There are a large number of synthetic polymers which can be crosslinked into 3D networks. The selection of a polymer matrix for hydrogel preparation must take into account the hierarchy of water solubilising groups: –OH, –COOH, $–COO^-$, >C=O, $>CHNH_2$, $–CONH_2$, $–SO_3H$, etc., present on the polymer backbone [8]. Water in the hydrogels is essential for maintaining the structure and physical properties of the hydrogel. The interaction between water and polymer is very crucial in determining the overall performance of a hydrogel system. The impact of solvent and polymer on each other is crucial in determining the phase transitions, transport properties and occupancy of water in the hydrogel network [10, 20].

1.1 Ambiphillic and Complex Hydrogel Networks

With the ever-increasing demand for hydrogels, innovative designs have led to the development of hydrogels with superior structural and functional properties. The use of block co-polymers with alternating hydrophilic and hydrophobic polymer domains results in hydrogels with microphase separation. These microphase separated hydrogels find great potential in biological applications. Interpenetrating networks (IPNs) are another way of achieving higher mechanical stability in hydrogel structures [6, 22, 25]. IPNs consist of a binary system in which the polymers are individually crosslinked to achieve microdomains [24]. Poly (ethylene oxide) (PEO) star polymers with a few long arms have been shown to have remarkable swelling abilities [13]. Nanocomposite hydrogels possess nano-sized fillers within the polymer matrix which could impart reinforcement to the polymer network [27].

1.2 Techniques for Investigating States of Components in a Hydrogel

Various experimental methods have been explored to study the physical manifestation of water in polymers. The physical properties and structure of water are usually assessed from binding sites in the polymer and by geometrical confinements [8]. The presence of boundaries and interfaces in the polymer matrix reduces the degrees of freedom as well as the natural order that can be observed in the bulk phase of water. A number of factors are taken into account while evaluating the behaviour of water within the hydrogel system. Bound, unbound/free water as well as freezability and inability to freeze the water is taken into account [11].

NMR studies investigate the difference in property of the various states of water present within the hydrogel matrix [15]. This technique enables detailed investigation of the morphology, molecular organization, interactions and internal mobility of the components of a hydrogel system [26]. Low temperature NMR helps to investigate bound–water dynamics that are closely associated with the hydrogel matrix [8]. NMR and dielectric studies often take into account that the behaviour of water molecules directly bound to the polymer chains (bound water) is significantly different from the behaviour of water that is surrounded by other water molecules (free water).

Raman spectroscopy (RS) has been widely used to study the molecular orientation of water. Molecular vibrations used as a probe in RS have relaxation times ($T = 10$–13–10–‘4 s) that are comparable to the rotational rearrangement of liquid water molecules ($T = 10$–11–10–12 s) [17]. Raman spectrum is sensitive to changes in the structure of water and its small structural domains in the hydrogel network.

Differential Scanning Calorimetry (DSC) provides direct thermal analytic data of the hydrogels. This analysis provides insights into the physical and chemical changes that occur as a result of heat evolved or absorbed during the heating and cooling cycles [16]. The changes in glass transition and crystallization temperatures can be easily followed with the help of this technique [9].

Dilatometry and electrical conductivity measurements are used to study the shrinkage or expansion of hydrogels over a specified range of temperature. It gives an insight into the total volume change as a result of physical or chemical changes [5].

Specific conductivity studies can be carried out using an impedance bridge. The electrical conductivity thus obtained can be used to investigate the correlation between the water content present in the hydrogels and other measurable variables such air permeability [4].

Dielectricrelaxation spectroscopy (DRS) can be used to study the correlation between structural and physical properties of the hydrogel. This technique is very sensitive in determining the critical water contents in the hydrogel system. These values can be obtained from the changes in water or the hydrogel matrix behaviour [14].

Thermally stimulated depolarization current (TSDC) technique is useful in determining the transitions that occur as a function of changes in mobility at the molecular scale. It is favoured over other thermal analyses due to its high sensitivity. The electrical properties of the hydrogel can be determined through the measurement of thermal relaxation effects [3].

Microscopy especially electron microscopy provides valuable information on the surface morphology and pore structures present in the hydrogels [8].

Studies on diffusion and swelling characteristics of hydrogels can be studied in order to fine tune the design of a hydrogel matrix in order to obtain ideal diffusion control of solute diffusion.

Theoretical methods are employed for hydrogels when the needs for exploring details in an experiment are limited by the resolving ability of the experimental set up. Network structure formation is usually determined by using kinetic models, statistical models and Monte Carlo simulations. Kinetic models, which are mean field models usually, determine the overall properties of the system [21]. The statistical and Monte Carlo models predict in-depth, the network properties and provide detailed insights into the sol and gel states [2, 7].

Such theoretical simulation experiments help to determine the stability, degradation and failure of hydrogel structure. Molecular dynamics (MD) simulation methods have been carried out extensively to determine various aspects of state, structure and dynamics of the binary hydrogel system [30].

1.3 Properties of Water in Hydrogels

Water is primarily responsible for determining the macroscopic states and properties of hydrogels. The state of water in hydrogels in not uniform as it is constrained by the polymer. In the hydrogels matrix, a fraction of water exists in at least three known states such as water bound to the polymer which is non-freezing, another fraction exists as weakly bound which can freeze and another fraction exists as unbound water which is capable of freezing at 0 °C [11]. All these states of water are in turn dependent on the type and amount of solute present. Salinity, pH and the structural property of the solutes affects water behaviour in the hydrogels. The physicochemical attributes of hydrogels depend on the properties of water such as its domain size (including micro and nano-sized domains), electroconductivity and density [8, 11].

The hydrogen bond network among water molecules has been shown to lead to anomalous behaviour in the static and dynamic properties within the polymer network. Such anomalies are investigated using simulation studies such as molecular dynamics (MD) or Monte Carlo (MC) methods. The swelling behaviour of hydrogels is governed by a variety of non-ideal thermodynamic schemes. Swelling in a hydrogel matrix is a complex play between the thermodynamic compatibility between the polymer and water which is counteracted by the crosslinks in the hydrogel, which tries to prevent water absorption by the system [23].

1.4 Properties of Polymer in Hydrogels

The polymer in a hydrogel network comprises about 5–10% of the total hydrogel volume and it acts as a structural scaffold to hold the water inside the network [14]. Some of the properties of the hydrogels are attributed to their pendant polymeric group such the polarity, crystalline nature and supramolecular structure [23]. The transport properties of the hydrogels are influenced by the changes induced in the solvent due to the presence of polymer [20]. The polymer is known to enhance the viscosity of the solvent within the hydrogel matrix and it is dependent on the nature of the solvent [18]. Various simulation and diffusion experiments indicate that water has limited mobility in hydrogels due to the modification of H-bond network structure and dynamics by the polymer [20]. A study involving PVA-water system indicated that the solvation depended on the hydrogen bonds between the polymer and water molecules and the polymer also induced water clustering within hydrogel networks [19]. Raman spectroscopy studies have revealed that the presence of ionic groups in the polymer side chains tends to disrupt the H-bonding between the water molecules leading to unfavourable orientations around the ionic groups of the polymer. However, the presence of hydrophobic side chains tends to make H-bonding between the water molecules stronger and leads to the formation of a stable hydration shell around the hydrophobic polymer chains [17].

It has been observed that polymers of synthetic origin show better mechanical properties due to their complex structural conformations. These conformations lead to higher glass transition temperatures and chain motion is usually restricted below these temperatures [31]. MD simulations of a binary system involving PVA and water indicated that both the components played a crucial role in determining the glass transition properties [30].

2 Conclusion

The design and development of hydrogels has been evolving and continues to reflect the fast paced developments in various fields of science and technology. The simpler hydrogels of yesterday are being replaced by stimuli sensitive and complex structured hydrogels which can perform countless physical, chemical and biological functions. Chemical modification of existing materials to attach or detach various functional groups from the polymer backbones can help create innumerable variations of hydrogels. These complex hierarchical structures are the future for various biomedical applications such as tissue engineering and targeted drug delivery. The complexity of the hydrogel network and their thermodynamic states determines various properties such as diffusivity, chemical/biological interactions, molecular sieve diameter and overall stability.

It is expected that there will be advancements in this field to churn out hydrogels that are technological superior to the currently available ones. The ease of production and modification will be considered as the benchmark for future applications; this will enable fast and easy synthesis of tailor made hydrogels to suit individual needs. With the increasing complexity in the design of hydrogels, sophisticated analysis techniques will also develop simultaneous to thoroughly investigate such complicated networks. This will also witness the fine tuning of existing models for network predication and probably the development of newer simulation models for studying complex hydrogel structures. Research and development in this field is likely to lead to marked improvement in the quality of life for a worker in an industry as well a patient suffering from a chronic illness.

References

1. Ahmed EM (2015) Hydrogel: preparation, characterization, and applications: a review. J Adv Res 6:105–121
2. Anseth KS, Bowman CN (1994) Kinetic gelation model predictions of crosslinked polymer network microstructure. Chem Eng Sci 49:2207–2217
3. Armenia E, Spera V, Barbucci R (2018) Microarchitecture of water confined in hydrogels. Hydrogels. CRC Press, pp 9–39
4. Austin DT, Champeney DC (1995) A technique for measuring the alternating current electrical conductivity of hydrogels. J Br Contact Lens Assoc 18:115–118
5. Choi S, Jhon MS, Andrade JD (1977) Nature of water in synthetic hydrogels: III. Dilatometry, specific conductivity, and dielectric relaxation of poly (2, 3-dihydroxypropyl methacrylate). J Colloid Interface Sci 61:1–8
6. Deshpande AA, Pahari S, Menon SK, Badiger MV, Rajamohanan P, Wadgaonkar PP, Roy S, Tonelli C (2018) Mechanism of the formation of microphase separated water clusters in a water-mediated physical network of perfluoropolyether tetraol. Soft Matter 14:2339–2345
7. Flory PJ, Rehner J Jr (1943) Statistical mechanics of cross-linked polymer networks I. Rubberlike elasticity. J Chem Phys 11:512–520
8. Gun'ko V, Savina I, Mikhalovsky S (2017) Properties of water bound in hydrogels. Gels 3:37
9. Hofer K, Mayer E, Johari G (1990) Glass-liquid transition of water and ethylene glycol solution in poly (2-hydroxyethyl methacrylate) hydrogel. J Phys Chem 94:2689–2696
10. Hsu T-P, Ma DS, Cohen C (1983) Effects of inhomogeneities in polyacrylamide gels on thermodynamic and transport properties. Polymer 24:1273–1278
11. Jhon MS, Andrade JD (1973) Water and hydrogels. J Biomed Mater Res 7:509–522
12. Kamoun EA, Fahmy A, Taha TH, El-Fakharany EM, Makram M, Soliman HM, Shehata H (2018) Thermo-and pH-sensitive hydrogel membranes composed of poly (*N*-isopropylacrylamide)-hyaluronan for biomedical applications: influence of hyaluronan incorporation on the membrane properties. Int J Biol Macromol 106:158–167
13. Keys KB, Andreopoulos FM, Peppas NA (1998) Poly (ethylene glycol) star polymer hydrogels. Macromolecules 31:8149–8156
14. Konsta A, Daoukaki D, Pissis P, Vartzeli K (1999) Hydration and conductivity studies of polymer–water interactions in polyacrylamide hydrogels. Solid State Ionics 125:235–241
15. Kyritsis A, Pissis P, Ribelles JG, Pradas MM (1995) Polymer-water interactions in poly (hydroxyethyl acrylate) hydrogels studied by dielectric, calorimetric and sorption isotherm measurements. Polym Gels Netw 3:445–469
16. Lee HB, Jhon MS, Andrade JD (1975) Nature of water in synthetic hydrogels. I. Dilatometry, specific conductivity, and differential scanning calorimetry of polyhydroxyethyl methacrylate. J Colloid Interface Sci 51:225–231
17. Maeda Y, Tsukida N, Kitano H, Terada T, Yamanaka J (1993) Raman spectroscopic study of water in aqueous polymer solutions. J Phys Chem 97:13903–13906

18. Mikosch W, Dorfmüller T, Eimer W (1994) Rotational diffusion in polyacrylamide gels as a function of solvent quality. J Chem Phys 101:11052–11059
19. Müller-Plathe F (1998) Microscopic dynamics in water-swollen poly (vinyl alcohol). J Chem Phys 108:8252–8263
20. Netz PA, Dorfmüller T (1998) Computer simulation studies on the polymer-induced modification of water properties in polyacrylamide hydrogels. J Phys Chem B 102:4875–4886
21. Okay O (1999) Formation of macroporous styrene–divinylbenzene copolymer networks: theory vs. experiments. J Appl Polym Sci 74:2181–2195
22. Pan Y, Wang J, Cai P, Xiao H (2018) Dual-responsive IPN hydrogel based on sugarcane bagasse cellulose as drug carrier. Int J Biol Macromol 118:132–140
23. Peppas N, Huang Y, Torres-Lugo M, Ward J, Zhang J (2000) Physicochemical foundations and structural design of hydrogels in medicine and biology. Annu Rev Biomed Eng 2:9–29
24. Rault J, Lucas A, Neffati R, Monleón Pradas M (1997) Thermal transitions in hydrogels of poly (ethyl acrylate)/poly (hydroxyethyl acrylate) interpenetrating networks. Macromolecules 30:7866–7873
25. Shah KR (1987) Microphase separated hydrogels for controlled release of bioactive materials. Google Patents
26. Shapiro YE (2011) Structure and dynamics of hydrogels and organogels: an NMR spectroscopy approach. Prog Polym Sci 36:1184–1253
27. Suvina V, Krishna SM, Nagaraju D, Melo J, Balakrishna RG (2018) Polypyrrole-reduced graphene oxide nanocomposite hydrogels: a promising electrode material for the simultaneous detection of multiple heavy metal ions. Mater Lett 232:209–212
28. Tanaka M (2018) Hydrogel preparation and characterisation derived from chitosan and amino functional monomers for biomedical applications. J Mater Chem B 6:5115
29. Wang Y, Cao Z, Wu J, Ma C, Qiu C, Zhao Y, Shao F, Wang H, Zheng J, Huang G (2018) Mechanically robust, ultrastretchable and thermal conducting composite hydrogel and its biomedical applications. Chem Eng J 360:231
30. Wu C (2010) Cooperative behavior of poly (vinyl alcohol) and water as revealed by molecular dynamics simulations. Polymer 51:4452–4460
31. Yoshida H, Hatakeyama T, Hatakeyama H (1993) Characterization of water in polysaccharide hydrogels by DSC. J Therm Anal 40:483–489

Chapter 7
Hybrid Nanohydrogels: Design and Applications

Luis Valencia, Andrea Aguilar-Sánchez, Javier Enríquez, and Ramón Díaz

Abstract Hydrogels are composed of three-dimensional cross-linked polymer networks with hydrophilic nature, which can therefore absorb large quantities of water within the spaces available among the polymer chains. Hydrogels can provide good mechanical support and/or a hydrated environment that offer good cytocompatibility and controlled release of molecules. During the last decade, vast amount of research has been focused in the development of hybrid nanohydrogels which include the incorporation of a secondary nanosized component to the hydrogel matrix in order to provide additional reinforcement or tailor a specific application such as imparting biological functions in tissue engineering, drug delivery and gene therapies. This chapter provides a fresh insight into some of the recent developments in hybrid nanohydrogels, describing some physical and chemical cross-linking approaches to form strong networks. Moreover, the use of synthetic and biological molecules to impart desired properties is also described, focusing mainly in tissue engineering and drug delivery applications.

1 Introduction

Hydrogels are three-dimensional, cross-linked water soluble polymer networks which can adsorb a large amount of water or biological fluids without dissolving [1]. This is possible due to the polar hydrophilic groups in their structures that are hydrated when in contact with water, creating a primary bound with it. The high water retention capacity of hydrogels provides a similar physio-chemical environment to

L. Valencia (✉)
Materials Technology and Chemistry, Alfa Laval Tumba AB, SE-14782 Tumba, Sweden
e-mail: luisalexandro.valencialopez@alfalaval.com

A. Aguilar-Sánchez
Department of Materials and Environmental Chemistry, Frescativägen 8, SE-10691 Stockholm, Sweden

J. Enríquez · R. Díaz
Research Center for Applied Chemistry, Enrique Reyna 140, 25294 Saltillo, Mexico

J. Jose et al. (eds.), *Nano Hydrogels*, Gels Horizons: From Science to Smart Materials,
https://doi.org/10.1007/978-981-15-7138-1_7

native extracellular membranes, and therefore, hydrogels exhibit high biocompatibility, which have made them a great deal of research focus during the last decades, especially for tissue engineering and drug delivery applications.

Recently, great attention has been centered toward the use of nanohydrogels, which, as the name stipulates it, are three-dimensional polymer networks that have embedded nanoparticles either acting as cross-linkers and therefore enhancing the mechanical robustness of the hydrogels or introducing functionality due to their high surface area and versatility of functionalization, as well as the possibility of encapsulating bioactive compounds. Within the scope of this chapter, it is not possible to cover all relevant aspects of hybrid nanohydrogels, and therefore, the focus will be to demonstrate some of the recently published works on hybridization of hydrogels toward advanced mechanical reinforcement and for tailoring specific functions for tissue engineering and drug delivery applications.

1.1 Design of Hybrid Nanohydrogels

Due to the ambiguity of the terms "hybrid" and "nanocomposite" and the wide misuse of these terms in the literature nowadays, it is necessary to begin this chapter by defining whether the materials fall into hybrids or not. The most accepted definition of a hybrid (from the material's chemistry perspective) is a material that combines two or more components which are blended on the molecular scale with chemical bonds between them [2]; In the way that the materials complement each other, acting synergistically to have new functions which the component materials do not possess individually.

Recently, hybrid nanohydrogels have gained significant interest, as they represent an excellent opportunity for the design and development of nanostructured materials. Different hybridization strategies can be used to provide mechanical reinforcement to a matrix, creating hybrid networks, where the secondary component is a nanoparticle chemically or physically bonded to the polymer network [3]. Moreover, hybridization of inert polymer networks with bio(macro) molecules can also provide physical support for cell growth and enhance the cell adhesion and cell proliferation, which is essential for tissue engineering applications for instance [4]. Also, specific functionalities can be tailored by hybridization of a hydrogel network with loaded nanoparticles, where high concentrations of active compounds can be encapsulated and released [5].

The physical properties and therefore targeted applications of the hybrid nanohydrogels essentially depend on two aspects:

- The composition of the secondary phase (nanocellulose, silica nanoparticles, graphene, etc.)
- The mechanism of network formation arising from the type of interaction between the polymer chains and the nanoparticles (chemically or physically cross-linked).

For physically cross-linked hydrogels, the gel is formed via hydrophobic, electrostatic or hydrogen bonding interactions, forming semi-permanent links among the polymer chains inside the network [6]. On the other hand, chemical cross-linking uses covalent bonding to prepare permanent hydrogels, which although it requires another level of chemical modification, it provides greater mechanical stability [3] and allows the tuning of variables such as gelation-time and gel pore size. Moreover, chemically cross-linked hydrogels guarantee adsorption of water/or bioactive compounds without any dissolution [6].

2 Hybridization of Hydrogels Toward Advanced Mechanical Reinforcement

Despite the many advantages aforementioned, in most hydrogels, a high water-uptake comes with an inherent fragility, which limits their usability in many applications [7]. Different strategies have been developed in order to produce hydrogels with high mechanical performance, such as (i) double network hydrogels [8], (ii) hydrophobic association [9], (iii) composite hydrogels using microparticles [10] and (iv) hybridization of hydrogels. Among them, there has been a growing interest in hybrid nanohydrogels during the last decade, where the incorporated nanoparticles can act as cross-linkers through covalent bonding or physical interactions, resulting in hybrid nanohydrogels that overcome the limitations related with conventional cross-linked hydrogels, such as structural heterogeneity and mechanical fragility [7]. The improvement in their performance related to mechanically stiff and highly elastomeric network in the nanocomposite hydrogels networks is attributed to the interactions between the polymer chains and nanoparticles [11], which enables the transfer of mechanical force within the cross-linked network resulting in enhanced mechanical strength and toughness [11].

Carbon-based nanomaterials such as graphene and carbon nanotubes (CNTs) have been the most promising and widely studied candidates for mechanical reinforcement of hydrogels. Graphene in its purest form exists in a single 2D monolayer of sp^2 carbon atoms arranged in a hexagonal arranged crystal lattice. The carbon–carbon sigma bonds in the graphene structure give rise to exceptional properties that are appropriate for reinforcement of hydrogels. Faghihi et al. [12], have combined the advantages of graphene oxide (GO) and poly(acrylic acid)/gelatin in the fabrication of nanohydrogels, and the results exhibited that the addition of GO significantly increased the Young's modulus and maximum stress of hydrogels. Regarding CNTs, this type of fillers, classified in multi-wall (MWCNT) or single-wall (SWCNT), is very effective in terms of high specific surface area and excellent mechanical properties, especially toughness [13]. Zhang et al. [13], synthetized high strength MWCNTs/cellulose hydrogels from NaOH/urea aqueous solution cross-linked by epichlorohydrin. The swelling testing showed that the equilibrium swelling ratio decreased with the increment of MWCNTs content. Additionally, the incorporation of

MWCNTs into cellulose hydrogel networks improved both thermal and mechanical properties.

Another important reinforcement additive of hydrogels is naturally occurring aluminosilicate clays, such as halloysite (HNTs). These nanotubes have a diameter of ca. 50 nm and length between 500 and 1000 nm [14]. Their inner surface is composed of aluminol groups (AL–OH) positively charged to capture the negatively charged molecules in the lumen, whereas the outer surface contains silanol groups (Si–OH), negatively charged to facilitate adhesion of positively charged molecules [15]. Park et al. [16], prepared hybrid nanohydrogels composed of HNTs and hyaluronic acid (HA) via photo-cross-linking of HA and HNTs modified with vinyl groups. The compressive mechanical properties of the hybrids revealed that the hydrogels exhibited a nonlinear behavior attributed to the strain stiffening of the polysaccharide-based hydrogels and the fracture stress increased with increment of HNTs content up to 10%.

Another important kind of nanofiller for hydrogels is nanocellulose, including both cellulose nanocrystals (CNC's) and cellulose nanofibers (CNF's). CNCs are rod-like crystalline structures that have a diameter between 5 and 30 nm (depending on the source and extraction method) and length >100 nm. Due to its characteristics, such as high aspect ratio, low density, outstanding mechanical properties and highly reactive surface, CNCs have been considered as one of the most important candidates to modify the mechanical behavior of hydrogels. Yang et al. [17] obtained and evaluated nanohydrogels reinforced by CNCs from two different sources and therefore different aspect ratios. They found from uniaxial tensile measurements that the values of aspect ratios and non-permanent interactions between the fillers and matrix dominated the reinforcement. Also, they argue that the improvement in modulus of the hydrogels is correlated to the volume of the constrained polymer, where the CNCs impart significant enhancement to the entanglement network. Yang et al. [18] also carried out the mechanical reinforcement using CNCs in hydrogels based on poly(acrylamide) (PAM) with multiple cross-links. They observed that the hybrid CNC-PAM hydrogel exhibited higher Young's modulus and higher fracture strength than the PAM reference, without CNC's; and the nanohydrogel suffered greater deformation by increasing the content of CNCs were the effective physical interactions in the network promoted an increase in the fracture strength.

On the other hand, cellulose nanofibers (CNFs) are also promising reinforcement additives for hydrogels. Varying depending on their biological origin, CNF shaves a high aspect ratio 4–20 nm wide and >1 μm of length, consisting of alternating crystalline and amorphous domains of cellulose [19]. CNFs can form a rigid network in different matrices, subsequently benefiting their mechanical properties. Wang et al. [20], mechanically reinforced hydrogels of gelatin with the incorporation of CNFs, where the reinforcement was associated to the formation of a stiff three-dimensional network of CNFs, physically cross-linked with gelatin via electrostatic interactions and entanglement. CNFs have also been used as a reinforcement additive of polyvinyl alcohol (PVA) hydrogels. PVA chains are strong, tough and highly stretchable polymer chains, which can entangle cellulose nanofibrils, CNF acting as physical cross-linker to maintain mechanical integrity [21]. Likewise when the hydrogels were stretched, the fracture of PVA and disintegration of the hydrogen bonds occurred, dissipating great amount of energy, and maintaining the stretchability, yielding excellent mechanical properties to the nanohydrogels [22].

3 Hybrid Nanohydrogels for Tissue Engineering Applications

Tissue engineering is the combination of cells, engineering and materials science which aim to restore, preserve or enhance tissue functions. Tissue can be engineered in different ways, one of the most convenient methods is to use three-dimensional tissue scaffolds for the formation of new viable tissue. Here, cells from the type of tissue that needs to be regenerated are incorporated to the scaffold for their delivery in vivo, in the way that the scaffold provides a space for new tissue formation and controls its structure and function. This technique is used to fabricate soft tissues such as cartilage, ligament, tendon, artery or hard tissues such as bones.

During the last years, nanohydrogels have demonstrated to be a promising option for the fabrication of polymer scaffolds for tissue engineering [23] because of their high water content, swellability and permeability. These specific characteristics provide a good media that benefit the diffusion of oxygen, nutrients and waste inside the structure of the scaffold, which is necessary as an environment for cell encapsulation and a successful tissue regeneration [24]. However, it is still a challenge to find the most suitable composition of the material, as it has to mimic the role of the extracellular matrix in a way that the body reacts as if it was real tissue [23].

3.1 Chemically Cross-Linked Hybrid Nanohydrogels for Tissue Engineering

There are different approaches to chemically cross-linking hydrogels, where a typical method involves the addition of a cross-linking agent consisting of small reactive molecules that promote the network formation, such as glutaraldehyde, glyceraldehyde, formaldehyde, gossypol, tannic acid, among others [25]. For instance, Tanpichai et al. [26] successfully prepared poly(vinyl alcohol) (PVA/CNCs hydrogels using glutaraldehyde (GA) as a cross-linker. In this case, GA induced the cross-linking reaction of the hydroxyl groups in PVA chains and CNCs. As a result, the addition of CNCs decreased the creep elasticity due to restriction of the polymer chains, but without affecting the swelling ratio and thermal stability. The hydrogels exhibited promising properties for tissue engineering, such as high strength, elasticity and water-holding capacity.

Another way to chemically cross-link hybrid nanohydrogels is via photo-cross-linking, in which a photoinitiator decomposes when exposed to UV light, generating

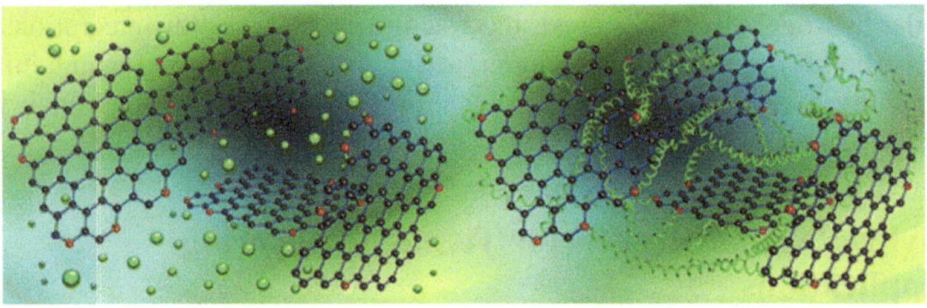

Fig. 1 Schematic model of GPO hydrogel formation. Left: before polymerization. Green balls are the monomer molecules. Right: after polymerization. The green spirals are the polymer chains, and the red balls are the peroxyl groups [28]

free radicals that react with the hydrogel displaying polymerizable groups such as acrylate or methacrylate, which can be cross-linked. The mild conditions necessary to trigger this type of cross-linking make it advantageous in tissue engineering [4].

One example of this approach is the preparation of chitosan-based hydrogels reinforced with nano-graphene oxide (nGO). Feng et al. functionalized chitosan and nGO with photocurable methacrylategroups to produce mechanically enhanced hydrogels that were cross-linked using BAPO-OH as photoinitiator, which is active at wavelengths longer than 350 nm, avoiding any possible damage of cells within the scaffold structure. The mechanical performance was increased as the content of M–*n*GO increased, and therefore, it was demonstrated that the low mechanical properties of chitosan-based photocured hydrogels can be improved via hybridization [27].

Liu et al. [28] functionalized GO/PA sheets by radiation-induced peroxidation to obtain graphene peroxide (GPO). This functionalization enhanced the interactions between GPO and PAM. In this work, the hybrid nanohydrogels were obtained via in situ free radical polymerization using GPO as polyfunctional initiator and cross-linking center between the polymer chains and the GO sheets. This combination resulted in a mechanically stiff and elastomeric hydrogel, which potentially can be used in tissue engineering. A schematic model of GPO hydrogel formation is shown in Fig. 1.

3.2 Physically Cross-Linked Nanohydrogels for Tissue Engineering

Secondary interactions, such as hydrophobic, electrostatic or hydrogen bonding interactions, form the network in physically cross-linked hydrogels, where semi-permanent junction among the polymer chains is obtained without the need of additional cross-linkers or initiators. Nevertheless, a major drawback is the lower mechanical robustness of the physically cross-linked hydrogels, as well as their easy dissolution, and strong response to stimuli such as pH, temperature and ionic strength.

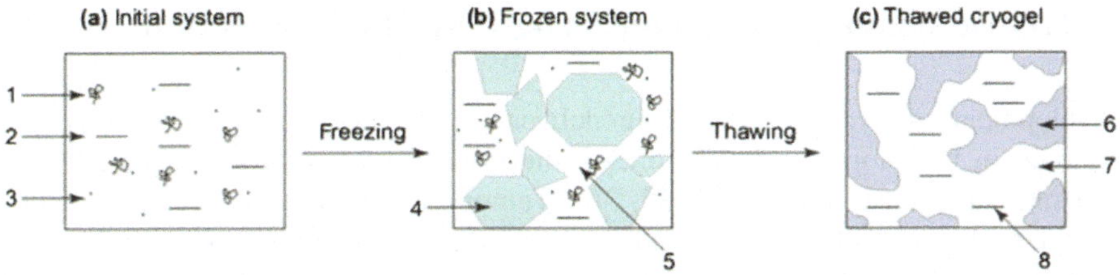

Fig. 2 Different stages that the hydrogel undergoes during the freeze/thaw process. The initial system consists of (1) polymer macromolecules in the solution, (2) solvent and (3) low molecular solutes. The frozen system contains (4) polycrystals of frozen solvent and (5) unfrozen liquid microphase. After thawing, the system includes a polymeric network (6), macropores (7) and solvent (8) [30]

Physical cross-linking of hydrogels can be carried out via crystallization induced by freeze–thaw cycles, where the cross-linking occurs due to the presence of crystalline regions. The polymer solution undergoes gelation reactions, resulting in a hydrogel with a heterogeneous phase that is formed due to the freezing (crystallization). The solubility of the polymer changes when the water converts into ice, which generates regions rich in polymer and regions lacking polymer [29]. The polymer-rich regions eventually turn into polymeric chains, joined by hydrogen bonds, which structure remains after thawing [30]. The different stages that the hydrogel undergoes during the freeze–thaw process are represented in Fig. 2.

Butylina et al. [31] prepared hybrid nanohydrogels of PVA/CNCs via crystallization induced by freeze–thaw cycles. The resulting materials exhibited better compressive properties as a function of incorporated CNCs. On the contrary, the increase in number of freeze–thaw cycles from 3 to 5 negatively affected the compressive properties of materials. Zhang et al. [32], freeze-thawed PVA/GO hydrogels via physical cross-linking through hydrogen bonding between GO and PVA, demonstrate a significant improvement in tensile and compressive strength, compared to pure PVA hydrogels.

Abouzeid et al. [33] cross-linked TEMPO-oxidized cellulose nanofibers (TOCNF)/sodium alginate (SA) hydrogels using calcium chloride as ionic cross-linker prior to 3D printing. The hydrogels exhibited excellent compressive properties compared to pure SA and pure TOCNF showing promising properties for bone tissue scaffolds.

Gaharwar et al. [34] physically cross-linked poly(ethylene oxide)/silica nanoparticles to form hybrid nanohydrogels without the addition of a photo/chemical initiator. The nanohydrogels were vigorously mixed so that the silicate interacted with the polymer chains and formed a fully exfoliated network. Afterward, the swollen hydrogel was subjected to shearing and solvent evaporation. Dense films were obtained, with tunable mechanical properties depending on the silicate concentration. Moreover, a shear-thinning behavior was observed, which is potentially useful for injectable hydrogels for minimally invasive tissue engineering.

4 Hybrid Nanohydrogels for Drug Delivery Applications

Development of hydrogels for drug delivery applications has been extensively explored in the biomedical field during the last decades, growing at an accelerated rate since early reports [5, 35, 36]. Tumors as targets in cancer treatments, wound healing, ophthalmology and other similar applications have been a main focus in research related to nanohydrogels for drug delivery. Nanohydrogels are very promising structures due to the combination of great swelling capacity, elasticity and biocompatibility [37–39], which are inherent properties of all hydrogels but complemented via hybridization with loaded nanoparticles, where high concentrations of bioactive compounds can be encapsulated and released in a controlled manner upon biodegradation or by responding to external stimuli such as temperature [40], pH [41] or a magnetic field [42]. Moreover, nanosized hydrogel particles can be developed as well, which have higher possibility to transit through the different physiological barriers without being easily eliminated by the spleen or liver, for example, longer permanence in the blood stream, etcetera [43, 44].

4.1 Hybrid Nanohydrogels Based on Natural Polymers for Drug Delivery Applications

Natural polymers have been widely used in controlled drug delivery, due to their biocompatibility, biodegradability, nontoxicity and abundance of surface functional groups [45, 46]; being polysaccharides (such as cellulose, chitosan or dextran) and proteins (such as gelatin, collagen or fibrin) the main natural sources. Li et al. [47] reported the preparation of 5-fluorouracil-loaded nanohydrogels by using the sodium salt of the carboxymethyl cellulose (SCMC) and lysozyme (Ly), an antimicrobial enzyme, separately dissolving the drug and the SCMC, followed by mixing both solutions at different SCMC:Ly ratios at 80 °C. 5-fluorouracil-loaded spherical nanohydrogels were obtained with an average hydrodynamic diameter of 214 nm and a swelling ratio about 5. The in vitro release tests showed a slower release in a simulated gastric fluid (pH 1.2) than in a simulated intestinal fluid (pH 7.4), which implies a protection effect of the drug by the nanohydrogels in the stomach ensuring a sustained release in intestines. In a similar study, Li et al. [48] reported methotrexate-loaded nanohydrogels prepared from carboxymethyl cellulose (CMC) and Ly at different ratios following a similar procedure to that described above by Zhu et al., but in this case, the drug was dissolved in the Ly solution and added dropwise to the CMC solution. In this case, the nanohydrogles presented a regular spherical shape with an average hydrodynamic diameter of 123 nm. The in vitro release tests showed a much higher toxicity of the loaded nanohydrogels in HepG2 and MCF-7 cells than that of free methotrexate, which was attributed to the fact that loaded nanostructures could easily enter the interior of the cells by their small diameters and generate a cytotoxic effect on cancerous cells. Another contribution of Li et al. [49] was the encapsulation of doxorubicin in nanohydrogels prepared in a similar procedure than those described for 5-fluorouracil but in this case using SCMC/low density lipoprotein (LDL), a biological assembly responsible for transporting cholesterol around the body, as components. Spherical-shaped nanohydrogels were also reported with average diameter around 90 nm and a zeta potential of −35 mV. This last characteristic favored the loaded stage of the cationic anticancer drug resulting in a loading efficiency of 98%. The release of the drug from the loaded hydrogel was pH-dependent releasing faster at mildly acidic environments that under physiological pH conditions.

Chitosan, the second most abundant natural polymer, have also been extensively used for drug encapsulation in hydrogels. Zhang et al. [50] reported the preparation of chitosan-based luminescent/magnetic hybrid nanogels with average sizes about 160 nm by direct gelation of chitosan, cadmium telluride quantum dots and superparamagnetic iron oxide, which were loaded with insulin favored by the abundant amino groups from chitosan through conjugating via hydrogen bonds. Insulin release was promoted under physiological pH conditions (7.4) compared to mildly acidic conditions (5.3) explained by the more favorable solubility of insulin at pH 7.4. Zhou et al. [51] designed a nanohydrogel based on chitosan-poly(methacrylic acid) network containing immobilized cadmium selenide quantum dots with hydrodynamic diameters below 174 nm, for controlled drug delivery applications, among other applications like tumor cell imaging. Temozolomide was the anticancer drug loaded in these nanostructures, which was controlled released by a modification of the physicochemical environment of embedded quantum dots for converting chemical/biochemical signals to optical signals, this effect prompted by the pH-induced volume phase transition that can undergo the nanohydrogels.

Dextran is another important polysaccharide with multiple applications, most of them in the biomedical area, formed by a complex branched polysaccharide constituted by units of glucose with α-1,6 glycosidic linkages and with branches from α-1,3 linkages. Swain et al. [52] designed a novel biocompatible and stimuli responsive nanohydrogels constituted by polyacrylamide/dextran and decorated with 20 nm silver particles, which were efficiently dispersed throughout the nanohydrogel network. The function of silver nanoparticles was to increase the swelling and water retention properties of the nanohydrogels at specific pH values. The hydrogels showed the capacity to efficiently load ornidazole, an antibiotic drug. The nanohydrogels were prepared by polymerizing acrylamide in the presence of dextran, using methylene bis-acrylamide as cross-linker followed by incorporation of silver nanoparticles by treatment with silver nitrate followed by reduction reaction with sodium borohydride. The in vitro release of ornidazole was 98.5% at 6 h. Dou et al. [53] reported the preparation of dextran/polyacrylic acid (PAA)-based nanohydrogels with application in anticancer drugs delivery, using a redox sensitive disulfide group for cross-linking the chains. Doxorrubicine, as anticancer drug, was incorporated to ~98 nm nanohydrogels by conjugation through an acid-labile hydrazine bond. The in vitro and in vivo studies revealed that the hydrogels exhibited a dual pH/redox responsiveness on controlled doxorrubicine release, less toxicity of loaded nanohydrogels in comparison with free doxorrubicine, an excellent

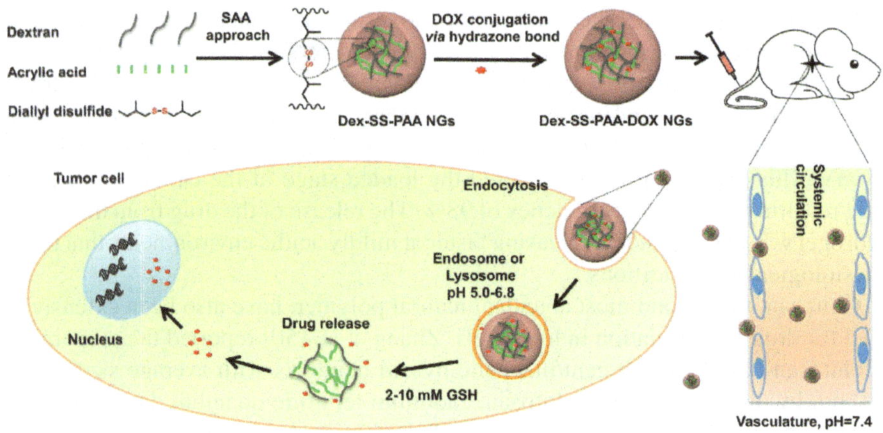

Fig. 3 Schematic illustration depicting the fabrication of the nanohydrogels, as well as their subsequent loading with doxorrubicine and their tumor-microenvironment sensitive drug release behaviors

growth inhibition of MDA-MB-231 tumors. Figure 3 shows the schematic illustration of nanohydrogels formation, the subsequent loading with doxorrubicine and their tumor-microenvironment sensitive drug release behaviors.

Some natural gums have also been used to design nanohydrogels with drug delivery applications. In this sense, Ghaemy et al. [54] designed a hydrogel based on tragacanth gum, incorporating functionalized multi-walled carbon nanotubes as secondary component and indomethacine as the drug loaded, while Torchilin et al. [55] prepared a hydrogel based on gellan gum, integrating through chemical links the prednisolone, an anti-inflammatory drug, and physically entrapping the paclitaxel, an anticancer drug, for obtaining a multi drug delivery nanohydrogel based on gellan gum.

4.2 *Hybrid Nanohydrogels Based on Synthetic Polymers for Drug Delivery Applications*

Synthetic polymers are also very important in biomedical applications, as they can offer similar properties to natural polymers, but also providing the possibility to tailor-specific properties for specific applications, for example, controlling the molecular weight, cross-linking degree and precise control of functional groups. Popular synthetic polymers for the synthesis of hydrogels are acrylamide, the *N*-isopropylacrylamide (PNIPAm), acrylic acid, methacrylic acid and derivatives of both, which have the ability to respond to an external stimulus. Rashidi et al. [56] reported the preparation of nanohydrogels from the in situ polymerization of *N*-isopropylacrylamide in a solution containing magnetic nanoparticles (Fe_3O_4), using

APS as initiator and a hybrid starch-maleate as cross-linker. The thermo- and pH-sensitive magnetic nanohydrogels were then loaded with mitoxantrone, an anti-cancer drug. Figure 4a shows the schematic representation for the preparation of the magnetic nanohydrogels, while Fig. 4b shows digital images of starch-maleate magnetic nanoparticles stable ferrofluid, magnetic nanohydrogels dispersion and magnetic response of nanohydrogels.

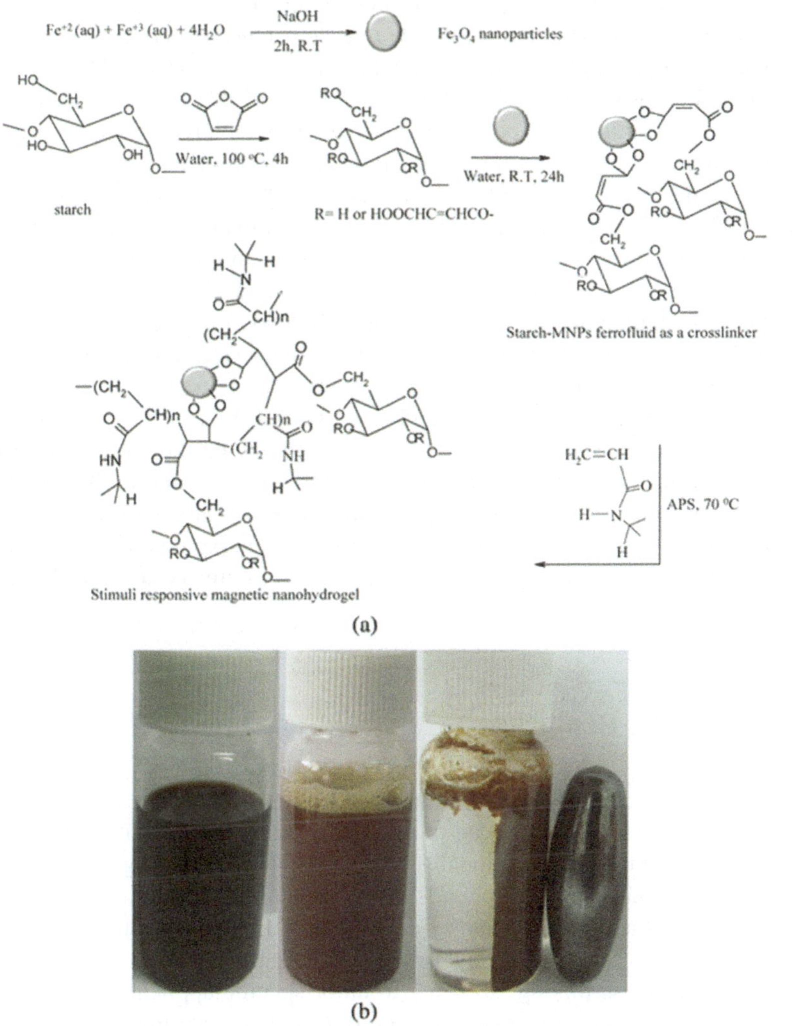

Fig. 4 **a** Schematic description for the preparation of magnetic nanohydrogels; **b** digital images of starch-maleate-magnetic nanoparticles stable ferrofluid, magnetic nanohydrogles dispersion and magnetic response of nanohydrogels (left to right)

Hamishenkar et al. [57] also worked with PNIPAm-based nanohydrogels containing Fe_3O_4 nanoparticles for loading anticancer drugs. In this case, the total components of the pH and thermal responsive hydrogels were a poly(*N*-isopropylacrylamide-*co*-itaconic anhydride) copolymer, poly(ethylene glycol) and the Fe_3O_4 nanoparticles. Doxorrubicine was the anticancer drug used in this study. The loaded nanohydrogels presented a regular spherical shape with an average diameter about 20 nm. The in vitro release studies revealed that the highest drug release was at 41 °C and a pH of 5.3, while at physiological conditions (37 °C and a pH of 7.4), the materials exhibited negligible release values. Moreover, doxorrubicine-loaded nanohydrogels presented higher cytotoxicity effects against HeLa cells than free drug, which was explained by the slow release of the loaded anticancer drug. Kim et al. [58] worked with polyacrylamide-based nanohdyrogels loaded with the 5-Fluorouracil as anticancer drug. The hydrogels were prepared through a in situ free radical polymerization including green tea extract (80% polyphenols) as secondary component, N, N'-methylenebisacrylamide as cross-linker and potassium persulfate as initiator. The presence of green tea molecules in the nanohydrogels improved their water–uptake ability and the stabilization of the magnetic nanoparticles in the networks. The nanohydrogels were subsequently loaded with iron ions (Fe^{2+}/Fe^{3+}) via a swelling method, followed by the conversion of iron ions into magnetic nanoparticles of about 10 nm in the nanohydrogel network via treatment with ammonia solution. The nanohydrogels were then loaded with 5-fluorouracil, showing encapsulation efficiencies ranging from 43 to 81% depending on the presence or absence of an external magnetic field, which was also studied as variant in the release tests resulting in a slightly higher percentage of drug release when the external magnetic field was used. These nanohydrogels present both superparamagnetic and biocompatible properties and are good candidates for drug delivery or other biomedical applications.

5 Concluding Remarks

The introduction of a secondary nanosized component into a hydrogel matrix, forming hybrid nanohydrogels, can provide mechanical reinforcement or the possibility to yield additional functionality such as imparting biological functions or encapsulation of bioactive compounds that can be encapsulated and released upon biodegradation of application of an external stimuli. Depending on the desired properties of the hydrogels, different hybridization strategies can be followed via chemical or physical cross-linking, allowing to tailor-specific applications. Some of the most prominent uses of nanohydrogels are in tissue engineering and drug delivery applications, which are further discussed in the following chapters.

References

1. Ahmed EM (2015) Hydrogel: Preparation, characterization, and applications: a review. J Adv Res 6:105–121. https://doi.org/10.1016/j.jare.2013.07.006
2. Zou H, Wu S, Shen J (2008) Polymer/Silica nanocomposites: preparation, characterization, properties . Chem Rev 108:3893–3957. https://doi.org/10.1021/cr068035q
3. Hennink WE, van Nostrum CF (2012) Novel crosslinking methods to design hydrogels. Adv Drug Deliv Rev 64:223–236
4. Hunt JA, Chen R, van Veen T, Bryan N (2014) Hydrogels for tissue engineering and regenerative medicine. J Mater Chem B 5319–5338
5. Hoare TR, Kohane DS (2008) Hydrogels in drug delivery: progress and challenges. Polymer (Guildf) 49:1993–2007. https://doi.org/10.1016/j.polymer.2008.01.027
6. Parhi R (2017) Cross-linked hydrogel for pharmaceutical applications: a review. Adv Pharm Bull 7:515–530. https://doi.org/10.15171/apb.2017.064
7. Dong W, Huang C, Wang Y, Sun Y, Ma P, Chen M (2013) Superior mechanical properties of double-network hydrogels reinforced by carbon nanotubes without organic modification. Int J Mol Sci 14:22380–22394. https://doi.org/10.3390/ijms141122380
8. Chen Q, Chen H, Zhu L, Zheng J (2015) Fundamentals of double network hydrogels. J Mater Chem B 3:3654–3676. https://doi.org/10.1039/C5TB00123D
9. Geng Y, Lin XY, Pan P, Shan G, Bao Y, Song Y, Wu ZL, Zheng Q (2016) Hydrophobic association mediated physical hydrogels with high strength and healing ability. Polymer (Guildf) 100:60–68. https://doi.org/10.1016/j.polymer.2016.08.022
10. Visser J, Melchels FPW, Jeon JE, Van Bussel EM, Kimpton LS, Byrne HM, Dhert WJA, Dalton PD, Hutmacher DW, Malda J (2015) Reinforcement of hydrogels using three-dimensionally printed microfibres. Nat Commun 6:1–10. https://doi.org/10.1038/ncomms7933
11. Gaharwar AK, Peppas NA, Khademhosseini A (2014) Nanocomposite hydrogels for biomedical applications. Biotechnol Bioeng 441–453
12. Faghihi S, Karimi A, Jamadi M, Imani R, Salarian R (2014) Graphene oxide/poly(acrylic acid)/gelatin nanocomposite hydrogel: experimental and numerical validation of hyperelastic model. Mater Sci Eng C 38:299–305. https://doi.org/10.1016/j.msec.2014.02.015
13. Zhang Y, Huang R, Peng S, Ma Z (2015) MWCNTs/cellulose hydrogels prepared from NaOH/urea aqueous solution with improved mechanical properties. J Chem. 10.1155/2015/413497
14. Lvov Y, Wang W, Zhang L, Fakhrullin R (2015) Halloysite clay nanotubes for loading and sustained release of functional compounds. Adv Mater 28:1227–1250. https://doi.org/10.1002/adma.201502341
15. Tao D, Higaki Y, Ma W, Takahara A (2015) Halloysite nanotube/polyelectrolyte hybrids as adsorbents for the quick removal of dyes from aqueous solution. Chem Lett 44:1572–1574. https://doi.org/10.1246/cl.150727
16. Park K-L, Ma W, Higaki Y, Takahara A (2017) Mechanically enhanced hyaluronic acid hybrid hydrogels with halloysite nanotubes. Chem Lett 46:1217–1219. https://doi.org/10.1246/cl.170484
17. Yang J, Zhao J-J, Xu F, Sun R-C (2013) Revealing strong nanocomposite hydrogels reinforced by cellulose nanocrystals: insight into morphologies and interactions. ACS Appl Mater Interfaces 5:12960–12967. https://doi.org/10.1021/am403669n
18. Yang J, Han CR, Zhang XM, Xu F, Sun RC (2014) Cellulose nanocrystals mechanical reinforcement in composite hydrogels with multiple cross-links: correlations between dissipation properties and deformation mechanisms. Macromolecules 47:4077–4086. https://doi.org/10.1021/ma500729q
19. Miao C, Hamad WY (2013) Cellulose reinforced polymer composites and nanocomposites: a critical review. Cellulose 20:2221–2262. https://doi.org/10.1007/s10570-013-0007-3
20. Wang W, Zhang X, Teng A, Liu A (2017) Mechanical reinforcement of gelatin hydrogel with nanofiber cellulose as a function of percolation concentration. Int J Biol Macromol 103:226–233. https://doi.org/10.1016/j.ijbiomac.2017.05.027

21. Bian H, Wei L, Lin C, Ma Q, Dai H, Zhu JY (2018) Lignin-containing cellulose nanofibril-reinforced polyvinyl alcohol hydrogels. ACS Sustain Chem Eng 6:4821–4828. https://doi.org/10.1021/acssuschemeng.7b04172
22. Yang X, Abe K, Biswas SK, Yano H (2018) Extremely stiff and strong nanocomposite hydrogels with stretchable cellulose nanofiber/poly(vinyl alcohol) networks. Cellulose 25:6571–6580. https://doi.org/10.1007/s10570-018-2030-x
23. Lee KY, Mooney DJ (2001) Hydrogels for tissue engineering. Chem Rev 101:1869–1879. https://doi.org/10.1021/cr000108x
24. Shirzaei Sani E, Portillo-Lara R, Spencer A, Yu W, Geilich BM, Noshadi I, Webster TJ, Annabi N (2018) Engineering adhesive and antimicrobial hyaluronic acid/elastin-like polypeptide hybrid hydrogels for tissue engineering applications. ACS Biomater Sci Eng 4:2528–2540. https://doi.org/10.1021/acsbiomaterials.8b00408
25. Chen Y, Zhou X, Lin Q, Jiang D (2014) Bacterial cellulose/gelatin composites: in situ preparation and glutaraldehyde treatment. Cellulose 21:2679–2693
26. Tanpichai S, Oksman K (2016) Cross-linked nanocomposite hydrogels based on cellulose nanocrystals and PVA: mechanical properties and creep recovery. Compos Part Appl Sci Manuf. https://doi.org/10.1016/j.compositesa.2016.06.002
27. Feng Z, Hakkarainen M, Grützmacher H, Chiappone A, Sangermano M (2019) Photocrosslinked chitosan hydrogels reinforced with chitosan-derived nano-graphene oxide. Macromol Chem Phys 1900174. 10.1002/macp.201900174
28. Liu J, Chen C, He C, Zhao J, Yang X, Wang H (2012) Synthesis of graphene peroxide and its application in fabricating super extensible and highly resilient nanocomposite hydrogels. ACS Nano 6:8194–8202
29. Mihranyan A (2013) Viscoelastic properties of cross-linked polyvinyl alcohol and surface-oxidized cellulose whisker hydrogels. Cellulose 20:1369–1376
30. Zhang H, Zhang F, Wu J (2013) Physically crosslinked hydrogels from polysaccharides prepared by freeze thaw technique. React Funct Polym 73:923–928
31. Butylina S, Geng S, Oksman K (2016) Properties of as-prepared and freeze-dried hydrogels made from poly(vinyl alcohol) and cellulose nanocrystals using freeze-thaw technique. Eur Polym J 81:386–396. https://doi.org/10.1016/j.eurpolymj.2016.06.028
32. Zhang L, Zhipeng W, Xu C, Li Y, Gao J, Wang W, Liu Y (2011) High strength graphene oxide/polivinyl alcohol composite hydrogels. J Mater Chem 21:10399–10406
33. Abouzeid RE, Khiari R, Beneventi D, Dufresne A (2018) Biomimetic mineralization of three-dimensional printed alginate/TEMPO-oxidized cellulose nanofibril scaffolds for bone tissue engineering. Biomacromol 19:4442–4452
34. Gaharwar AK, Kishore V, Rivera C, Bullock W, Wu C-J, Akkus O, Schmidt G (2012) Physically crosslinked nanocomposites from silicate-crosslinked PEO. Macromol Biosci 12:779–793
35. Agrahari V, Agrahari V, Mitra AK (2016) Nanocarrier fabrication and macromolecule drug delivery: challenges and opportunities. Ther Deliv 7:257–278. https://doi.org/10.4155/tde-2015-0012
36. Dai H, Chen Q, Qin H, Guan Y, Shen D, Hua Y, Tang Y, Xu J (2006) A temperature-responsive copolymer hydrogel in controlled drug delivery. Macromolecules 39:6584–6589. https://doi.org/10.1021/ma060486p
37. Joglekar M, Trewyn BG (2013) Polymer-based stimuli-responsive nanosystems for biomedical applications. Biotechnol J 8:931–945. https://doi.org/10.1002/biot.201300073
38. Dalwadi C, Patel G (2015) Application of nanohydrogels in drug delivery systems: recent patents review. Recent Pat Nanotechnol 9:17–25. https://doi.org/10.2174/187221050966150101151521
39. Wu H-Q, Wang C-C (2016) Biodegradable smart nanogels: a new platform for targeting drug delivery and biomedical diagnostics. Langmuir 32:6211–6225. https://doi.org/10.1021/acs.langmuir.6b00842
40. Sattari M, Fathi M, Daei M, Erfan-Niya H, Barar J, Entezami AA (2017) Thermoresponsive graphene oxide—starch micro/nanohydrogel composite as biocompatible drug delivery system. BioImpacts 7:167–175. https://doi.org/10.15171/bi.2017.20

41. Roointan A, Farzanfar J, Mohammadi-Samani S, Behzad-Behbahani A, Farjadian F (2018) Smart pH responsive drug delivery system based on poly(HEMA-co-DMAEMA) nanohydrogel. Int J Pharm 552:301–311. https://doi.org/10.1016/j.ijpharm.2018.10.001
42. Jaiswal MK, Gogoi M, Dev Sarma H, Banerjee R, Bahadur D (2014) Biocompatibility, biodistribution and efficacy of magnetic nanohydrogels in inhibiting growth of tumors in experimental mice models. Biomater Sci 2:370–380. https://doi.org/10.1039/C3BM60225G
43. Duncan R, Gaspar R (2011) Nanomedicine(s) under the Microscope. Mol Pharm 8:2101–2141. https://doi.org/10.1021/mp200394t
44. Chen X, Cheng X, Soeriyadi AH, Sagnella SM, Lu X, Scott JA, Lowe SB, Kavallaris M, Gooding JJ (2014) Stimuli-responsive functionalized mesoporous silica nanoparticles for drug release in response to various biological stimuli. Biomater Sci 2:121–130. https://doi.org/10.1039/C3BM60148J
45. Yadav P, Yadav H, Shah VG, Shah G, Dhaka G (2015) Biomedical biopolymers, their origin and evolution in biomedical sciences: a systematic review. J Clin Diagn Res 9:21–25. https://doi.org/10.7860/JCDR/2015/13907.6565
46. Gopi S, Amalraj A, Sukumaran NP, Haponiuk JT, Thomas S (2018) Biopolymers and their composites for drug delivery: a brief review. Macromol Symp 380:1800114. https://doi.org/10.1002/masy.201800114
47. Zhu K, Ye T, Liu J, Peng Z, Xu S, Lei J, Deng H, Li B (2013) Nanogels fabricated by lysozyme and sodium carboxymethyl cellulose for 5-fluorouracil controlled release. Int J Pharm 441:721–727. https://doi.org/10.1016/j.ijpharm.2012.10.022
48. Li Z, Xu W, Zhang C, Chen Y, Li B (2015) Self-assembled lysozyme/carboxymethylcellulose nanogels for delivery of methotrexate. Int J Biol Macromol 75:166–172. https://doi.org/10.1016/j.ijbiomac.2015.01.033
49. He L, Liang H, Lin L, Shah BR, Li Y, Chen Y, Li B (2015) Green-step assembly of low density lipoprotein/sodium carboxymethyl cellulose nanogels for facile loading and pH-dependent release of doxorubicin. Colloids Surf B Biointerfaces 126:288–296. https://doi.org/10.1016/j.colsurfb.2014.12.024
50. Shen J-M, Xu L, Lu Y, Cao H-M, Xu Z-G, Chen T, Zhang H-X (2012) Chitosan-based luminescent/magnetic hybrid nanogels for insulin delivery, cell imaging, and antidiabetic research of dietary supplements. Int J Pharm 427:400–409. https://doi.org/10.1016/j.ijpharm.2012.01.059
51. Wu W, Shen J, Banerjee P, Zhou S (2010) Chitosan-based responsive hybrid nanogels for integration of optical pH-sensing, tumor cell imaging and controlled drug delivery. Biomaterials 31:8371–8381. https://doi.org/10.1016/j.biomaterials.2010.07.061
52. Prusty K, Swain SK (2018) Nano silver decorated polyacrylamide/dextran nanohydrogels hybrid composites for drug delivery applications. Mater Sci Eng C 85:130–141. https://doi.org/10.1016/j.msec.2017.11.028
53. Wang H, Dai T, Zhou S, Huang X, Li S, Sun K, Zhou G, Dou H (2017) Self-assembly assisted fabrication of dextran-based nanohydrogels with reduction-cleavable junctions for applications as efficient drug delivery systems. Sci Rep 7:40011
54. Badakhshanian E, Hemmati K, Ghaemy M (2016) Enhancement of mechanical properties of nanohydrogels based on natural gum with functionalized multiwall carbon nanotube: study of swelling and drug release. Polymer (Guildf) 90:282–289. https://doi.org/10.1016/j.polymer.2016.03.028
55. D'Arrigo G, Navarro G, Di Meo C, Matricardi P, Torchilin V (2014) Gellan gum nanohydrogel containing anti-inflammatory and anti-cancer drugs: a multi-drug delivery system for a combination therapy in cancer treatment. Eur J Pharm Biopharm 87:208–216. https://doi.org/10.1016/j.ejpb.2013.11.001
56. Fathi M, Entezami AA, Arami S, Rashidi M-R (2015) Preparation of N-Isopropylacrylamide/itaconic acid magnetic nanohydrogels by modified starch as a crosslinker for anticancer drug carriers. Int J Polym Mater Polym Biomater 64:541–549. https://doi.org/10.1080/00914037.2014.996703
57. Poorgholy N, Massoumi B, Ghorbani M, Jaymand M, Hamishehkar H (2018) Intelligent anticancer drug delivery performances of two poly(N-isopropylacrylamide)-based magnetite

nanohydrogels. Drug Dev Ind Pharm 44:1254–1261. https://doi.org/10.1080/03639045.2018.1442845

58. Jayaramudu T, Raghavendra GM, Varaprasad K, Raju KM, Sadiku ER, Kim J (2016) 5-Fluorouracil encapsulated magnetic nanohydrogels for drug-delivery applications. J Appl Polym Sci 133:43921. https://doi.org/10.1002/app.43921

Chapter 8
Cross-Linking, Modular Design and Self-assembly in Hydrogels

Smitha Benny, Jiya Jose, and Sabu Thomas

Abstract Gels can be recognised as a stiff but flexible, soft everyday material. They survive the "inversion test", it is solid-like rheology that defies the character of the gel. Low-molecular-weight gels can be classified into organogels and hydrogels based on its constitution. All these gels have wide range of applications in the fields of biomedical engineering and pharmaceutical formulation. Hydrogels are highly tuneable viscoelastic hydrophilic polymers with 3D networks of cross-linking. Despite being mostly liquid, they have solid-like rheology due to its cross-linking. They are highly water-swellable polymer networks with water imbibing properties which gives them the flexibility to mimic natural tissues. The cross-linking is stabilised via interactions including Van der Waals, covalent bonding and hydrogen bonding. Hydrogels are formed by gelators of low molecular weight and exhibit colloidal properties. Stimuli-responsive nature of supramolecular gels can be utilised in targeted drug delivery systems. Natural polymeric hydrogels have a trending application in modern medicine due to its profound implication in sensing, targeted drug delivery, controlled release of a bio-active substance, etc. These gelators assemble by noncovalent interactions like π-π interactions and hydrogen bonding. The properties of hydrogels can be tuned by changing the external stimuli. These polymeric materials that can show both effector and sensor functions can be used to mimic the natural system, thereby fabricating intelligent systems. This chapter gives brief introduction on gels, following the different type of light molecular weight. Guanosine-based hydrogels and its applications are also discussed further.

S. Benny
School of Chemical Sciences, Mahatma Gandhi University, Kottayam, Kerala 686560, India

J. Jose (✉) · S. Thomas
International and Inter University Centre for Nanoscience and Nanotechnology, Mahatma Gandhi University, Kottayam, Kerala 686560, India
e-mail: jiyajose@gmail.com

J. Jose et al. (eds.), *Nano Hydrogels*, Gels Horizons: From Science to Smart Materials,
https://doi.org/10.1007/978-981-15-7138-1_8

1 Gel Formation

Gels can be compared with a solid matrix that immobilises a liquid component by surface tension effects (Fig. 1).

Gels can be categorised based on its liquid phase as organogels and hydrogels. The common methodology for the synthesis of gels is by dissolving a low percentage (0.1–5 wt.%) of gelator molecule in an appropriate heated solvent. Upon cooling below the temperature of gelation (T_{gel}), the affinity between gelator and liquid phase decreases and the former self-assembles into a three-dimensional (3D) entangled network of solid, immobilising the liquid phase through strong intermolecular forces, allowing it to support its own weight without collapsing.

Gels can be further subcategorised into two different classes based on the nature and type of interaction as chemical gels and physical gels. In chemical gels the cross linking is via covalent bonds [2–4]. While noncovalent interactions like van der Waals forces, hydrogen bonds and Coulombic interactions maintain the fibrous network of a physical gel and due to these interactions, they are thermally reversible. Because their networks are covalently linked and essentially permanent, chemical gels swell or shrink when exposed to an external stimulus. Conversely, physical gels are held together by reversible, noncovalent forces and can often be degraded by appropriate stimuli [5–9] (Fig. 2).

In hydrogels, where polar groups which are generally highly solvated, the gelation process is generally dominated by hydrophobic effects. Directional hydrogen bonding and dipolar interactions tend to dominate in the case of organic gels [11].

1.1 Low-Molecular-Weight Gelators

Supramolecular gels are a type of physical gel in which noncovalent interactions like hydrogen bonding and van der Waals interactions help in the association of fibrous network in order to frame various building blocks. This association could principally include the noncovalent cross-linking of polymers. Supramolecular gels are mainly referred to gels made from "low-molecular-weight" gelators (LMWG), compounds with molecular weight less than 3000 Da, while, in polymer gels, most of the solid

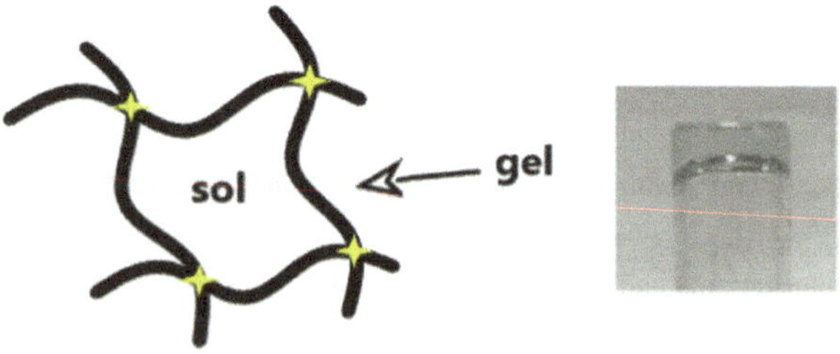

Fig. 1 Gels maintain solid-like rheology by establishing a fibrous network (gel) that immobilises the liquid phase (sol) [1]

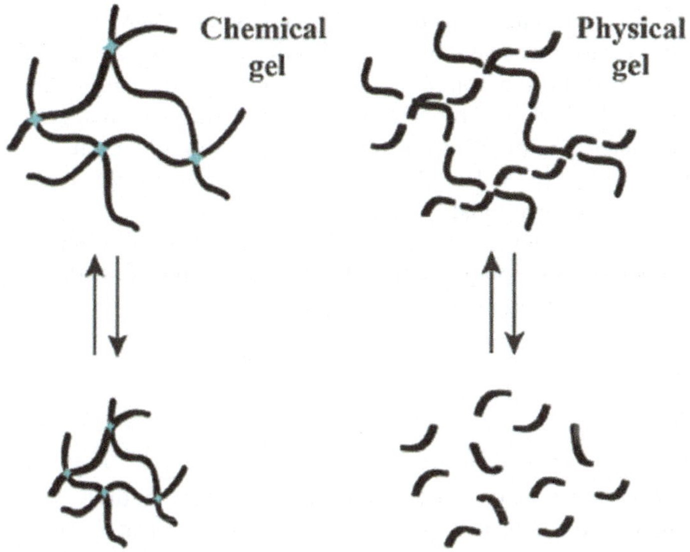

Fig. 2 Chemical gels can swell or shrink since the network or cross-linking is covalently linked and permanent when an external stimulus is applied. Physical gels get easily degraded with an appropriate stimulus since they are held together by reversible, noncovalent forces [10]

components establish themselves via covalent bonding. There is a microphase separation through molecular recognition pathways and self-assembly in LMW gelators. Molecular gelation mostly proceed via nucleation mechanism rather than the isodesmic process, that is, the process of gelation is hierarchical and stepwise. The molecular building blocks at first forms a one-dimensional nucleus, followed by nuclear growth to form fibres and larger aggregates, which can branch and bundle [10]. The entanglement of these fibres to a 3D mesh is referred to as a self-assembled fibrillar network (Safin) (Fig. 3).

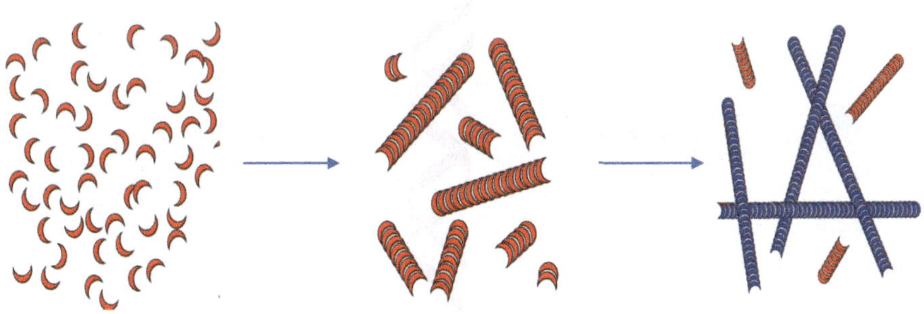

Fig. 3 Molecular gelation most often occurs via a nucleation process, in which the LMW gelator assembles to form a self-assembled fibrillar network (SAFiN) [10]

While gelation can sometimes occur by just mixing the LMW gelator with solvent at ambient temperature, more often than not, heating the sample is required to dissolve the gelator. Cooling the solution results in a supersaturated solution that then forms the gel. Because the gelation process involves reversible, multistep assembly, the resulting gel material is often responsive to various stimuli and, thus, is attractive for many applications [5–8, 10, 12–14]. The LMWGs are very versatile due to its diverse structure and functionality. There are numerous examples of multicomponent LMW gelating systems [15]. The molecular gels have been made from metal coordination complexes, polyaromatics [16, 17], dendrimers [18, 19], poly urea [1, 20] and quaternary ammonium salts [21].

1.2 LMGO

Gels are colloidal in nature, and LMNOs appear to have entirely versatile architecture including tapes, sheets, rods derived by the hierarchical assembly of gelator molecule which is facilitated by the physical molecular interactions such as hydrogen bonding, van der Waals forces, p–p stacking, London dispersion forces and electrostatic interactions [22, 23]. The mechanism of fibre formation was depicted successfully by Estroff and Hamilton in 2001. They individually characterised the primary, secondary and tertiary structure of the fibrous assemblies. Fibres form a network which is responsible for gelation via series of assembly. Initially, the assembly into the primary nanostructure is driven by one-dimensional interaction on the molecular level (Fig. 4).

Molecular interactions are essential for the formation of 1D fibres rather than other structures. But the gelation is determined by the delicate balance between the molecules ability to dissolve and aggregate into solution. The interactions are

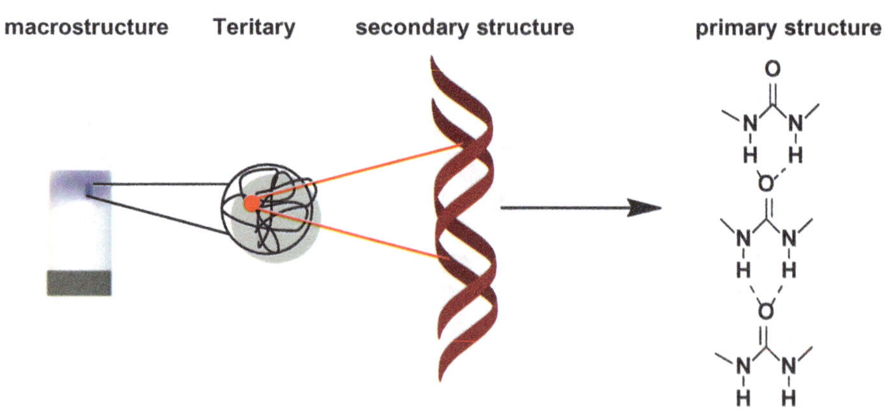

Fig. 4 Primary, secondary, tertiary and macrostructure of a self-assembled physical network [13]

mostly noncovalent such as hydrogen bonding helps in the self-assembly while the weak interactions in the aqueous environment play an important role in anisotropic and aggregation in water. Gelation requires a continuous network of fibres which is achieved by cross-linking which results in the fibre branching, fibre enlargement and trapping in the mobile phase [24–28]. It was proposed by Terech and Weiss that gelation in organic media happens via attractive forces that are largely dipolar, and in case of metal coordinate bonds, it may involve specific intermolecular hydrogen bonding.

The formation of fibres is via three steps: initially, fibre nucleation, repeated crystalline fibre branching and fibre growth. Within the fibres, the packing is primarily determined by a balance between weak. The arrangement or packing between the fibres is primarily by the balance between the weak physical interactions as with the hydrogels including forces such as intermolecular hydrogen bonding, London dispersion forces, electrostatic forces and p–p stacking. In contrast to the traditional crystallisation, in self-assembled fibrillar networks (SAFINs), there is only growth among one axis of the three-dimensional structure similar to the pattern with radial arms initiating from the core in a Cayley tree structure. Several models have been developed to explain the transition of amphiphilic gelator molecules from their molecular to primary and secondary aggregate structures. But the small number of studies reported do not offer a single mechanism for self-assembly. Unidirectional formation of the thin branched fibres into 3D networks occurs due to anisotropic interactions via aggregation and the minimisation of the large surface energy that results from individual fibre formation [29–34].

1.3 Hydrogels

Peppas defined hydrogels as macromolecular networks which are swollen in biological fluids or water. Having various possible definitions hydrogels can be classified based on the nature and type of network into three, namely entangled networks, networks formed by secondary interactions and covalently cross-linked networks. These intelligent materials are sensitive and can respond to various chemical and physical changes including the pH [34–37], electrical field strength [38–40], ionic strength [41, 42], magnetic stimuli [43, 44], heat [33, 45–47] and ultrasound irradiation [48–51]. The basic principles, the structural features of gelators, the influence of solvents and role of noncovalent interactions, and properties of gels are discussed below.

The permanent network is formed by covalent cross-linking which allows the free diffusion of water, enhancing the mechanical properties of the gel [52–55].

Hydrogels may undergo minute change in environmental conditions with a larger change in physicochemical properties, sol–gel phase transition, degradation and shape transformation. Ordinary hydrogels when compared to the smart ones undergo only the swelling–deswelling process depending upon the availability of water in the system. Hydrogels turn out to be smart when it has additional properties over the basic properties like a swelling–deswelling. The environmental factor or the external stimuli can be chemical (pH, ion type, ionic strength and solvent), physical (temperature, electricity, magnetic field, ultrasound and pressure) or biological (enzyme, antibody and glucose). Despite having similar properties and appearance, polymeric hydrogels differ from supramolecular hydrogels in various subtle ways.

Unlike the polymeric hydrogels that originate from a randomly cross-linked network made of strong covalent bonds, hydrogels are the consequence of molecular self-assembly driven by weak, noncovalent interactions among hydro-gelators in water. This subtle yet fundamental difference not only renders more ordered molecular arrangement in the supramolecular hydrogels but also manifests itself in the process of hydrogenation. While simple swelling usually confers a polymeric hydrogel, a stimulus or a triggering force is necessary to bias thermodynamic equilibrium for initiating the self-assembly process or phase transition to obtain a supramolecular hydrogel. Therefore, there are many forms of stimuli or triggers for manipulating weak interactions. For the transition from a non-gel state to a hydrogel to occur, the free energy must be negative. Thus, the overall impact of the stimuli or triggers usually is negative ΔH or positive ΔS or both, which can be achieved by either physical methods (e.g. changing the temperature, applying ultrasound or modulating the ionic strength) or chemical methods (e.g. pH change, chemical or photochemical reactions, redox and catalysis) [56].

Due to the diverse applications in various fields of science, water gelating compounds (hydro-gelators) have been studied extensively. Moreover, low-molecular-weight hydro-gelators (LMWH) are preferred over their polymeric counterparts due to its thermo-reversible nature and rapid response to external stimuli and intermolecular associations within the three-dimensional network of the self-assembly. The type of interactions in the association is noncovalent in nature including the van der Waals interactions, dipole–dipole interactions, hydrogen bonding and interactions, p–p interactions.

2 Nucleobases

Self-assembly and molecular recognition properties of nucleobases, nucleosides and nucleic acids play a quintessential role in the formation of molecular gels. These N-bases have the ability to form hydrogen bonds and to π-stack, these are some the fundamental interactions that have the potential to control the structure and function of DNA and RNA assemblies.

These interaction possibilities make them capable for supramolecular assemblies; based on this nature, numerous molecular gels are synthesised from nucleobases, nucleosides and nucleic acids (Fig. 5).

Nucleobases are nitrogen-containing heterocycles which are the basic components of the nucleosides, nucleotides and nucleic acids. These five nitrogen bases are classified into two categories purines (including adenine A and guanine G) and pyrimidines (uracil U, thymine T and cytosine C). They differ in the basic structure

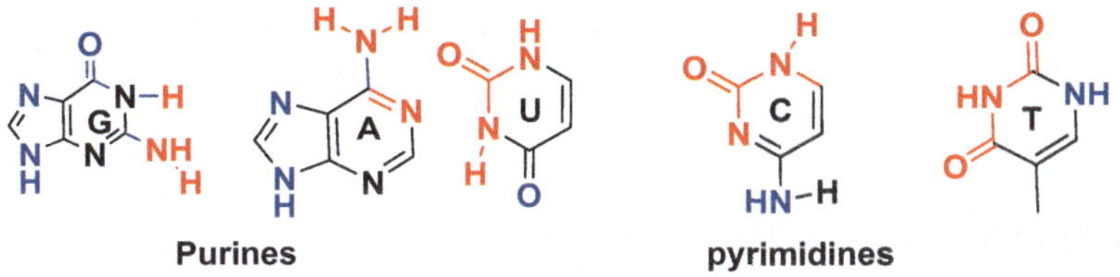

Fig. 5 Purines and pyrimidines

and the number of hydrogen bonding ability. Purines have multiple hydrogen bonding possibilities, while the pyrimidine bases have a single edge of the three hydrogen bond donors and acceptors. The aromatic nature of these nucleobases gives the ability to p-stack (Fig. 6).

The ribose sugar present in the nucleosides and nucleotides can also be a factor for the supramolecular structure and function. The nitrogen bases are attached to the ribose sugar via N-glycosidic linkage which results in the formation of a nucleoside (Fig. 7).

The phosphorylation of the nucleoside results in the formation of nucleotide which are the building blocks of nucleic acids. These nucleic acid polymers are RNA and DNA. The phosphate anion part of the nucleotide enhances electrostatic interactions. The most prominent noncovalent interaction is the base pairing between these nucleotides [1]. The complementary nucleobase pairs, adenine–uracil (thymine T in DNA) and guanine-cytosine form two and three hydrogen bonds, respectively. If we

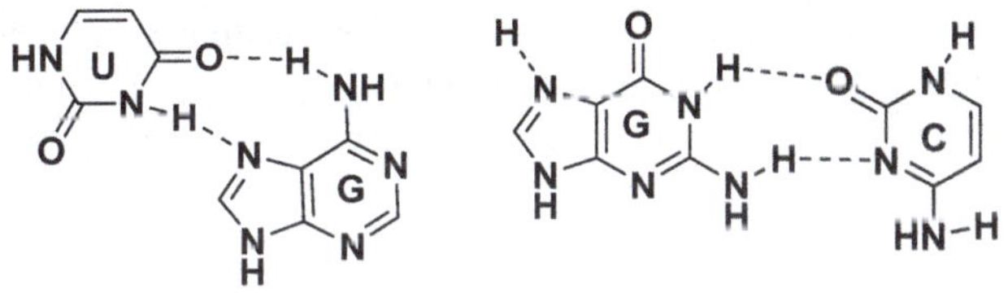

Fig. 6 Hoogsteen interaction

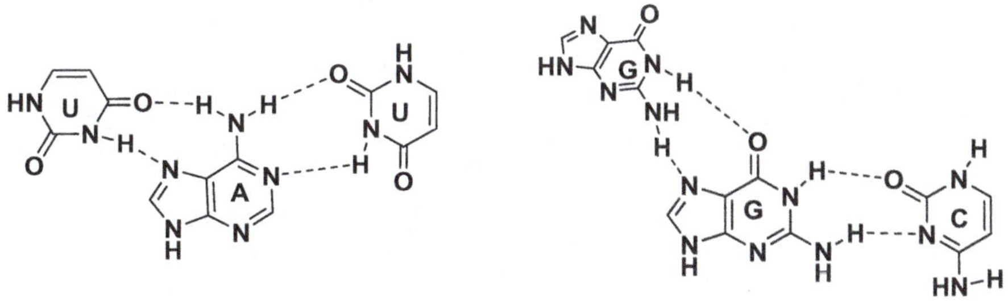

Fig. 7 Base triplets

consider base pairs in which at least two hydrogen bonds are formed, there are 28 base pairing motifs possible among the four nucleobases [53–57].

3 Guanosine-Based Hydrogels

Guanosine is a natural nucleoside that has the capability to homodimerise and unique self-assembly properties (Fig. 8).

Guanosine contains natural nucleobase purine that can provide multiple edges for hydrogen bonding interactions, improving its self-assembly properties. Guanosine and its derivatives self-assemble into dimmers, sheets and ribbons. Non-canonical base pairing can lead to the formation of macrocycles. Mostly, G-based hydrogels are based on the supramolecular assembly of macrocyclic G-quadrant units. The stacking of the quadret units can lead to the formation of G-quadruplex which can extend its network to form hydrogels. G-quadret can bind with mono or divalent ions form G8-M sandwiched structure. The gelation process of G-wires is driven by branching, physical cross-linking ad lateral aggregation. The gel network can be easily broken down by disrupting the supramolecular assemblies using appropriate external stimuli. This reversible nature guanosine-based hydrogels make them stimuli-responsive "smart" biomaterials. G4K+ borate hydrogels can be used to deliver the cargo molecule [58] (Fig. 9).

The multistep hierarchical nucleation process helps in the sol–gel transitions which can hydrogenate the guanosine. In gelation, guanosine or its derivatives are heated to dissolve the gelator, and cooling of this homogenous solution can give rise to the formation of a metastable state that do not free flow leading to the synthesis of self-supported hydrogel. All the process of heating and cooling guanosine is associated through Hoogsteen-type hydrogen bonding and forms a planar aromatic G-quadret

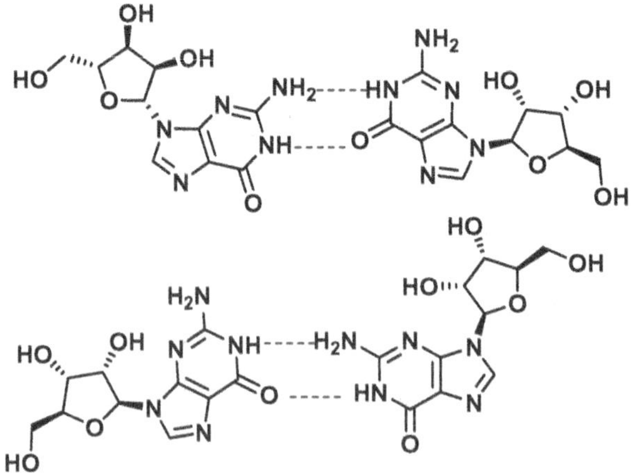

Fig. 8 Guanosine quadruplex

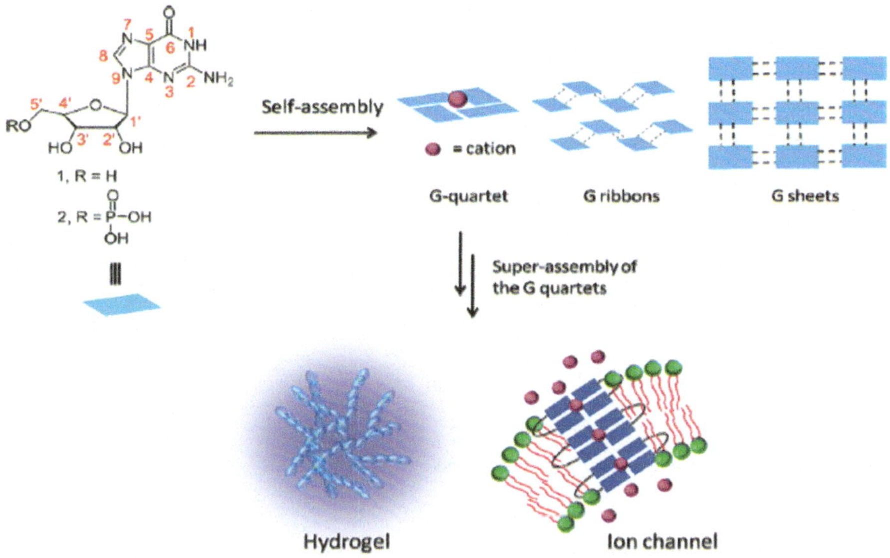

Fig. 9 Schematic illustration of hierarchical assemblies formed by guanosine derivatives [58]

that stacks upon each other and grows into G-wires. The process like physical cross-linking, aggregation and branching of G-wires is the driving force to the gelation process. The building block of these G-wires is the guanosine tetrad which is formed via Hoogsteen hydrogen bonding between each of the guanosines and its neighbours. The gelation and gel formation in solutions of individual guanosine compounds are widely studied since a long time using visual detection, bulk physical measurements, circular dichroism spectroscopies and absorption, light scattering, X-ray diffraction, neutron scattering, and NMR [51, 59, 60].

Supramolecular models studied on the basis of results have columnar structures formed by the self-assembly of G-quadrets through stacking and stabilised by the metal ion that is centrally located and coordinated to eight oxygen atoms in guanines [12, 15, 61–63].

An alternative model was proposed in which the GMP monomers associated by the Hoogsteen hydrogen bonding form a helical network which is further stabilised base stacking of two cations. In either of the cases, the concentration of guanosine increases and organises itself into higher ordered, anisotropic liquid crystalline phases with hexagonal organisation. The biological significance of G-quartet structures formed by G-rich sequences of DNA and RNA and the implications of guanosine self-assembly for the origin of life triggers the interest in guanosine. A second area of interest has been the enantiomeric selectivity exhibited by lipophilic derivatives of guanosine. The potential applications of guanosine gels in the broader arenas of nanotechnology and biotechnology are worth exploring due to the reversibility, tunability, aqueous solubility, physical stability, biocompatibility and chemical and chiral selectivity of the gels, as well as their potential for reversible encapsulation

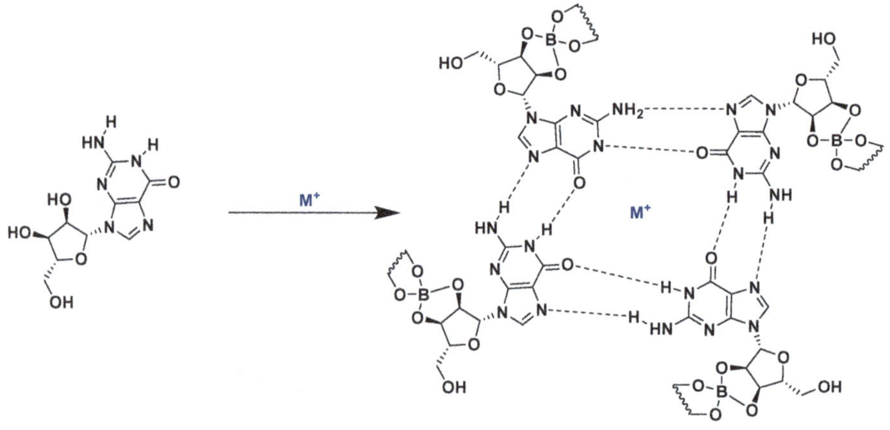

Fig. 10 K+ stabilised self-assembly of guanosine

and reversible introduction of functionality. It was recently discovered that guanosine gels formed by binary mixtures of the soluble 5-guanosine monophosphate (GMP) and relatively insoluble guanosine (Guo) in aqueous solution exhibit unique thermo-responsiveness that can be controlled by adjusting the Guo/GMP ratio, cation content and pH. At neutral pH and room temperature, GMP alone is too soluble in water to form firm gels, while Guo is too insoluble to form a stable gel even in the presence of high K+ concentrations. The present studies of GMP-Guo mixtures reveal, not surprisingly, that GMP helps to solubilise Guo while the insolubility of Guo promotes gelation at lower concentrations of GMP (Fig. 10).

Many guanine nucleosides and nucleotides were subsequently found to form hydrogels through the formation of similar helical arrangements. In the two decades that followed, the implications of pH on GMP assemblies and the role of stabilisation played by alkali cations were both established. In recent years, the interest in G-quadruplex structures has heightened due to the potential biological implications of these suprastructures (i.e. as a pertinent motif for fragile X syndrome, gene expression and telomerase inhibition). Additionally, the structural composition of G4-quartets and higher order assemblies has been extensively characterised through advanced solution and solid-state NMR techniques.

4 Biological Applications

The major goal of synthesising supramolecular hydrogels is to develop systems that can be effective for biological applications. Appropriate external stimuli can be used to disrupt the supramolecular assemblies to break down gel network. Owing to this reversible nature, guanosine-based hydrogels have been considered as stimuli-responsive "smart" biomaterials. Small molecular cancer drugs are not target specific and can cause systemic toxicity. Guanosine-based systems have the same goals to accomplish, while the high concentration of the K+ which is helpful in gelation.

These are ideal for biomedical applications, there have been some significant advances towards utilising these materials for tissue scaffolding and drug delivery. Recently, Rowan and co-workers showed that hydrogels formed with 8-methoxy-20,30,50-tri-O-methylguanosine derivative could not only form gels at physiological concentrations of monovalent cation. Reports suggest that guanosine-based gels could indeed be promising for tissue scaffolding applications [13, 55].

5 Conclusion

Hydrogels are soft and versatile materials that can form a three-dimensional network which encapsulate large amount of water. This versatility is attained from its three-dimensional gel matrix which consists of cross-linked polymer. The gels are standardised by noncovalent interactions including van der Waals, covalent bonding, electrostatic interactions, dipole–dipole interactions and hydrogen bonding. Supramolecular smart hydrogels are stimuli responsive and can be used in targeted drug delivery systems. Guanosine-based hydrogels have a tandem amount of importance in the field of water purification and drug delivery systems. Exploration of potential applications of guanosine gels has only recently begun to attract interest, with the major focus on columnar "G-wires" and layered thin films of guanosine "nanoribbons" as molecular wires for nanoelectronics and tissue scaffolding applications. Recent studies have focused primarily on developing novel guanosine-based gelators, improving the lifetime stability of guanosine hydrogels and utilising these materials for biomedical and drug delivery applications.

References

1. Beginn U, Sheiko S, Möller M (2000) Macromol Chem Phys 201:1008–1015
2. Lee KY, Mooney DJ (2001) Chem Rev 101:1869
3. Xing B, Yu CW, Chow KH, Ho PL, Fu D, Xu B (2002) J Am Chem Soc 124:14846
4. Kouwer PH, Koepf M, Le Sage VA, Jaspers M, van Buul AM, Eksteen-Akeroyd ZH, Woltinge T, Schwartz E, Kitto HJ, Hoogenboom R (2013) Nature 493:651–655
5. Zweep N, van Esch JH (2014) Functional molecular gels, pp 1–29
6. Weiss RG, Terech P (eds) (2006) Molecular gels, materials with self-assembled fibrillar networks. Springer, Dordrecht
7. Nishinari K (2009) Gels: structures, properties, and function. In: Tokita M, Nishinari K (eds), vol 136. Springer, pp 87–94
8. Fages F (2005) Low molecular mass gelators. Springer, Berlin
9. Peters GM, Davis JT (2016) Chem Soc Rev 45:3188
10. De Greef TFA, Smulders MMJ, Wolffs M, Schenning APHJ, Sijbesma RP, Meijer EW (2009) Chem Rev 109:5687–5754
11. Shi C, Huang Z, Kilic S, Xu J, Enick RM, Beckman EJ, Carr AJ, Melendez RE, Hamilton AD (1999) Science 286:1540

12. Hirst AR, Escuder B, Miravet JF, Smith DK et al (2008) High-tech applications of self-assembling supramolecular nanostructured gel-phase materials: from regenerative medicine to electronic devices. Angew Chem Int Ed 47:8002–8018
13. Skilling KJ, Citossi F, Bradshaw TD, Ashford M, Kellam B, Marlow M (2014) Insights into low molecular mass organic gelators: a focus on drug delivery and tissue engineering applications. Soft Matter 10:237–256
14. Liu XY, Li J-L (2013) Soft fibrillar materials: fabrication and applications. Wiley-VCH, Weinheim
15. Babu SS, Praveen VK, Ajayaghosh A (2014) Functional π-gelators and their applications. Chem Rev 114:1973–2129
16. Yagai S (2011) Supramolecular soft material. In: Nakanishi T (ed). Wiley, Hoboken, pp 77–95
17. Piepenbrock M, Lloyd GO, Clarke N, Steed JW (2010) Chem Rev 110:1960–2004
18. Hirst R, Smith DK (2005) Top Curr Chem 256:237–273
19. Soler M, Newkome GR (2012) Supramolecular chemistry: from molecules to nanomaterials. In: Gale PA, Steed JW. Wiley, pp 3283–3319
20. Fages F, Vögtle F, Zinic M (2005) Top Curr Chem 256:77–131
21. Schoonbeek FS, van Esch JH, Hulst R, Kelloggand RM, Feringa BL (2000) Chemistry 6:2633–2643
22. de Loos M, Ligtenbarg AGJ, van Esch J, Kooijman H, Spek AL, Hage R, Kellogg RM, Feringa BL (2000) Eur J Org Chem 3675–3678
23. Graham T (1861) Philos Trans R Soc Lond 151:183–224
24. Lloyd DJ (1926) Colloid Chem 1:767
25. Raeburn J, Cardoso A, Adams D (2013) Chem Soc Rev 42:5143–5156
26. Smith M, Williams RJ, Tang C, Coppo P, Collins RF, Turner ML, Saiani A, Ulijn RV (2008) Adv Mater 20:37–41
27. Braun H-G, Cardoso AZ (2012) Colloids Surf B 97:43–50
28. Israeachvili I, Wennerstrom H (1992) J Phys Chem 96:520–531
29. Aggeli A, Nyrkova IA, Bell M, Harding R, Carrick L, McLeish TCB, Semenov AN, Boden N (2001) Proc Natl Acad Sci USA 98:11857–11862
30. Liu XY (2005) Low molecular mass gelators: design, self-assembly, function. In: Fages F (ed), vol 256, pp 1–37
31. Liu XY, Sawant PD (2001) Appl Phys Lett 79:3518–3520
32. Liu XY, Sawant PD (2002) Angew Chem Int Ed 41:3641–3645
33. Liu XY, Sawant PD (2002) Adv Mater 14:421–426
34. Richter A, Paschew G, Klatt S, Lienig J, Arndt K-F, Adler H-JP (2008) Sensors 8:561–581
35. Cheng E, Xing Y, Chen P, Yang Y, Sun Y, Zhou D, Xu L, Fan Q, Liu D (2009) Angew Chem Int Ed 48:7660–7663
36. Marcombe R, Cai S, Hong W, Zhao X, Lapusta Y, Suo Z (2010) Soft Matter 6:784–793
37. Zhou SL, Matsumoto S, Tian HD, Yamane H, Ojida A, Kiyonaka S, Hamachi I (2005) Chem Eur J 11:1130–1136
38. Guiseppi-Elie A (2010) Biomaterials 31:2701–2716
39. Kulkarni RV, Sa B (2009) J Bioact Compat Polym 24:368–384
40. Kulkarni RV, Biswanath SA (2007) J Appl Biomater Biomech 5:125–139
41. Zhang RS, Tang MG, Bowyer A, Eisenthal R, Hubble J (2005) Biomaterials 26:4677–4683
42. Zhao B, Moore JS (2001) Langmuir 17:4758–4763
43. Traitel T, Kost J, Lapidot SA (2003) Biotechnol Bioeng 84:20–28
44. Liu T-Y, Hu S-H, Liu K-H, Liu D-M, Chen S-Y (2008) J Control Release 126:228–236
45. Liang Y-Y, Zhang L-M, Jiang W, Li W (2007) ChemPhysChem 8:2367–2372
46. Liu XY, Sawant PD, Tan WB, Noor IBM, Pramesti C, Chen BH (2002) J Am Chem Soc 124:15055–15063
47. Maeda S, Kato T, Kogure H, Hosoya N (2015) Appl Phys Lett 106:171909
48. Asmarandei I, Fundueanu G, Cristea M, Harabagiu V, Constantin M (2013) J Polym Res 20:293
49. Lee SC et al (2013) Adv Drug Deliv Rev 65:17–20

50. Wang QQ, Kong M, An Y, Liu Y, Li JJ, Zhou X, Feng C, Li J, Jiang SY, Cheng XJ, Chen XG (2013) J Mater Sci 48:5614–5623
51. Wichterle O, Lím D (1960) Hydrophilic gels for biological use. Nature 185:117–118
52. Rokita B, Rosiak JM, Ulanski P (2009) Macromolecules 42:3269–3274
53. Blackburn GM, Gait MJ, Loakes D, Williams DM (eds) (2006) Nucleic acids in chemistry and biology. Royal Society of Chemistry, Cambridge
54. Soyfer VN, Potaman VN (1995) Triple-helical nucleic acids. Springer, New York
55. Davis JT (2004) Angew Chem Int Ed 43:668–698
56. Du X et al (2015) Chem Rev 115:13165–13307
57. Balasubramanian S, Neidle S (eds) (2006) Quadruplex nucleic acids. Royal Society of Chemistry, Cambridge
58. Bhattacharyya T, Saha P, Dash J (2018) ACS Omega 3:2230–2241
59. Du X, Zhou J, Shi J, Xu B (2015) Supramolecular hydrogelators and hydrogels: from soft matter to molecular biomaterials. Chem Rev 115:13165–13307
60. Sangeetha NM, Maitra U (2005) Supramolecular gels: functions and uses. Chem Soc Rev 34:821–836
61. Datta S, Bhattacharya S (2015) Multifarious facets of sugar-derived molecular gels: molecular features, mechanisms of self-assembly and emerging applications. Chem Soc Rev 44:5596–5637
62. Buerkle LE, Rowan SJ (2012) Supramolecular gels formed from multi-component low molecular weight species. Chem Soc Rev 41:6089–6102
63. Estroff LA, Hamilton AD (2004) Water gelation by small organic molecules. Chem Rev 104:1201–1218

Chapter 9
Hydrogel as Bio-Ink for Organ Regeneration

Hemand Aravind, Blessy Joseph, and Sabu Thomas

Abstract An organ is an organ; nothing other can replace it or act as it. That is why there is an increasing medico-demand for tissue-engineered tissues and organs. Scientific world presently looking for alternative fabrication approaches to develop tissues and organs as conventional techniques is not capable of fabricating constructs with required structural, mechanical, and biological complexity. In such a condition, 3D bioprinting offers great potential to fabricate highly complex constructs with precise control of structure, mechanics, and biological matter, especially cells and extracellular matrix components. 3D bioprinting is an additive manufacturing approach that utilizes a "bioink" to fabricate devices and scaffolds in a layer-by-layer manner. 3D bioprinting allows printing of a cell suspension into a tissue construct with or without a scaffold support. The most common bioinks are cell-laden hydrogels, decellularized ECM-based solutions, and cell suspensions. In this chapter, an effort is taken to briefing hydrogels with particular focus on bioink design requirements. We also present the current state of the art in bioink design including the challenges and future directions.

Keywords Bio-fabrication · Tissue engineering · Regenerative medicine · Hydrogel · Cell printing · Extracellular matrix

1 Introduction

One of the promising and emerging multidisciplinary fields of bioengineering is tissue engineering, and its contribution comes majorly on two areas: (i) developing new methods to repair, regenerate, and replace damaged tissues and organs

H. Aravind
Department of Chemistry, Aromatic and Medicinal Plant Research Station, Eranakulam, Kerala, India

B. Joseph · S. Thomas (✉)
International and Inter University Centre for Nano Science and Nanotechnology, Mahatma Gandhi University, PD Hills (PO), Kottayam, Kerala 686 560, India
e-mail: sabuthomas@mgu.ac.in

J. Jose et al. (eds.), *Nano Hydrogels*, Gels Horizons: From Science to Smart Materials,
https://doi.org/10.1007/978-981-15-7138-1_9

and (ii) Constructing in vitro tissue models to better understand tissue development, disease development, and screen mode of action of new drugs [1–6]. In our changed social health status, more people are vulnerable to serious diseases which are directly affecting vital organs like kidney, liver, heart, pancreases, etc. In spite of latest advances in tissue engineering, there is a continuous lack of tissues and organs for transplantation and a shortage for tissue models for drug discovery and testing [7]. Extensively long waiting lists for organ transplantation exist all around the world. According to U.S. Department of Health and Human Services, as of June 2017, around 120,000 patients are in need of lifesaving organ transplant in the USA while only about 5200 donors are available. Also, while the number of transplants performed every year since 2003 has been somehow constant, the number of patients waiting at the year-end has been growing [8]. Under these circumstances, scientists are eager to find alternative ways to compensate for this shortage of organ. Unfortunately, conventional techniques, such as porogen-leaching, injection molding, and electrospinning, are generally recognized as the bottleneck due to limited control over scaffold architecture, composition, pore shape, size, and distribution [9–11]. 3D bioprinting is an actively studied method in tissue engineering since it shows effective control over scaffold fabrication and cell distribution. Printing resolution of 3D bioprinting techniques is 10–10,000 mm which is a wide range showing flexibility of bioprinting compared to other assembly methods such as molding and porous scaffolds. 3D bioprinting enables fabrication of scaffolds, devices, and tissue models with high complexity [9, 11–14]. 3D printing enables creation of tissues from commonly used medical images (such as X-ray, magnetic resonance imaging, and computerized tomography scan) using computer-aided design. Custom and patient-specific design, on-demand fabrication, high structural complexity, low-cost, and high-efficiency are some of the major advantages of 3D printing and such things making it very attractive for medicine [15, 16].

3D bioprinting is a technology to fabricate constructs from living cells with or without a carrier material in a layer-by-layer manner [9, 11, 12, 17, 18]. The material that is printed is referred to as a "bioink," which can be defined as an ink formulation that allows printing of living cells. Here, we would like to note that many of the biomaterial ink formulations are not suitable for cell printing. For instance, polycaprolactone (PCL) and poly(lactic acid) (PLA) are the most widely used biomaterials in 3D printing. However, they could only be printed at elevated temperatures in the form of a polymer melt or when dissolved in organic solvents as a polymer solution. Therefore, they are not considered as bioinks in this review, as both approaches are not suitable for live cell printing [19, 20]. In this paper, we discuss one among the most commonly used bioinks, cell-laden hydrogels [16, 21–23] and give the current state of the art in bioink design with challenges and future directions. A brief description and comparison of the bioprinting methods with particular focus on bioink design requirements are also given.

2 3D Bioprinting Technologies

3D printing technology is a promising innovative concept in tissue engineering; instead of using 2D structures with numerous limitations, nowadays scientists can use 3D scaffolds for cell studies. 3D bioprinting is comparatively manageable and cell friendly as it is required to allow cell printing, and of course this requirements restricted the number of 3D printing techniques that are appropriate for bioprinting (Fig. 1) [13, 24]. At present, the 3D printing technology available in industry can print a wide range of materials by using diverse ink formulations [16]. Fused deposition modeling (FDM) is a 3D printing technique pioneered in the 1990s by Stratasys, and presently, it is the trade mark of company. The company continues to be a leader in manufacturing 3D printers all over the world. Alternatively, the 3D printers that are based on this technology are also called as fused filament fabrication (FFF), plastic jet printing (PJP) or material extruding printers, which is the generic name for these 3D printers. Fused deposition modeling (FDM) is an extrusion-based printing and utilizes synthetic thermoplastics and their composites with ceramics and metals [25]. Because of its best performance at high temperature (140–250 °C) in melt state, it eliminates FDM as an option for bioprinting. Direct ink writing (DIW) is also an extrusion-based printing widely utilized in meso- and micro-scales and allows extrusion of high viscosity solutions, hydrogels, and colloidal suspensions [14]. DIW allows printing of cell suspensions and/or aggregates with or without a carrier. Inkjet printing is another technology for cell printing. The processing principle is deposition of polymeric solutions, colloidal suspensions, and cell suspensions, with relatively low viscosities [<10 cP (mPa s)] at relatively high shear rates (10^5–10^6 s^{-1}) in the form droplets (~50 μm in diameter) [26–29]. As compared to extrusion-based bioprinters, inkjet bioprinters are not readily available. Drop-on-demand printing that is one of the inkjet printing technologies enables the printing of complex and precise sections of living tissues or organs on the culture substrates utilizing cells and/or biomaterials as bioinks [30, 31]. Selective laser sintering utilizes metals, ceramics, polymers, and composites in powder form (10–150 μm in diameter) and is not suitable for bioprinting. In this technique, a directed laser beam locally melts either directly the powder or a polymeric binder onto the bed surface [32]. Layers of fresh powder are continuously supplied after each layer is created. Stereolithography (SLA) requires

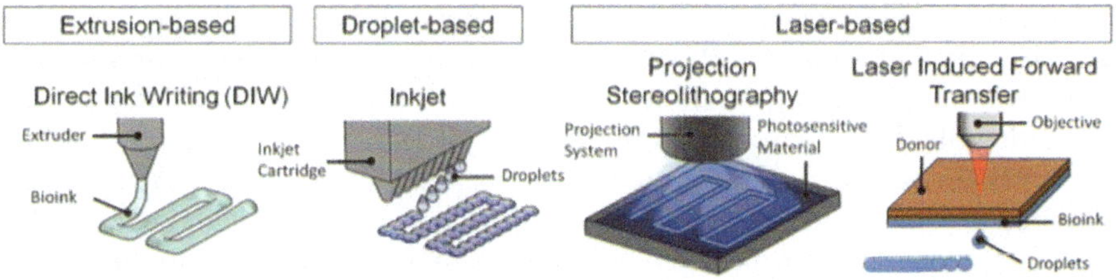

Fig. 1 3D bioprinting techniques for bioprinting of tissues and organs. Figure with permission from Miller and Burdick [43]. Copyright 2016, American Chemical Society reproduced

a viscous photocurable polymer solution or a prepolymer, which is exposed to a directed light (such as UV or laser) to spatially cross-link the solution [33]. SLA could potentially be considered for printing live cells as long as a cell-laden prepolymer formulation is used and the photocuring takes place in a mild, cell-friendly condition, which is the two major issues for SLA in bioprinting [34–36]. When 3D printing technologies are considered for bioprinting, the most commonly used technologies are DIW and inkjet printing [13, 14]. In addition to these technologies, laser-induced forward transfer (LIFT) is also shown to be suitable for bioprinting [37–42]. In this technique, ink solution is coated onto a glass slide and coated with a laser absorption layer (metal or a metal oxide). Laser is directed to the laser absorption layer with an ablation spot size between 40 and 100 μm in diametercreating a local pressure to eject the ink layer to the substrate.

3 Bioink Design

An ultimate bioink formulation should gratify certain material and biological requirements. Material properties are printability, mechanics, degradation, and functionalizability. Biological requirements mainly include biocompatibility, cytocompatilibilty, and bioactivity. When material properties are considered, printability is the most important constraint. Printability encompasses two parts: (i) the processability of the bioink formulation and (ii) the print fidelity associated with the mechanical strength of the printed construct to self-sustain a 3D structure post-printing. Depending on the printing process, printability could potentially involve solution viscosity, surface tension, and cross-linking properties. Viscosity is a crucial parameter for a bioink formulation as it affects both the print fidelity and cell encapsulation efficiency. High viscosity polymer solutions are less likely to flow easily so that the printed structure could hold its shape at longer times post-printing. However, they require higher pressures to flow, limiting the gage size and smallest achievable print size (mainly for DIW). In this regard, Tirella et al. [44] investigated the processing window for alginate hydrogels using pressure-assisted microfabrication (DIW technique). They successfully developed a 3D phase diagram showing the interplay between bioink viscosity, print velocity, and applied pressure to obtain high print reliability [44]. The bioink formulation is preferred to have a tunable viscosity to be compatible with different bioprinters. For instance, bioinks for inkjet or droplet-based bioprinters have viscosity values close to 10 mPa s [29]; the viscosity of bioinks for extrusion-based DIW bioprinting ranges from 30 to 6×10^7 mPa s [13, 14, 45]; for laser-assisted bioprinting, the bioink viscosity is in the range of 1–300 mPa s [45, 46]. For high viscosity bioinks used in extrusion and droplet-based print, the shear-thinning feature is desired to compensate for the high shear stress associated with high viscosity. The overall mechanics, i.e., achievable stiffness, is important not only to create self-supporting constructs but also to control and direct cellular behavior. Degradation is important for the functional amalgamation of the printed construct in vivo by enabling cells to gradually replace the construct with their ECM. Both the bioink and the degradation products should not contain materials that induce inflammatory host response when implanted. Functionalizability is required to incorporate biochemical cues, i.e., bioactivity, to direct cellular behavior, such as adhesion, migration, and differentiation. In addition to biocompatibility and cytocompatibility, high cell viability, both prior- and post-printing, is crucial for the ink formulation. In addition to bioink design, a recent study showed the importance of the print substrate for live cell inkjet printing. In this work, computational and experimental studies confirmed that the stiffness of the print substrate directly influences the impact forces acting on the droplet, which affects the overall cell survival [47]. Below we will discuss the commonly used bioinks including current state of the art in ink design.

4 Established Bioinks

The most commonly used bioinks for tissue and organ printing are cell-laden hydrogels, decellularized extracellular matrix (dECM)-based solutions, and cell suspensions (Fig. 2). Cell-laden hydrogels are particularly attractive due to their tunable properties and their ability to recapitulate the cellular microenvironment [48]. ECM-based bioink formulations or decellulerized tissue inks are an emerging field due to their inherent bioactivity and ease of formulation into a printable bioink [49]. Cell suspension inks based on cell aggregates are a viable option to create scaffold-free biological constructs [50, 51].

5 Cell-Laden Hydrogels

Cell-laden hydrogels are the most commonly used bioinks as they can be easily formulated for extrusion-based (DIW), droplet-based (inkjet), and laser-based (SLA and LIFT) bioprinting technologies. Cell-laden hydrogel bioink formulations utilize natural hydrogels such as agarose, alginate, chitosan, collagen, gelatin, fibrin, and hyaluronic acid (HA), as well as synthetic hydrogels such as pluronic (poloxamer) and poly(ethylene glycol) (PEG), or blends of both. Natural hydrogels offer inherent bioactivity except for agarose and alginate and display a structural resemblance to ECM. For instance, fibrin and collagen hydrogels with inherent filamentous structure display strain-stiffening property, mimicking the nonlinear elastic behavior of the soft tissues in our body [54, 55]. Synthetic hydrogels permit but do not promote cellular function, yet there are many ways to tether bioactive cues into synthetic hydrogels [56]. When compared to natural hydrogels, synthetic hydrogels generally offer tunable mechanical properties. Many natural polymers (such as gelatin and HA) have functionalizable backbone side chains enabling them to be functionalized with chemical moieties to induce cross-linking (chemical- and/or photo-cross-linking) or additional bioactivity [57]. Blends of synthetic and natural polymers have been used to develop mechanically tunable hydrogels with user-defined bioactivity. Finally, the

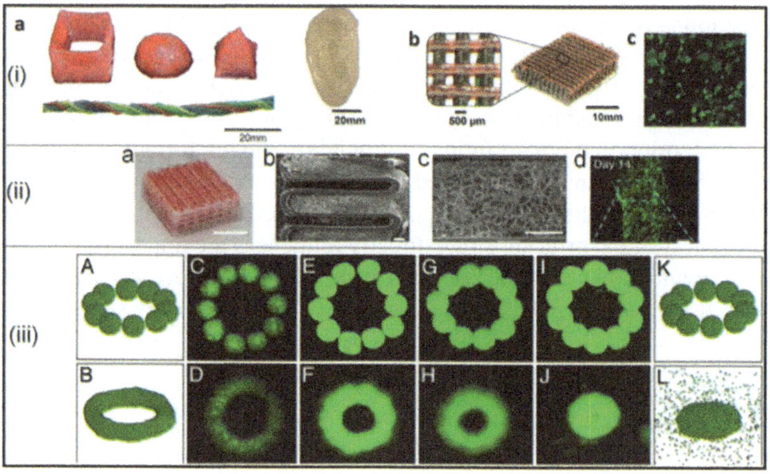

Fig. 2 **i** 3D printed constructs in various forms (**a**, **b**) using poly(ethylene glycol)–alginate–nanoclay hydrogels. Red food dye was incorporated into some of the bioink formulations for visibility. Live/dead assay of cells (**c**) in a collagen infused mesh from (**b**). Reprinted with permission from Hong et al. [52]. Copyright 2015, John Wiley and Sons. **ii** Tissue construct printed from decellularized extracellular matrix (dECM) (**a**), SEM images of hybrid constructs from dECM supported with polycaprolactone framework (**b**, **c**), and fluorescent images of cells (**d**). Scale bars are 5 mm for (**a**), 400 μm for (**b**, **c**), and 100 μm for (**d**). Adapted with permission from Pati et al. [49]. Copyright 2014, Nature Publishing Group. **iii** Cell aggregate (500-μm average diameter) configurations in simulations (**A**, **B**, **K**, **L**) and experiments. **C–J** correspond to cell aggregates embedded in a neurogel with RGD fragments (**C**, **D**) and collagen gels of concentration 1.0 mg/ml (**E**, **F**), 1.2 mg/ml (**G**, **H**), and 1.7 mg/ml (**I**, **J**). Figure adapted with permission from [53]. Copyright 2004, National Academy of Sciences

mechanical properties and/or bioactivity can also be tuned by incorporating small amounts of nanoparticles into bioink formulation [58].

Usually, all hydrogel bioink formulations require printing of a polymer solution followed by subsequent cross-linking. This requires a highly viscous polymer solution (polymer wt% >3%) and rapid cross-linking to develop self-supporting structures. There are two forms of cross-linking: physical and chemical cross-linking. Physical cross-linking is a non-chemical approach that utilizes hydrophobic interactions, ionic interactions, and hydrogen bonding. Chemical cross-linking relies on the formation of covalent bonds, which could be a radical polymerization (such as photo-cross-linking) or Michael-type addition reaction. The chemically cross-linked hydrogels form a mechanically robust network as compared to the physically cross-linked hydrogels, which is particularly important for the stem cell behavior including differentiation [59, 60]. Recently, hydrogels have been defined as two- or multi-component systems consisting of a three-dimensional network of polymer chains and water that fills the space between macromolecules. Depending on the properties of the polymer (polymers) used, as well as on the nature and density of the network joints, such structures in an equilibrium can contain various amounts of water; typically in the swollen state, the mass fraction of water in a hydrogel is much higher than the mass fraction of polymer. In practice, to achieve high degrees of swelling, it is common to use synthetic polymers that are water-soluble when in non-cross-linked form.

Hydrogels may be synthesized in a number of "classical" chemical ways. These include one-step procedures like polymerization and parallel cross-linking of multifunctional monomers, as well as multiple step procedures involving synthesis of polymer molecules having reactive groups and their subsequent cross-linking, possibly also by reacting polymers with suitable cross-linking agents. The polymer engineer can design and synthesize polymer networks with molecular-scale control over structure such as cross-linking density and with tailored properties, such as biodegradation, mechanical strength, and chemical and biological response to stimuli [61].

Pluronic and PEG are the most common synthetic polymers for bioprinting. Pluronic, a poloxamer-based triblock copolymer composed of two hydrophobic groups between a water-soluble group, has been widely used in extrusion-based bioprinting as it gels at room temperature but flows at temperatures below 10 °C. However, it is not very stable and erodes within hours. Thus, it is generally used as a supporting material [62]. Lewis Lab took an advantage of this property and printed pluronic within a photopolymerizable hydrogel to create micro-channels [63]. Müller et al. [64] developed an acrylated pluronic to create UV cross-linked stable gels post-printing [64]. The most common forms of PEG for bioinks are PEG-diacrylate (PEG-DA) and PEG-methacrylate, which are suitable for extrusion-based, droplet-based, and laser-based printing technologies [52, 65, 66]. PEG is hydrophilic and not adhesive to proteins and cells; therefore, it requires blending with other natural polymers or functionalization with biochemical cues. It is possible to form strong robust hydrogels using PEG-based polymers. For instance, Hockaday et al. [67] printed aortic valve geometries using PEG-DA hydrogels blended with alginate and achieved tenfold range in elastic modulus from ~5 to ~75 kPa [67]. Hong et al. [52] reported D printing of tough and biocompatible, cell-laden PEG–alginate–nanoclay hydrogels infused with collagen [68]. Rutz et al. [69] developed partially cross-linked PEG-based multi-material bioink formulations with tunable viscosity to enhance print fidelity and secondary cross-linking ability to stabilize the constructs [69].

Alginate is one of the most commonly used natural polymers to formulate bioinks for inkjet and DIW printing. For inkjet printing, calcium chloride is jetted onto alginic acid solution [70]. For extrusion-based printing, alginate is printed as a viscous solution, and the constructs are exposed to $CaCl_2$ solution to induce post-printing cross-linking. Alginate is not cell adhesive, thus it is generally blended with other natural polymers (e.g., gelatin and fibrinogen) to induce cell adhesion and biological activity [71–75]. Note that the majority of the natural polymers are used as a component of bioink formulation. HA and gelatin that have been utilized extensively in the form of functionalized polymers thus fall into the synthetic polymer category, which is discussed below.

Gelatin is commonly used in the form of gelatin methacryloyl (GelMA)-based hydrogel for DIW [76, 77]. Lim et al. [74] recently reported a visible light photo-cross-linking system to minimize the oxygen inhibition in photopolymerized GelMA hydrogels [74]. They reported higher print fidelity and cell viability for ruthenium/sodium persulfate visible photo-initiator as compared to UV photo-initiator Igracure 2959. Similar to gelatin, HA has been modified in many ways to create cell-laden bioinks [78–80]. For instance, Burdick Lab reported HA-based supramolecular hydrogels cross-linked by cyclodextrin–adamantane host–guest interactions, which are capable of shear-thinning and self-healing [78]. The non-covalent bonds allow direct writing of inks into support gels. HA hydrogels were developed to display both shear-thinning behavior due to guest–host bonding and stabilization post-printing via UV-induced covalent cross-linking [80]. Supramolecular hydrogels are particularly attractive for extrusion-based printing as they could flow under shear and self-heal immediately after printing, leading to high print fidelity. In addition to guest–host bonding, self-assembling peptides [81] and polypeptide–DNA hydrogels [82] are other emerging candidates for bioink design.

6 Nanoparticle-Reinforced Hydrogels

Nanocomposite hydrogels are found to be more superior to conventional hydrogels in terms of stability, mechanical strength, and stiffness. Hybrid ink of monomer (*N*-acryloyl glycinamide) (NAGA) and nanoclay (Laponite XLG) was developed by Zhai et al. suitable for 3D printing. The printed pregel NAGA-clay fine-tuned to form PNAGA clay composite hydrogel scaffold by polymerizing with UV light radiation. The prepared scaffolds supported osteogenic differentiation of primary rat osteoblast (ROB) cells. Moreover they facilitated the regeneration of new bone in tibia defects of rats [83]. Water immersion studies were performed, and it was concluded that even after immersion for months, the scaffold was stable and did not show further swelling activity. Thus, it was confirmed that addition of nanoclay into PNAGA had no influence on hydrogen bonding interactions. The mechanical properties was analyzed in terms of bearing external load investigated by pressing the sample with car wheel and hand folding as shown in Fig. 3.

Nanoparticles show great promise for purification and removal of toxins. This strategy have been used to fabricate toxification device that mimic liver lobule microstructure. The matrix poly(ethylene glycol) diacrylate (PEGDA) allows the efficient trapping of toxins while polyacetylene nanopartciles sense and attract toxins [84]. The ability to produce patient-specific implants is a major attraction of 3D printing or additive manufacturing. It has enabled the design of complex architectures required for hearing aids. A team of researchers developed bionic ear using alginate hydrogel matrix (Fig. 4). The matrix pre-seeded with viable chondrocytes was then 3D printed along with silver nanoparticle-infused silicone solutions. The printed bionic ear possessed enhanced auditory sensing for radio frequency reception

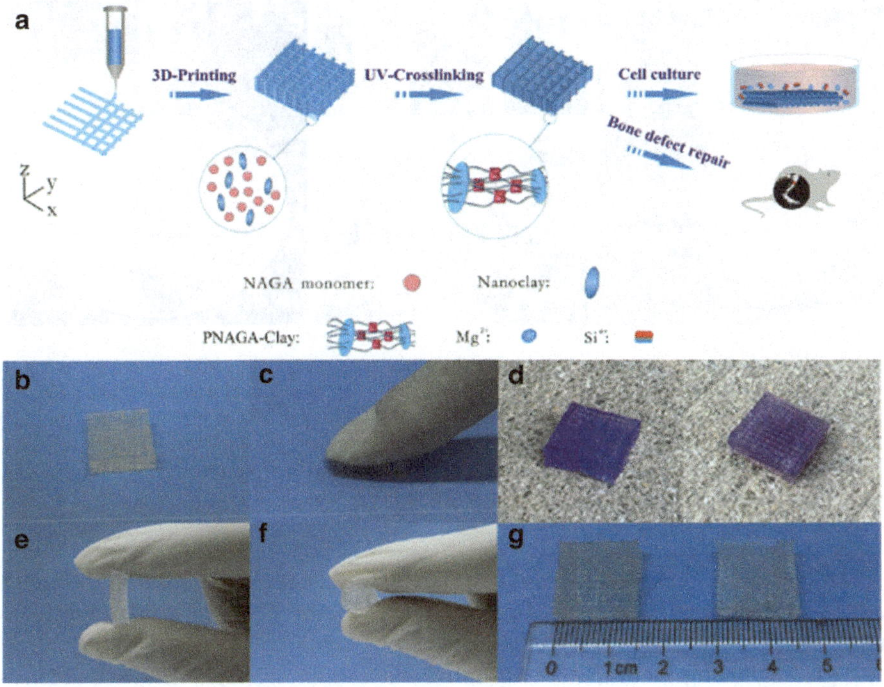

Fig. 3 Procedure of 3D-printing PNAGA-clay scaffold (**a**) and photographs of PNAGA20%-clay scaffolds showing their ability to resist finger compression (**b** and **c**), car wheel pressing (**d** left and right denote before and after pressing), and hand folding (**e** and **f**). The scaffold is very stable even after immersing in water for a long time (**g** and left and right denote before and after water immersion for 3 months). The scaffolds used for the car wheel pressing experiment were stained with gentian violet. Reproduced with permission from [83]. Copyright © 2017, American Chemical Society

and moreover the printing process had no adverse effect on the viability of the cells [85].

Hydrogels based on cellulose are widely known for their availability, biocompatibility, and efficient cell encapsulation [86]. Nanocellulose containing hydrogels have shown good cell growth and cell viability. NFC-alginate bioink was used to print auricular constructs along with chondrocytes [87]. The chondrocyte cells proliferated and cartilage specific extracellular matrix was seen around the cells.

7 Summary and Future Perspectives

3D printing has a strong potential to become a common fabrication technique in medicine as it enables fabrication of modular and patient-specific scaffolds and devices, and tissue models, with high structural complexity and design flexibility

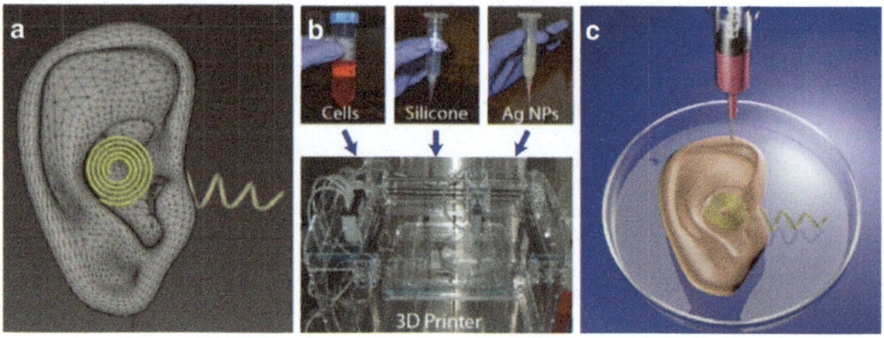

Fig. 4 Three-dimensional interweaving of biology and electronics via additive manufacturing to generate a bionic ear. (**a**) CAD drawing of the bionic ear. (**b**) (top) Optical images of the functional materials, including biological (chondrocytes), structural (silicone), and electronic (AgNP-infused silicone) used to form the bionic ear. (Bottom) a 3D printer used for the printing process. (**c**) Illustration of the 3D printed bionic ear. Reproduced with permission from [85]. Copyright © 2013, American Chemical Society

[5, 9, 62, 88–91]. There is a significant interest in designing novel bioink formulations toward the goal of achieving the "ideal" bioink for each bioprinting technology [45]. Cell-laden hydrogels are the most common bioinks, offering novel strategies including multi-material printing, shear-thinning capability, and sequential cross-linking toward self-supporting constructs. Decellularized extracellular matrix (dECM)-based bioinks provide an alternative approach utilizing decellularized tissues, yet the processing of decellularized tissue increases the cost of the bioinks. Cell aggregate printing enables direct printing of cells into tissue constructs, but the size of these constructs is currently limited as the process requires large quantities of cells. In addition to bioink development, there is also need for bioprinters with high resolution, which is particularly important to develop vascularized constructs. Considering future perspectives, supramolecular hydrogels with reversible cross-linking mechanism [79] and stimuli-responsive materials for biomimetic 4D printing [92] are potentially the most interesting candidates for bioink design. Four-dimensional (4D) printing is an emerging as a fascinating method to fabricate stimuli-responsive 3D structures with wide applications in organ engineering and tissue regeneration. The concept introduced in 2013 has gained much popularity, and several hydrogel-based inks have been developed for 4D printing. Much of the works focus on altering the shape of the 3D printed materials in response to temperature change or water absorption [93]. 4D printing may provide a novel platform for biomedical studies of functional synthetic tissues and organs. Significant efforts are required to design highly robust hydrogels having shape memory effect. Development of such hydrogels are still in the infant stage. There are still many hurdles to overcome when considered for biomedical applications, since biocompatibility and biodegradability is a major concern when tissue engineering is concerned. Finally, there are still many regulatory challenges to move the 3D bioprinted constructs into clinic.

References

1. Griffith LG, Naughton G (2002) Tissue engineering—current challenges and expanding opportunities. Science (80–). https://doi.org/10.1126/science.1069210
2. Benam KH, Dauth S, Hassell B, Herland A, Jain A, Jang K-J, Karalis K, Kim HJ, MacQueen L, Mahmoodian R, Musah S, Torisawa Y, van der Meer AD, Villenave R, Yadid M, Parker KK, Ingber DE, Engineered in vitro disease models. Annu Rev Pathol. https://doi.org/10.1146/annurev-pathol-012414-040418
3. Tibbitt MW, Rodell CB, Burdick JA, Anseth KS (2015) Progress in material design for biomedical applications. Proc Natl Acad Sci. https://doi.org/10.1073/pnas.1516247112
4. Nguyen D, Hägg DA, Alma F, Ekholm J, Brants C, Kalogeropoulos T, Zaunz S, Concaro S, Brittberg M, Lindah A, Gatenholm P, Enejder A (2017) Cartilage tissue engineering by the 3D bioprinting of iPS cells in a nanocellulose/alginate bioink. Sci Rep 7:1–10. https://doi.org/10.1038/s41598-017-00690-y
5. Zhang YS, Duchamp M, Oklu R, Ellisen LW, Langer R, Khademhosseini A (2016) Bioprinting the cancer microenvironment. ACS Biomater Sci Eng. https://doi.org/10.1021/acsbiomaterials.6b00246
6. Langer R, Vacanti J (1993) Tissue engineering. Science (80–):260, 920–926. https://doi.org/10.1126/science.8493529
7. Bajaj P, Schweller RM, Khademhosseini A, West JL, Bashir R (2014) 3D biofabrication strategies for tissue engineering and regenerative medicine. Annu Rev Biomed Eng. https://doi.org/10.1146/annurev-bioeng-071813-105155
8. https://optn.transplant.hrsa.gov (n.d.)
9. Murphy SV, Atala A (2014) 3D bioprinting of tissues and organs. Nat Biotechnol. https://doi.org/10.1038/nbt.2958
10. Groen N, Guvendiren M, Rabitz H, Welsh WJ, Kohn J, De Boer J (2016) Stepping into the omics era: opportunities and challenges for biomaterials science and engineering. Acta Biomater. https://doi.org/10.1016/j.actbio.2016.02.015
11. Shafiee A, Atala A (2016) Printing technologies for medical applications. Trends Mol Med. https://doi.org/10.1016/j.molmed.2016.01.003
12. Mandrycky C, Wang Z, Kim K, Kim DH (2016) 3D bioprinting for engineering complex tissues. Biotechnol Adv. https://doi.org/10.1016/j.biotechadv.2015.12.011
13. Ozbolat IT, Moncal KK, Gudapati H (2017) Evaluation of bioprinter technologies. Addit Manuf. https://doi.org/10.1016/j.addma.2016.10.003
14. Ozbolat IT, Hospodiuk M (2016) Current advances and future perspectives in extrusion-based bioprinting. Biomaterials. https://doi.org/10.1016/j.biomaterials.2015.10.076
15. Guillemot F, Mironov V, Nakamura M (2010) Bioprinting is coming of age: report from the international conference on bioprinting and biofabrication in bordeaux (3B'09). In: Biofabrication. https://doi.org/10.1088/1758-5082/2/1/010201
16. Guvendiren M, Molde J, Soares RMD, Kohn J (2016) Designing biomaterials for 3D printing. ACS Biomater Sci Eng. https://doi.org/10.1021/acsbiomaterials.6b00121
17. Dababneh AB, Ozbolat IT (2014) Bioprinting technology: a current state-of-the-art review. J Manuf Sci Eng. https://doi.org/10.1115/1.4028512
18. Cui H, Nowicki M, Fisher JP, Zhang LG (2017) 3D bioprinting for organ regeneration. Adv Healthc Mater. https://doi.org/10.1002/adhm.201601118
19. Jose RR, Rodriguez MJ, Dixon TA, Omenetto F, Kaplan DL (2016) Evolution of bioinks and additive manufacturing technologies for 3D bioprinting. ACS Biomater Sci Eng. https://doi.org/10.1021/acsbiomaterials.6b00088
20. Munaz A, Vadivelu RK, St John J, Barton M, Kamble H, Nguyen NT (2016) Three-dimensional printing of biological matters. J Sci Adv Mater Dev. https://doi.org/10.1016/j.jsamd.2016.04.001
21. Levato R, Visser J, Planell JA, Engel E, Malda J, Mateos-Timoneda MA (2014) Biofabrication of tissue constructs by 3D bioprinting of cell-laden microcarriers. Biofabrication. https://doi.org/10.1088/1758-5082/6/3/035020

22. Jakus AE, Rutz AL, Shah RN (2016) Advancing the field of 3D biomaterial printing. Biomed Mater. https://doi.org/10.1088/1748-6041/11/1/014102
23. Panwar A, Tan LP (2016) Current status of bioinks for micro-extrusion-based 3D bioprinting. Molecules. https://doi.org/10.3390/molecules21060685
24. Ozbolat IT, Peng W, Ozbolat V (2016) Application areas of 3D bioprinting. Drug Discov Today. https://doi.org/10.1016/j.drudis.2016.04.006
25. Turner BN, Strong R, Gold SA (2014) A review of melt extrusion additive manufacturing processes: I. Process design and modeling. Rapid Prototyp J. https://doi.org/10.1108/RPJ-01-2013-0012
26. Mironov V, Boland T, Trusk T, Forgacs G, Markwald RR (2003) Organ printing: computer-aided jet-based 3D tissue engineering. Trends Biotechnol. https://doi.org/10.1016/S0167-7799(03)00033-7
27. Wilson WC, Boland T (2003) Cell and organ printing 1: protein and cell printers, Anat Rec Part A Discov Mol Cell Evol Biol. https://doi.org/10.1002/ar.a.10057
28. Nakamura M, Kobayashi A, Takagi F, Watanabe A, Hiruma Y, Ohuchi K, Iwasaki Y, Horie M, Morita I, Takatani S (2006) Biocompatible inkjet printing technique for designed seeding of individual living cells. Tissue Eng. https://doi.org/10.1089/ten.2005.11.1658
29. Gudapati H, Dey M, Ozbolat I (2016) A comprehensive review on droplet-based bioprinting: past, present and future. Biomaterials. https://doi.org/10.1016/j.biomaterials.2016.06.012
30. Nishiyama Y, Nakamura M, Henmi C, Yamaguchi K, Mochizuki S, Nakagawa H, Takiura K (2009) Development of a three-dimensional bioprinter: construction of cell supporting structures using hydrogel and state-of-the-art inkjet technology. J Biomech Eng. https://doi.org/10.1115/1.3002759
31. Choi WS, Ha D, Park S, Kim T (2011) Synthetic multicellular cell-to-cell communication in inkjet printed bacterial cell systems. Biomaterials. https://doi.org/10.1016/j.biomaterials.2010.12.014
32. Shirazi SFS, Gharehkhani S, Mehrali M, Yarmand H, Metselaar HSC, Adib Kadri N, Osman NAA (2015) A review on powder-based additive manufacturing for tissue engineering: selective laser sintering and inkjet 3D printing. Sci Technol Adv Mater. https://doi.org/10.1088/1468-6996/16/3/033502
33. Skoog SA, Goering PL, Narayan RJ (2014) Stereolithography in tissue engineering. J Mater Sci Mater Med. https://doi.org/10.1007/s10856-013-5107-y
34. Elomaa L, Pan CC, Shanjani Y, Malkovskiy A, Seppälä JV, Yang Y (2015) Three-dimensional fabrication of cell-laden biodegradable poly(ethylene glycol-co-depsipeptide) hydrogels by visible light stereolithography. J Mater Chem B. https://doi.org/10.1039/c5tb01468a
35. Wang Z, Abdulla R, Parker B, Samanipour R, Ghosh S, Kim K (2015) A simple and high-resolution stereolithography-based 3D bioprinting system using visible light crosslinkable bioinks. Biofabrication. https://doi.org/10.1088/1758-5090/7/4/045009
36. Morris VB, Nimbalkar S, Younesi M, McClellan P, Akkus O (2017) Mechanical properties, cytocompatibility and manufacturability of chitosan: PEGDA hybrid-gel scaffolds by stereolithography. Ann Biomed Eng. https://doi.org/10.1007/s10439-016-1643-1
37. Barron JA, Spargo BJ, Ringeisen BR (2004) Biological laser printing of three dimensional cellular structures. Appl Phys A Mater Sci Process. https://doi.org/10.1007/s00339-004-2620-3.
38. Barron JA, Wu P, Ladouceur HD, Ringeisen BR (2004) Biological laser printing: A novel technique for creating heterogeneous 3-dimensional cell patterns. Biomed Microdevices. https://doi.org/10.1023/B:BMMD.0000031751.67267.9f
39. Ringeisen BR, Kim H, Barron JA, Krizman DB, Chrisey DB, Jackman S, Auyeung RYC, Spargo BJ (2004) Laser printing of pluripotent embryonal carcinoma cells. Tissue Eng. https://doi.org/10.1089/107632704323061843
40. Hopp B, Smausz T, Kresz N, Barna N, Bor Z, Kolozsvári L, Chrisey DB, Szabó A, Nógrádi A (2005) Survival and proliferative ability of various living cell types after laser-induced forward transfer. Tissue Eng. https://doi.org/10.1089/ten.2005.11.1817

41. Doraiswamy A, Narayan RJ, Lippert T, Urech L, Wokaun A, Nagel M, Hopp B, Dinescu M, Modi R, Auyeung RCY, Chrisey DB (2006) Excimer laser forward transfer of mammalian cells using a novel triazene absorbing layer. Appl Surf Sci. https://doi.org/10.1016/j.apsusc.2005.07.166
42. Koch L, Kuhn S, Sorg H, Gruene M, Schlie S, Gaebel R, Polchow B, Reimers K, Stoelting S, Ma N, Vogt PM, Steinhoff G, Chichkov B (2010) Laser printing of skin cells and human stem cells. Tissue Eng Part C Methods. https://doi.org/10.1089/ten.tec.2009.0397
43. Miller JS, Burdick JA (2016) Editorial: special issue on 3D printing of biomaterials. ACS Biomater Sci Eng 2:1658–1661. https://doi.org/10.1021/acsbiomaterials.6b00566
44. Tirella A, Orsini A, Vozzi G, Ahluwalia A (2009) A phase diagram for microfabrication of geometrically controlled hydrogel scaffolds. Biofabrication. https://doi.org/10.1088/1758-5082/1/4/045002
45. Hölzl K, Lin S, Tytgat L, Van Vlierberghe S, Gu L, Ovsianikov A (2016) Bioink properties before, during and after 3D bioprinting. Biofabrication. https://doi.org/10.1088/1758-5090/8/3/032002
46. Guillotin B, Souquet A, Catros S, Duocastella M, Pippenger B, Bellance S, Bareille R, Rémy M, Bordenave L, Amédée J, Guillemot F (2010) Laser assisted bioprinting of engineered tissue with high cell density and microscale organization. Biomaterials. https://doi.org/10.1016/j.biomaterials.2010.05.055
47. Tirella A, Vozzi F, De Maria C, Vozzi G, Sandri T, Sassano D, Cognolato L, Ahluwalia A (2011) Substrate stiffness influences high resolution printing of living cells with an ink-jet system. J Biosci Bioeng. https://doi.org/10.1016/j.jbiosc.2011.03.019
48. Fedorovich NE, Alblas J, de Wijn JR, Hennink WE, Verbout AJ, Dhert WJA (2007) Hydrogels as extracellular matrices for skeletal tissue engineering: state-of-the-art and novel application in organ printing. Tissue Eng. https://doi.org/10.1089/ten.2006.0175
49. Pati F, Jang J, Ha DH, Won Kim S, Rhie JW, Shim JH, Kim DH, Cho DW (2014) Printing three-dimensional tissue analogues with decellularized extracellular matrix bioink. Nat Commun. https://doi.org/10.1038/ncomms4935
50. Forgacs G, Foty RA (2004) Biological relevance of tissue liquidity and viscoelasticity. In: Deutsch A, Howard J, Falcke M, Zimmermann W (eds) Function and regulation of cellular systems. Birkhäuser, Basel, pp 269–277
51. Marga F, Neagu A, Kosztin I, Forgacs G (2007) Developmental biology and tissue engineering. Birth Defects Res C Embryo Today. https://doi.org/10.1002/bdrc.20109
52. Wüst S, Müller R, Hofmann S (2015) 3D Bioprinting of complex channels—effects of material, orientation, geometry, and cell embedding. J Biomed Mater Res Part A. https://doi.org/10.1002/jbm.a.35393
53. Jakab K, Neagu A, Mironov V, Markwald RR, Forgacs G (2004) Engineering biological structures of prescribed shape using self-assembling multicellular systems. Proc Natl Acad Sci. https://doi.org/10.1073/pnas.0400164101
54. Gardel ML, Shin JH, MacKintosh FC, Mahadevan L, Matsudaira P, Weitz DA (2004) Elastic behavior of cross-linked and bundled actin networks. Science (80–). https://doi.org/10.1126/science.1095087.
55. Storm C, Pastore JJ, MacKintosh FC, Lubensky TC, Janmey PA (2005) Nonlinear elasticity in biological gels. Nature. https://doi.org/10.1038/nature03521
56. Guvendiren M, Burdick JA (2013) Engineering synthetic hydrogel microenvironments to instruct stem cells. Curr Opin Biotechnol. https://doi.org/10.1016/j.copbio.2013.03.009
57. Burdick JA, Prestwich GD (2011) Hyaluronic acid hydrogels for biomedical applications. Adv Mater. https://doi.org/10.1002/adma.201003963
58. Ribeiro M, de Moraes MA, Beppu MM, Garcia MP, Fernandes MH, Monteiro FJ et al (2015) Development of silk fibroin/nanohydroxyapatite composite hydrogels for bone tissue engineering. Eur Polym J, 66–77
59. Huebsch N, Arany PR, Mao AS, Shvartsman D, Ali OA, Bencherif SA et al (n.d.) Harnessing traction-mediated manipulation of the cell/matrix interface to control stem-cell fate. Nat Mater, 518–526

60. Khetan S, Guvendiren M, Legant WR, Cohen DM, Chen CS, Burdick JA (2013) Degradation-mediated cellular traction directs stem cell fate in covalently crosslinked three-dimensional hydrogels. Nat Mater. https://doi.org/10.1038/nmat3586
61. Burkert S, Schmidt T, Gohs U, Dorschner H, Arndt KF (2007) Cross-linking of poly(*N*-vinyl pyrrolidone) films by electron beam irradiation. Radiat Phys Chem. https://doi.org/10.1016/j.radphyschem.2007.02.024
62. Kang HW, Lee SJ, Ko IK, Kengla C, Yoo JJ, Atala A (2016) A 3D bioprinting system to produce human-scale tissue constructs with structural integrity. Nat Biotechnol. https://doi.org/10.1038/nbt.3413
63. Wu W, Deconinck A, Lewis JA (2011) Omnidirectional printing of 3D microvascular networks. Adv Mater. https://doi.org/10.1002/adma.201004625
64. Müller M, Becher J, Schnabelrauch M, Zenobi-Wong M (2015) Nanostructured pluronic hydrogels as bioinks for 3D bioprinting. Biofabrication. https://doi.org/10.1088/1758-5090/7/3/035006
65. Cui X, Breitenkamp K, Finn MG, Lotz M, D'Lima DD (2012) Direct human cartilage repair using three-dimensional bioprinting technology. Tissue Eng Part A. https://doi.org/10.1089/ten.tea.2011.0543
66. Hribar KC, Soman P, Warner J, Chung P, Chen S (2014) Light-assisted direct-write of 3D functional biomaterials. Lab Chip. https://doi.org/10.1039/c3lc50634g
67. Hockaday LA, Kang KH, Colangelo NW, Cheung PYC, Duan B, Malone E, Wu J, Girardi LN, Bonassar LJ, Lipson H, Chu CC, Butcher JT (2012) Rapid 3D printing of anatomically accurate and mechanically heterogeneous aortic valve hydrogel scaffolds. Biofabrication. https://doi.org/10.1088/1758-5082/4/3/035005
68. Hong S, Sycks D, Chan HFA, Lin S, Lopez GP, Guilak F, Leong KW, Zhao X (2015) 3D printing: 3D printing of highly stretchable and tough hydrogels into complex, cellularized structures. Adv Mater. https://doi.org/10.1002/adma.201570182
69. Rutz AL, Hyland KE, Jakus AE, Burghardt WR, Shah RN (2015) A multimaterial bioink method for 3D printing tunable, cell-compatible hydrogels. Adv Mater. https://doi.org/10.1002/adma.201405076
70. Boland T, Tao X, Damon BJ, Manley B, Kesari P, Jalota S, Bhaduri S (2007) Drop-on-demand printing of cells and materials for designer tissue constructs. Mater Sci Eng C. https://doi.org/10.1016/j.msec.2006.05.047
71. Xu T, Baicu C, Aho M, Zile M, Boland T (2009) Fabrication and characterization of bio-engineered cardiac pseudo tissues. Biofabrication. https://doi.org/10.1088/1758-5082/1/3/035001
72. Jia J, Richards DJ, Pollard S, Tan Y, Rodriguez J, Visconti RP, Trusk TC, Yost MJ, Yao H, Markwald RR, Mei Y (2014) Engineering alginate as bioink for bioprinting. Acta Biomater. https://doi.org/10.1016/j.actbio.2014.06.034
73. Zhao Y, Yao R, Ouyang L, Ding H, Zhang T, Zhang K, Cheng S, Sun W (2014) Three-dimensional printing of Hela cells for cervical tumor model in vitro. Biofabrication. https://doi.org/10.1088/1758-5082/6/3/035001
74. Lim KS, Schon BS, Mekhileri NV, Brown GCJ, Chia CM, Prabakar S, Hooper GJ, Woodfield TBF (2016) New visible-light photoinitiating system for improved print fidelity in gelatin-based bioinks. ACS Biomater Sci Eng. https://doi.org/10.1021/acsbiomaterials.6b00149
75. Pan T, Song W, Cao X (2016) 3D bioplotting of gelatin/alginate scaffolds for tissue engineering: influence of crosslinking degree and pore architecture on physicochemical properties. J Mater Sci Technol 32:889–900 (2016)
76. Bertassoni LE, Cardoso JC, Manoharan V, Cristino AL, Bhise NS, Araujo WA, Zorlutuna P, Vrana NE, Ghaemmaghami AM, Dokmeci MR, Khademhosseini A (2014) Direct-write bioprinting of cell-laden methacrylated gelatin hydrogels. Biofabrication. https://doi.org/10.1088/1758-5082/6/2/024105
77. Loessner D, Meinert C, Kaemmerer E, Martine LC, Yue K, Levett PA, Klein TJ, Melchels FPW, Khademhosseini A, Hutmacher DW (2016) Functionalization, preparation and use of cell-laden gelatin methacryloyl-based hydrogels as modular tissue culture platforms. Nat Protoc. https://doi.org/10.1038/nprot.2016.037

78. Highley CB, Rodell CB, Burdick JA (2015) Direct 3D printing of shear-thinning hydrogels into self-healing hydrogels. Adv Mater. https://doi.org/10.1002/adma.201501234
79. Rodell CB, MacArthur JW, Dorsey SM, Wade RJ, Wang LL, Woo YJ, Burdick JA (2015) Shear-thinning supramolecular hydrogels with secondary autonomous covalent crosslinking to modulate viscoelastic properties in vivo. Adv Funct Mater. https://doi.org/10.1002/adfm.201403550
80. Ouyang L, Highley CB, Rodell CB, Sun W, Burdick JA (2016) 3D printing of shear-thinning hyaluronic acid hydrogels with secondary cross-linking. ACS Biomater Sci Eng. https://doi.org/10.1021/acsbiomaterials.6b00158
81. Raphael B, Khalil T, Workman VL, Smith A, Brown CP, Streuli C, Saiani A, Domingos M (2017) 3D cell bioprinting of self-assembling peptide-based hydrogels. Mater Lett. https://doi.org/10.1016/j.matlet.2016.12.127
82. Li C, Faulkner-Jones A, Dun AR, Jin J, Chen P, Xing Y, Yang Z, Li Z, Shu W, Liu D, Duncan RR (2015) Rapid formation of a supramolecular polypeptide-DNA hydrogel for in situ three-dimensional multilayer bioprinting. Angew Chem Int Ed. https://doi.org/10.1002/anie.201411383
83. Zhai X, Ma Y, Hou C, Gao F, Zhang Y, Ruan C, Pan H, Liu WW (2017) 3D-printed high strength bioactive supramolecular polymer/clay nanocomposite hydrogel scaffold for bone regeneration. ACS Biomater Sci Eng 3:1109–1118
84. Gou M, Qu X, Zhu W, Xiang M, Yang J, Zhang K, Wei Y, Chen S (2014) Bio-inspired detoxification using 3d-printed hydrogel nanocomposites. Nat Commun. https://doi.org/10.1038/ncomms4774
85. Mannoor MS, Jiang Z, James T, Kong YL, Malatesta KA, Soboyejo WO, Verma N, Gracias DH, McAlpine MC (2013) 3D printed bionic ears. Nano Lett. https://doi.org/10.1021/nl4007744
86. Blessy Joseph NK, Maria HJ, Thomas S (2018) Nanocellulose: health care applications. In: Mishra M (ed) Encyclopedia of polymer applications. CRC Press, pp 1829–1852
87. Martínez H, Schwarz S, Rotter N, Gatenholm P (2016) Bioprinting 3D bioprinting of human chondrocyte-laden nanocellulose hydrogels for patient-specific auricular cartilage regeneration. Bioprinting 1–2:22–35. https://doi.org/10.1016/j.bprint.2016.08.003
88. Jang J, Yi HG, Cho DW (2016) 3D printed tissue models: present and future. ACS Biomater Sci Eng. https://doi.org/10.1021/acsbiomaterials.6b00129
89. Jang J, Kim TG, Kim BS, Kim SW, Kwon SM, Cho DW (2016) Tailoring mechanical properties of decellularized extracellular matrix bioink by vitamin B2-induced photo-crosslinking. Acta Biomater. https://doi.org/10.1016/j.actbio.2016.01.013
90. Jang J, Park HJ, Kim SW, Kim H, Park JY, Na SJ, Kim HJ, Park MN, Choi SH, Park SH, Kim SW, Kwon SM, Kim PJ, Cho DW (2017) 3D printed complex tissue construct using stem cell-laden decellularized extracellular matrix bioinks for cardiac repair. Biomaterials. https://doi.org/10.1016/j.biomaterials.2016.10.026
91. Kuo CY, Eranki A, Placone JK, Rhodes KR, Aranda-Espinoza H, Fernandes R, Fisher JP, Kim PCW (2016) Development of a 3D printed, bioengineered placenta model to evaluate the role of trophoblast migration in preeclampsia. ACS Biomater Sci Eng. https://doi.org/10.1021/acsbiomaterials.6b00031
92. Gladman AS, Matsumoto EA, Nuzzo RG, Mahadevan, L, Lewis JA (2016) Biomimetic 4D printing. Nat Mater 15. https://doi.org/10.1038/NMAT4544
93. Bakarich SE, Gorkin R, In Het Panhuis M, Spinks GM (2015) 4D printing with mechanically robust, thermally actuating hydrogels. Macromol Rapid Commun 36:1211–1217. https://doi.org/10.1002/marc.201500079

Chapter 10
Hydrogel Formulation as Efficient Drug Carrier and Delivery for Selected Skin Diseases

Ramakrishnan Kumar, Sujitha Ayyanar, Premkumar Jayaraj, Akella Sivaramakrishna, Sanjay Rajagopalan, Sampath Parthasarathy, and Rajagopal Desikan

Abstract During the last a few decades, the rapid proliferation in the prevalence of skin diseases has been a major unease for healthcare providers, and it is currently regarded as a global encumbrance and reflected as one of the reasons for rise in health-related spending. Nano-medicine has ascended as the most unique means to break the chain of spreading and eliminating the skin disease altogether. Nano-formulations (NFs) by means of advanced nanotechnology are in great need to address the subject. Lately, hydrogel- and nanogel-based drug delivery approaches have postured new projections to simulate the natural intelligence of many biological systems. Due to their select porous interpenetrating network scheme, hydrophobic drug fusion and stimulus sensitivity, hydrogels are considered as a remarkable potential in the area of targeted drug delivery systems. This chapter gives an outline of an effort to highlight the current trends in hydrogel-based drug carrier cum delivery systems for skin diseases like skin cancer, psoriasis and wound healing. This chapter also covers diverse formulations techniques using hydrogel like topical, subcutaneous, transdermal and comprising its pharmaceutical formulations. Future forecasts and prospects that are accessible for hydrogel-based formulations for various skin disorders are also discussed.

Keywords Polymer · Drug carrier · Formulations · Skin disorder · Topical cream · Diffusion · Swelling · Transdermal · Subcutaneous delivery · Wound healing

---

R. Kumar · S. Ayyanar · P. Jayaraj · A. Sivaramakrishna · R. Desikan (✉)
Department of Chemistry, School of Advanced Sciences, Vellore Institute of Technology, Vellore, Tamil Nadu 632014, India
e-mail: rajagopal.desikan@vit.ac.in

S. Rajagopalan
School of Medicine, Cardiovascular Research Institute, Case Western Reserve University, Cleveland, OH, USA

S. Parthasarathy · R. Desikan
Burnett School of Biomedical Sciences, University of Central Florida, Orlando, FL, USA

J. Jose et al. (eds.), *Nano Hydrogels*, Gels Horizons: From Science to Smart Materials,
https://doi.org/10.1007/978-981-15-7138-1_10

1 Introduction

Hydrogels, water-swollen crosslinked polymer networks have been broadly exploited as wound dressings, therapeutic glue patches, contact lenses and tissue-modifying material during the last 30–40 years [1, 2]. Essentially, hydrogels are considered as perfect vehicles for drug delivery in view of their favorable properties. Hydrogels are fully biocompatible since they hold a close structural similarity to the natural extracellular matrix (ECM). Also, their porous structure is valuable to clench drugs in large quantities. Hydrogels offer an aqueous environment similar to physiological environment that supports to hold drug in their dynamic forms and prevents them from degradation. This property helps hydrogel is being used extensively as tropical care vehicular medicine. Several reports on the application side of hydrogels have pointed out the benefits of hydrogels in the treatment of skin-related diseases, drug delivery medium for a wide variety of skin diseases like skin cancer, skin infection, acne, skin rashes, ringworm and wounds. For instance, dexpanthenol is used for the prevention and treatment of the skin ailments and also used as skin fortification [3, 4].

In recent times, drug delivery has been the most evolving and promising technology in the biomedical field. The physiochemical properties of the drugs are essential for formulation with hydrogels. Once the drug and hydrogels are formulated, it is used for the treatment of diseases by targeted drug delivery system [5–7]. As can be seen from Fig. 1, there are several types of hydrogels that are used for treating skin diseases. In particular, photosensitive hydrogels can be used to release the drugs at the required specific target when it is exposed to specific quantum of light. Reinforced hydrogels can be made by blending specific hydrogel polymers with therapeutically active and biocompatible ingredients to have improved delivery properties. In spite of extensive application in countless disease targets including skin disorders, hydrogels have some shortcomings when it is indecorously formulated or used as drug carrier or delivery medium [8, 9]. A notable problem is that the astonishing permeability of hydrogels makes a swift outflow of the bulk of their drug substances. This occurrence known as "burst release" may have drug concentrations more than the toxic level in vivo, leading to ineffectual drug treatment and objectionable adverse effects [10]. Henceforth, frequent strategies have been tried to comprehend unrelenting drug leaching out from hydrogels with decreased burst effect. These methods encompass the restriction of drugs to gel matrices through a fragmentable spacer and the amalgamation of biodegradable micro- and nanospheres aiding as carriers of drug component [11].

2 Formulation of Hydrogel

The process of formulating the active pharmaceutical ingredient (API) with hydrogel involves mixing of inactive yet biocompatible excipients to afford formulated therapeutic products. This encompasses of preparing the drug, as robust and endurable to

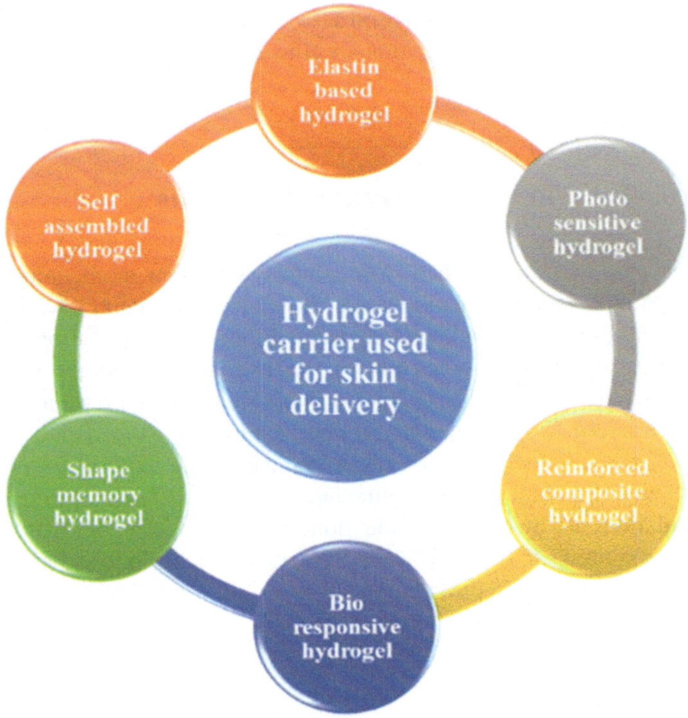
Elastin based hydrogel
Photo sensitive hydrogel
Reinforced composite hydrogel
Bio responsive hydrogel
Shape memory hydrogel
Self assembled hydrogel
Hydrogel carrier used for skin delivery

Fig. 1 Pictorial view of hydrogel carriers used for skin delivery

the patients. Suitably formulated therapeutic agents are administered by numerous mode of delivery [12]. For orally administered drugs, the route includes espousing the drug into a tablet or a capsule form. The drug has to be soluble in aqueous medium at a controlled rate, and the particle size and crystal form of the molecule are established. These drugs are scrutinized to guarantee that the encapsulated drug is safe and efficacious [13]. As a drug delivery vehicle, hydrogels are used as a transporter material, which can counteract at the site of gastrointestinal tract, colon, vagina and other body parts thus shielding the API from chemical degradation. It is capable of liberating the drug at the pre-requisite targeted site depending upon the targeted environment like pH or bonding interaction or chemical ionization of drug molecules [14–16]. Hydrogen bonding interactions between polymeric chain of hydrogel and glycoproteins in the mucosalining of the gastrointestinal tract makes the drug intangible of chemical transformation within GI tract. Formulation of drugs using hydrogel can also be prepared in the form of parenteral formulations or injectable formulations. These categories of formulations are used with the intravenous, subcutaneous, intramuscular and intra-articular administration [17]. Hydrogel-based topical formulations are also a vital type of formulation used in the skin-associated problems. In this technique, application of drugs on the required body surface like skin in the form of creams, gels, foams and ointments to treat the skin disorder [18]. Other topical medication comprises of formulation used as eye and ear drops. Powder form or paste formulation is used in dental application specifically for orthodontic or periodontics diseases [19].

3 Hydrogel as Carrier of Therapeutic Agents

Excruciating pain due to scratched skin conditions present momentous problems and woe to patients and clinicians. One of the main shortcomings with prevailing medication for these types of skin malady is the difficulty of application of medicine for wound dressing at the targeted places. An alternative approach is the use of skin lotions or other gels (hydrogel-loaded drugs) that may cure promptly with an unfailing release [20]. The selection of monomer for loading a therapeutic agent in the hydrogel matrix is an important step in developing hydrogel-API (active pharmaceutical ingredient) formulations. The main starting materials for preparing hydrogel-based formulations are by using suitable monomers which can hold the API till it is carried at the required site [21–23]. The polymers that are used for making hydrogel bio-compatible materials are provided in Table 1.

3.1 Cargo Loading

There are two methods commonly adopted for loading of drugs into hydrogels. In the first method, hydrogel is mixed with active pharmaceutical ingredient, an initiator and a crosslinker (if needed). Then, polymerization is carried out in situ and the drug is embedded within the polymer matrix. In the second method, on the other hand, the hydrogel is conceded to swell in the drug solution (refer Fig. 2). The loading of a drug into a hydrogel is influenced by various aspects viz. contact between polymer and solvent, cross-linking density of polymers, nature of the solvent, etc. These conditions affect the degree of swelling in a large extent [24, 25]. The loading of drug per unit mass of a polymer can be calculated using the following relation (Eq. 1)

$$\text{(Swollen polymer weight} - \text{Dry polymer weight)/(Polymer weight)} \quad (1)$$

3a *Diffusion controlled:* A very few applicable mechanisms are involved in drug delivery releases system. The Fick's law of diffusion is most widely applied in modeling this release. Two types of drug diffusion-controlled systems are used in hydrogel-drug delivery; (a) reservoir system is used in drug loading by an entrapment mechanism within a polymeric hydrogel membrane, and Fick's first law defines the drug delivery via the membrane system, (b) the matrix system is in an unstable state, thus the drug release happens by diffusion in a single-dimensional slap-shaped matrix, described by the second law of Fick's diffusion.

Table 1 Different types of the polymer are used pharma application

S.No.	Drug	Polymer	Application
1	Immobilized Antigen and Antibodies	Polyurethane, poly(ethylene glycol), poly(propyleneglycol) poly(vinyl pyrrolidone), polyethylene glycol and agar	Wound care treatment
2	Dextromethorphan Hydrobromide	Poly(vinyl pyrrolidone) Starch, poly(vinyl pyrrolidone), poly(acrylic acid)	Drug delivery and pharmaceutical formulation
3	Hyaluronic acid-tyramine	Collagen, fibrin, hyaluronic acid	Dental Materials
4	SR-rhGH	Other polymer material Hyaluronan	Tissue engineering, Implants
5	Vinylbenzyltrimethylammonium chloride (VBT) and p- sodium styrene sulphonate (SSS)	poly (vinyl methyl ether) (PVME) and poly (N-isopropyl acrylamide) (PNIPA) gels -	Injectable polymeric system
6	Peptide-based drug	Poly (vinyl methyl ether), poly(N-isopropyl acrylamide)	Technical products (cosmetic, pharmaceutical)
7	Polymer-based Drug	High-acyl gellan gum hydrogel	Rheological investigation
8	5-Fluorouracil	N-succinyl chitosan/Poly (acrylamide-co-acrylic acid) hydrogels	In vitro release of 5-fluorouracil (cancer drug releases)
9	Cellulose membrane	Semi-solid hydrogel ophthalmic, Loratadine-Loaded Thermoresponsive Hydrogel	ocular drug delivery (formulations and in vitro studies)
10	Camptothecin	Hydrogel on chitosan/β-glycerophosphate (β-GP)/β-cyclodextrin	Thermo-sensitive Hydrogel Containing Cyclodextrin

Based on the experimental evidence, it identifies that drug is evenly distributed across the hydrogel matrix used as a drug delivery system [26].

3b *Swelling controlled:* It is a release-controlled phenomenon. The swelling-controlled delivery applies when the diffusion of the drug is quicker than hydrogel bulge. If the polymer chains are soluble in water, erosion might also play a significant rate controlling role for drug release. Upon contact with aqueous media, liquid penetrates into the system, leading to steadily increasing water concentrations. As soon as the water content is high enough, the polymer chains start to disentangle from the network and diffuse through the liquid

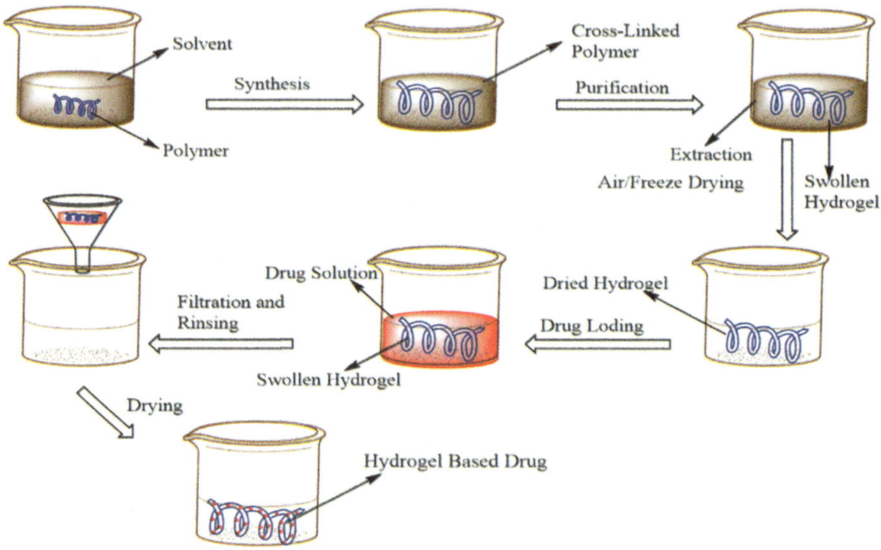

Fig. 2 Mechanism of the hydrogel-based drug delivery systems

unstirred boundary layer surrounding the device into the surrounding fluid [27]. For instance, the delivery of small molecule-based drugs on HPMC (hydroxypropyl methylcellulose) hydrogel tablets happens via swelling-controlled drug release concept [28].

3c *Chemically controlled:* In this method, the molecules are released during the chemical reactions happening inside a delivery matrix. Often times, reaction occurs by fragmentation of polymer chains through water or enzyme-mediated degradation and the released drugs can undergo either reversible or irreversible reactions arising between the polymeric network and releasable drug. It is further classified on the basis of reaction happening while drug release phase is on [29, 30].

1. Complete kinetically driven sustained release: The kinetically controlled and diffusion controlled are further classified into two types: (a) pendent chain (prodrugs) hydrogel network device covalently linked device via fragmentable spacer bonds, and the drug delivery is maneuvered by an approach with which spacer cleavage happens [31, 32]. In certain applications where an additional targeted delivery methodology is anticipated, it is necessary to project further enzymatically cleavable spacer bonds [33]. In surface eroding materials, drug delivery is controlled by the rate of surface erosion of the polymer matrix. In water-resistant polymeric network links, surface attrition happens when the fraction of water carried into the polymer is relatively slower than the rate of bond cleavage due to water molecule [34, 35]. However, the typically high water content of hydrogel, the eroding system was slow due to enzymatic degradation when the rate of the

enzyme reaction into the gel is not faster than the rate of enzymatic degradation systems. Surface eroding models directing at the delivery mechanism are established on hydrolytic degradation polymers [36, 37].

2. Diffusion-controlled system: Diffusion plays a vital part in many controlled drug delivery methods. Diffusion is the mass transport mechanism when other processes do not contribute to the control of drug release. The interactions between enzymes and the drugs, together with polymer degradation, control the diffusion and release of the drugs [38]. Diffusional mass transport is basically important for several processes in the body and nature as a whole. The primary concept is that a solute diffuses in a concentration gradient from region of higher concentration to nearby area of lower concentration. The diffusion equation can be solved when beginning and boundary conditions are given. Analytical approaches to the diffusion equation that are applicable to controlled drug release systems can be explained. The initial condition refers to the initial drug distribution in the system, before the release pathway begins. Boundary conditions imply to the fact that the conditions at the drug delivery system's boundaries during drug release; these specify drug concentrations or concentration gradients at the device's surfaces. The term "analytical solution" refers to an explicit mathematical expression satisfying the diffusion equation, along with the prescribed initial and boundary conditions. The analytical solution is used to calculate drug release from the delivery system as a function of time.

4 Topical Delivery

Topical drug delivery is a restrained drug delivery system which can be applied in the body via ocular, rectal, vaginal and skin as topical means. Skin is the easier stretchable organ on the human body for topical applications and is the central route of topical drug delivery system. This comprises the balanced method to topical formulations, principles of topical permeation and a simple factor of topical drug delivery systems. The scientific confirmation specifies that topical gel is a benign and active management for skin-related problems [39]. Effective components like desonide, a synthetic corticosteroid, are loaded in the hydrogel and used as an anti-inflammatory agent [40]. An antifungal formulation such as clotrimazole also developed by hydrogel formulation for vaginitis, which shows improved absorption than conventional creams [41].

The topical formulations are gel, cream, ointment, paste and lotion. For these types of formulation, drugs are prepared using hydrogel [42]. In this method, hydrogels have a crucial role like suspension agent, viscosity enhancer, thickening the gel as required in ointment or cream. For instance, Adapalene gel is a drug which is used for ACNE [43]; here carbomer 940, a minimally-toxic emulsion stabilizing agent, is added [44] for Adapalene gel drug formulations. Some of the topical drug delivery hydrogels are (i) polyethylene glycol (Lidocaine ointment) [45], (ii) Carbomer 940 (Adapalene gel) [43] and carbomer homopolymer type-C or PEG-400 (Voltaren gel) [46], and also, Carbopol-910, Carbopol-943, Carbopol-934P, Carbopol-940, Carbopol-941, etc., are used as various topical drug delivery systems [47, 48]. It offers thermodynamic stability to the drug, and it aided to increase topical drug availability, dermal permeation and skin flux with less toxicity [49].

5 Transdermal Drug Delivery

Drug delivery system to the skin disease is commonly directed for topical application of dermatological treatment of skin diseases or improvement of the skin care itself. Nowadays, the hydrogel-based systematic drug delivery path has been considered as a fitting method for the skin diseases. For this, transdermal technique is a right treatment for skin, and it is a systematic delivery of drugs as well [50]. Reasonable advantages of transdermal approach are that all drugs can be transported for the prolonged time at low cost and steady rate. The transdermal-based drug was easy to disconnected whenever it is required to do so by discarding the devices, and it can be a high water content property present in swollen hydrogels. The hydrogels can deliver the better acting ingredients for the skin diseases compare to conventional lotions and patches as shown in Fig. 3 [51]. Advantages of hydrogel-driven devices for transdermal drug delivery were projected by composite membranes of cross-linked polymer of PHEMA with nonwoven fabric polyester supported devices. It was suggested that the formulation-based liposome gel contains phosphatidylcholine liposomes. The liposome gel was considered as skin absorption activity of hydrocortisone, and it was expressed that hydrogels prepared from the copolymerization of bovine serum albumin (BSA) and PEG [52]. It contains over 96% of water which allows the hydrophilic and water-resistant pharmaceutical agents diffuse through polymer network. It was also asserted that it is the most likely application

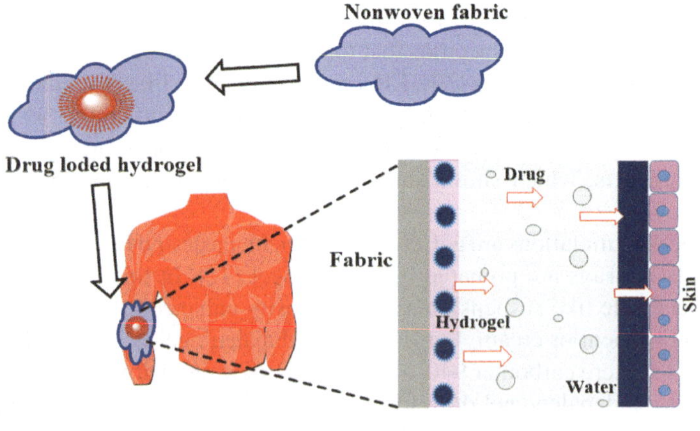

Fig. 3 Drug delivery through the skin epidermis by gel formation

of BSA-PEG hydrogels. Extensive studies on in situ photo-polymerizable hydrogels are synthesized from terminally diacrylate ABA block copolymers of lactic acid oligomers (A) and PEG (B) for barriers and specified drug delivery in a controlled manner. In recent times, studies in transdermal applications focus on electrically operated delivery, using iontophoresis and electroporation. Various hydrogel-oriented formulations have been investigated as a carrier for transdermal delivery to acquire the increased penetration of luteinizing releasing hormone, sodium nonivamide acetate, nicotine and enoxacin. Another method, a methylcellulose-mediated hydrogel was used as a viscous ultrasonic coupling medium for transdermal sonophoresis, resulting in an improved transfer of insulin and vasopressin by in vitro method across human skin [53].

6a *Formulation methods for Transdermal in Hydrogel* Transdermal is one of the methods of administration to deliver the drug across the skin, and it is to be applied as patches on the skin. The drug goes to epidermis and follows microcirculation of dermis [54]. The most common method for transdermal hydrogel formulations is to load the drug within hydrogel using topical drug delivery method [55] with the hydrogel loaded drug to make a shallow compartment from hollow ring-shaped device and drug-impermeable-backing membrane (laminated aluminum foil). A microporous tape of large area is stuck onto the impermeable-backing membrane to bring the transdermal patch in close interaction with the skin. The device is sealed by a release liner on the open side. The drug-loaded hydrogel formulation is tuned as per required ratio of drug and polymer [56]. The formulation for transdermal drug delivery is to load the drug in hydrogel matrix-type transdermal patches. The drug is prepared by solvent casting methodology using different ratio of hydrogels, surfactants or co-surfactants, emulsifier, with required additives, etc.

6 Subcutaneous Delivery

Substantial applications of hydrogel are also found to have in implantable therapeutics. The drug-loaded hydrogels inserted subcutaneously are revealed to arouse less objectionable body reactions, such as inflammation, carcinogenicity and immunogenicity. They are considered as biocompatible polymers due to their high water content and non-interference in the physiological activity in the human body. They also hold several encouraging properties like minimum mechanical irritation resulting to in vivo implantation. Also, their softness, elastic properties, inhibition of protein adsorption, cell adhesion arise from low interfacial tension between water and hydrogels make the subcutaneous delivery an easy method. It has wide suitability for specific drugs with hydrophilicity and molecular dimensions and has typical lotions to exploit, to discharge of incorporated drugs at the required site of action with time. Histological examination showed that the hydrogel was infused when incorporated subcutaneously into rats. Innumerable hydrogel formulations for subcutaneous delivery of anticancer drugs are also available. Prevalent reports on incorporated hydrogels are concentrated toward the assessment of recyclable systems. Later, two types of novel decomposable PEG hydrogels have been developed for the sustained release of proteins: The first option was developed by poly-condensation of bi-functional PEG and branched PEG polyols then hydrolysis of the ester linkages, the gel decompose into only PEG and PEG derivatives. The second type is PEG-oriented hydrogels with a functional group in which drug covalently linked to the hydrogel by an ester chemical bond [57]. The delivery of the drug is regulated by the hydrolysis of an ester bond between the hydrogel and the protein followed by diffusion of protein out of the hydrogel and by degradation of the gel. These hydrogels are designed on acrylate derivatives of dextran. Through this study, the use of hydrogels and the sustained release of the drug was completely understood.

7 Hydrogel for Melanoma, Psoriasis and Wound Healing

Drug delivery technology is aimed at the product efficiency, safety, convenience of the patient and compliance. The administration of drugs is commonly through the gastrointestinal tract, injections, inhalation, transdermal, topical and oral routes. In this section, we have focused on the drug delivery for the skin diseases. Because skin is the outermost organ and also the largest organ of the human body, it can be easily accessed for drug application. Skin diseases or skin problems are the emanate condition and burden for millions of people every day. Skin problems are due to various pathogens. Researchers in this area unraveled that dermatologic disorders are very less and commonly significance for the populations in many developing countries. There are numerous dermatological treatments that are available for skin-related problems.

A large amount of infectious diseases, associated with skin and hair follicles, might be due to bacteria, fungi and viral infection. These ailments are treated by therapeutic substances such as drugs and vaccines. An immense range of therapeutic indications that are covered by those substances are specially designed for skin or cutaneous administration. Even when the drugs have different molecular structure, they possess some common physicochemical characteristics, such as lipophilicity and poor aqueous solubility. The drugs should retain water partition coefficient value [log P] > 6.0. The drug formulation for delivery is to adequately manage therapeutic concentration in a reasonable time period and afford constant pharmacological action. Destitute drug insertion of skin limits their bioavailability and drugability. Here, hydrogels are used as a carrier molecule for the drug; it received attention owing to their efficiency to stimulate the penetration in the surface of the dermal region. The application of hydrogel-drug carrier system is able to produce effective drugs to the particular site in a proper manner. The drug-loaded hydrogel is based on the pharmacological system, which controls the release of therapeutic agents to the targeted region at the epidermal layer. Hydrogels show a high equilibrium water content (EWC) which provides the structure the ability to entrap water and subsequently water-soluble drugs. This characteristic makes hydrogels suitable for drug delivery systems [58].

7a ***Skin cancer***

New forms of treatments to aim disease target are essential while concurrently lessening the side effects produced due to foreign agents. To elude side effects, transdermal drug delivery systems seem as an encouraging alternate approach to carry antineoplastic agents. There are numerous benefits from using encapsulated antineoplastic agents; some of them are improved drug solubility, improved bioavailability, increased chemical stability, sustained drug release, extended half-life, non-specific organs or tissue dispersal, and lessening of the total dose required [59]. Altogether, the benefits delineated can help lessen adverse side effects to a dramatic degree. Bulky carrier-based drug delivery systems is a new area that has emerge due to the antagonistic side effects triggered by non-traditional therapies in patients with melanoma. These systems contest the cancerous cells, while destabilizing the adverse side effects. These categories of drug delivery systems hold drug carriers such as nanoparticles, dendrimers, cyclodextrins, liposomes and hydrogels that transport the bioactive antineoplastic drug inside the core/pocket/scaffold. Several types of drug delivery methodologies, such as the development of hydrogels based on natural and synthetic polymers as the drug carriers, have received distinct consideration. These biomaterials offer a stimulating opening for crafting innovative approaches of cancer therapy. Conventionally, paclitaxel (PTX) was administered intravenously to treat skin cancer. Nevertheless, since PTX could not discern among healthy cells and cancer cells, it has created countless undesirable side effects, occasionally resulting in the patient's death. Hence, to minimize the cytotoxicity and reduce side effects, targeted delivery of PTX to the cancerous cells, while not affecting the healthy cells, needs to be developed. Researchers have encapsulated the drug PTX in hydrogels [60]. However, additional efforts are essential to bring out studies on the efficacy of these hydrogel formulations in vitro and in vivo assays in melanoma.

Working on the encapsulation of the bioactive agents in hydrogel scaffolds and successive release, durable retention of 5-fluorouracil (5-Fu), an antineoplastic agent in a hydrogel based on polyethylene glycol, polycaprolactone and poly-L-lactic acid copolymers (MCL), within a tumor is achieved within hydrogel matrix [61]. It was revealed that single injection of 5-Fu-loaded MCL was found to be effective than repeated injections of free 5-Fu. This was confirmed by long-lasting retention of 5-Fu, which induced vital inhibition of tumor growth under in vitro and in vivo assays in melanoma [62]. Moreover, it was established that 5-Fu-loaded hydrogel could act as a biodegradable drug collection capable of offering continual release of 5-Fu after intratumoral injection, hence increasing the chemotherapeutic effect of 5-Fu while decreasing its systemic toxicity [63]. The tumors injected with saline or MCL survived to a great extent and several blood vessels (yellow arrow) amplified as the implantation time increased. Meanwhile, tumors injected with free 5-Fu (repeat) or 5-Fu-loaded MCL displayed on a surge in areas comprehending necrotic tissue that increased over time. These results designate that it is likely to employ formulations based on hydrogels as a new substitute for drug release platforms [64, 65].

7b ***Psoriasis***:

About 2% population is affected by psoriasis, a common skin disorder, affecting mostly adult population. It is considered as a prolonged inflammation of the skin described by erythematous scaly plaques [66]. Corticosteroid such as betamethasone (BD) is generally used comprehensively in topical medication for the treatment of mild to moderate psoriasis. However, the application of BD has practical shortcomings such as reduced permeability via skin which reduces its medicinal value at the requited site of action [67]. The foremost constraint stands in the hindered function of the skin, which is considered as one of the most impervious epithelia of the human body to exogenous substances. Consequently, the main tasks for a topical formulation are to offer an adequate rise in drug permeation into the skin, without causing any momentous non-reversible adjustment to the skin barrier function. The fabrication of a nano-carrier composite hydrogel formulation for enhanced patient amenability and topical drug delivery to psoriasis lesions was developed using methoxy—poly (ethylene glycol)—hexyl substituted poly (lactic acid) (mPEGhexPLA). mPEGhexPLA is a dual functional polymer which self-assembles to drug-loaded spherical nanostructures in an aqueous medium. These nanostructures have a passive, PEG-based surface with neutral to marginally negative net charge and a particle size <60 nm. Nano-carriers hold a large payload of the hydrophobic tacrolimus (TAC), which is an effective immune suppressive medicine. Prominently, TAC nano-carrier hydrogel composite formulation delivered considerably increased drug levels into inflamed skin permitting next-generation products with reduced drug dose and/or treatment frequency. The composite hydrogel was prepared by concentrated Carbopol® gels (1.2% (w/w)) at a batch size of 40 g. Carbopol® ETD 2020 (480 mg) was measured and spread into water for injectable to get a moderately swollen polymer. The pH was adjusted to 5.5 ± 0.2 with a NaOH solution (10% w/w). The gel was mixed well till the Carbopol® polymer was in its completely swollen state [68]. If essential, weight of the final gel was adjusted to 40 g with sterile water. 0.1% TAC composite hydrogels were prepared at a batch size of 40 g, by slow addition of 0.2% TAC mPEGhexPLA nano-carrier formulation (20 g) to the concentrated Carbopol® gel (20 g) under magnetic stirring. Lipid-, paraffin- or wax-based foundations are commonly used in semi-solid topical formulations of reduced soluble drugs. Further to cosmetic shortcomings, these products generally suffer from suboptimal dermal drug availability, due to an incomplete drug partitioning from the formulation base into the skin. It was validated that topical TAC hydrogel composite formulation carries increased drug doses into the skin, compared to a non-traditional ointment formulation. The inactive surface properties and small size of the nano-carrier system competently aid to overcome the skin barrier. When diluted below the threshold micellar concentration, the drug is released from the nano-carrier and forms a local depot in the skin. When the therapeutic efficiency of the hydrogel composite formulations was corresponding to commercially obtainable products in the existing in vivo study, product design prospects related with hydrogel-based formulations containing mPEGhexPLA nano-carriers, empower the development of ground-breaking topical composite dosage forms including foams, sprays or gels, with enhanced patient compliance. Increased solubilization and delivery capacity is anticipated to assist the generation of improved drug products with reduced dosing frequency or reduced drug dose [69].

7c ***Infected wound***

Wound healing method is the evolving new means to heal the impaired skin tissue with improved bio-friendly and bioactive materials. Skin-associated problems such as skin burn, skin ulcer and injured skin are non-affordable to treat for common people. Prosthetic tissue-engineered skin is made, but they are not ready to use due to high cost, and it would not always be matched by the patient. The wound healing applications have a parameter to regulate the wound contraction that can be assessed by this technique, considering that A0 is the original wound area, and A is the wound area at the time of biopsy: wound contraction % A0 − At/A0*100.

Several systems were studied, with or without chemicals to treat the skin alteration. Hyaluronic acid and gelatin are encouraging materials for the treatment due to their natural existence in human ECM of the skin tissues [70]. Other than these two materials, cellulose, alginate chitosan copolymers, chitosan–gelatin-honey copolymers and biphasic gelatin-silk systems are also used in this application [71, 72]. At present, many conventional products are on the market use, as a blend of definite materials and appropriate seeding of cells from innumerable origins. For example, applications of HYAFFTM esterified hyaluronic acid (HA) produced by FIDIA Limited; laser skin auto-graft, made up of an HA-membrane with keratinocytes, and hyalo-graft 3D, made with HA, with added fibroblasts. Table 2 represents some of the drug formulations that are adopted for various skin disorders.

8 Projections for Future Research

With the advancement in materials construction and engineering, variation of the in vivo efficacy of hydrogel nanoparticles is conceivable. With this groundwork, it is in the offing that, in the future, hydrogel nanoparticles with intended internal structures can be spawned for more adaptable drug delivery uses, including co-administration of multiple drugs. Indeed, a growing level of indication has clearly proposed that multi-drug therapies can provide an increased therapeutic benefit as related to single-drug remedial approach. This is demonstrated by a preceding study, in which double-walled polymeric microspheres are adopted to transport

Table 2 Some of the drugs formulation and its applications

S.no	Drug	Structure	Formulation	Application
1	Ketoconazole	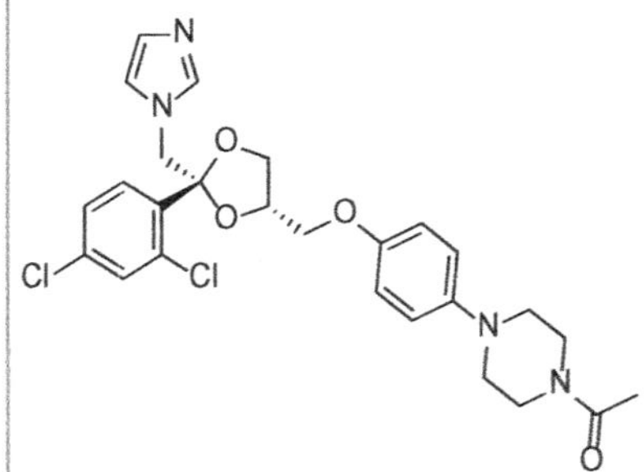	Topical / Transdermal	Antifungal
2	Sulconazole nitrate	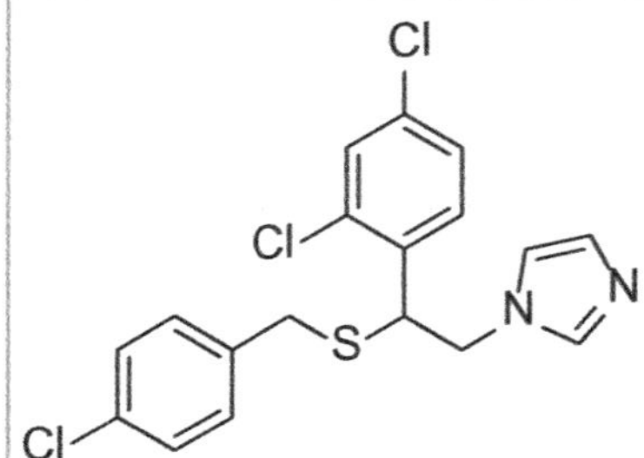	Topical / Transdermal/subcutaneous	Cutaneous dermatophytosis

(continued)

Table 2 (continued)

S.no	Drug	Structure	Formulation	Application
3	Miconazole nitrate	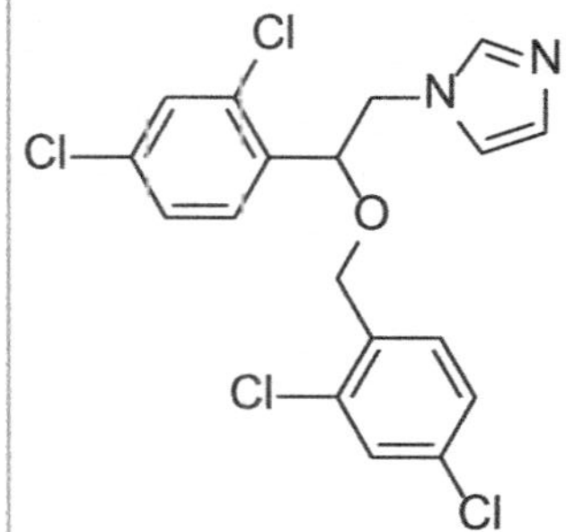	Topical / Transdermal/subcutaneous	Cutaneous dermatophytosis
4	Tacrolimus	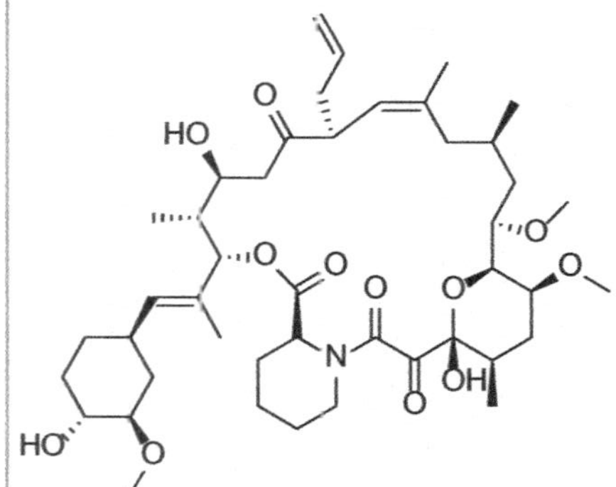	Topical / Transdermal/subcutaneous	Vitiligo, Atopic keratoconjunctivitis

(continued)

Table 2 (continued)

S.no	Drug	Structure	Formulation	Application
5	Tazarotene	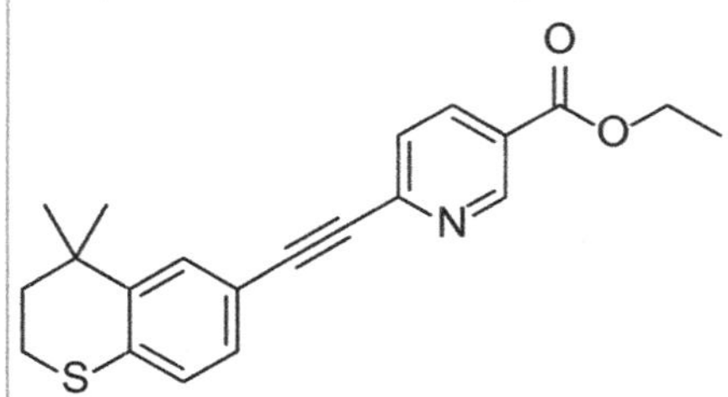	Topical / Transdermal	Psoriasis
6	Calcipotriol/betamethasone dipropionate combination	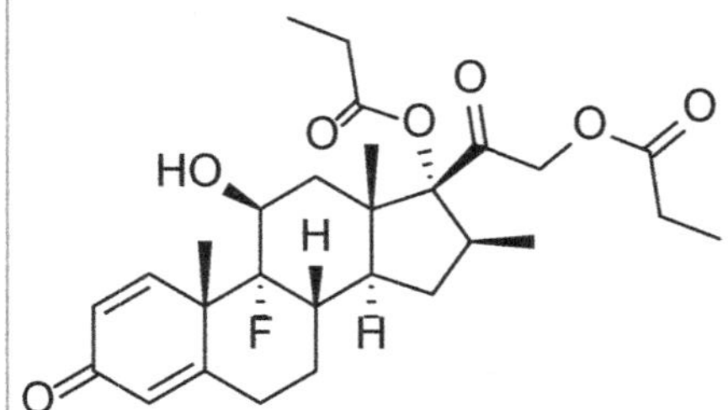	Topical / Transdermal	Psoriasis

(continued)

Table 2 (continued)

S.no	Drug	Structure	Formulation	Application
7	Calcipotriol	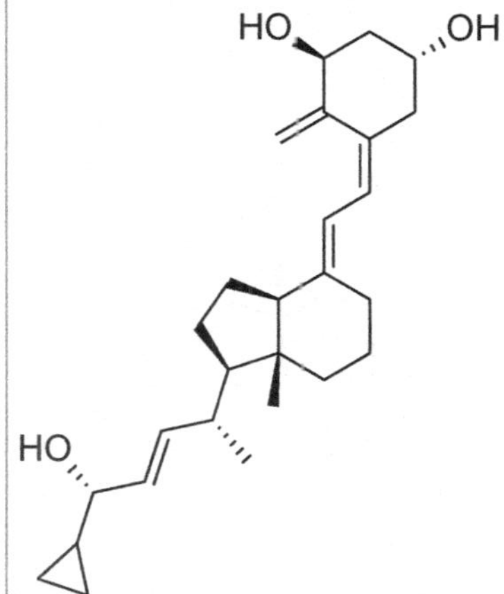	Topical / Transdermal	Psoriasis
8	Methotrexate	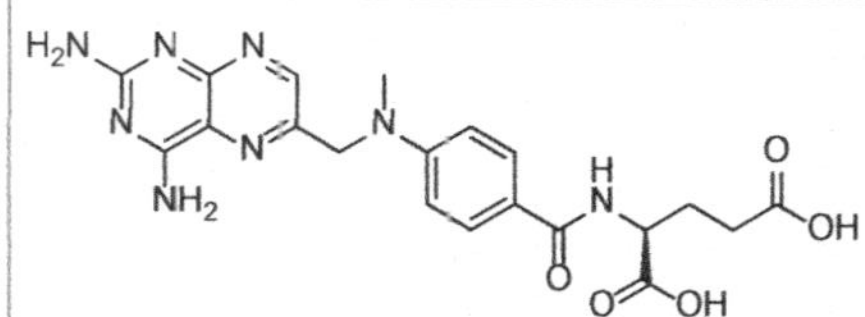	Topical / Transdermal/subcutaneous	Psoriasis

(continued)

Table 2 (continued)

S.no	Drug	Structure	Formulation	Application
9	Tazarotene	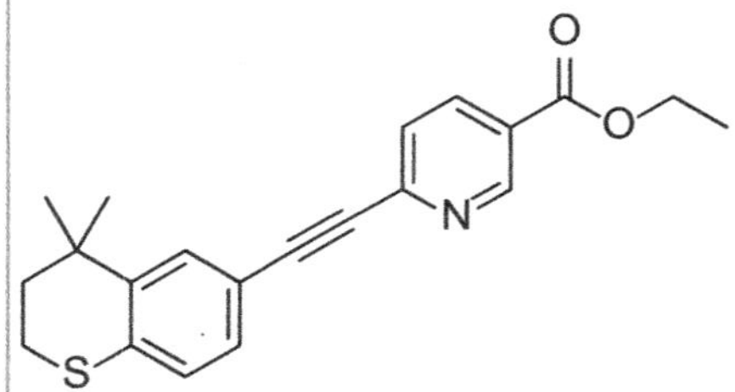	Topical / Transdermal/subcutaneous	Psoriasis
10	Calcipotriene	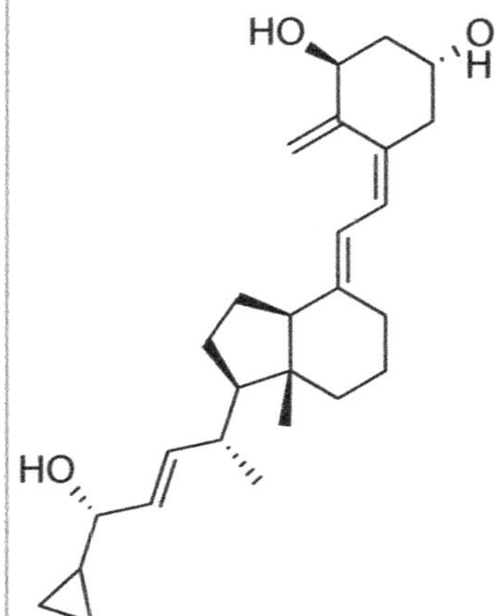	Topical / Transdermal/subcutaneous	Psoriasis

(continued)

Table 2 (continued)

S.no	Drug	Structure	Formulation	Application
11	Minoxidil	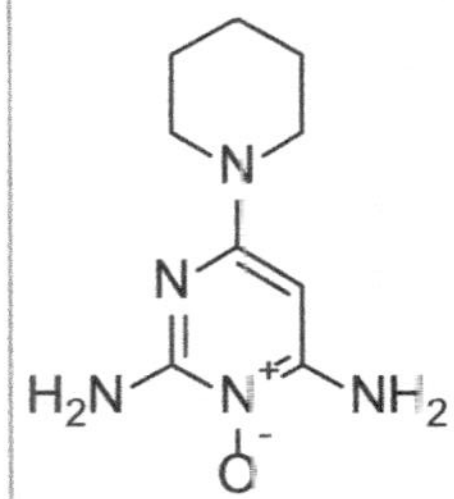	Propylene glycol--water-ethanol solutions, Topical / Transdermal	Androgenic alopecia
12	Miconazole	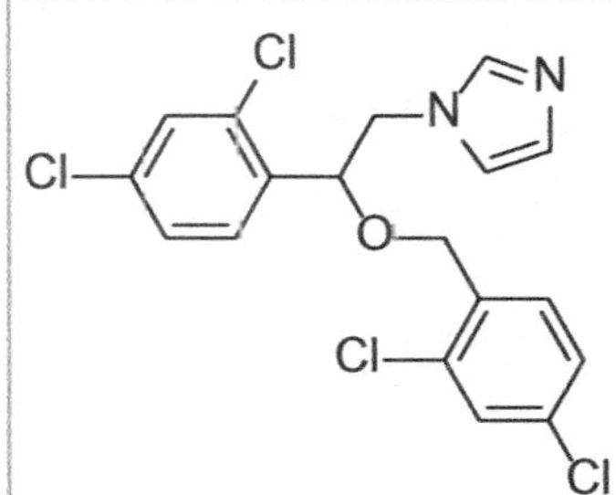	Powders, parenteral, gels, creams, and ointments, Topical / Transdermal/subcutaneous	Candida infections, fungal infections
13	Amphotericin B	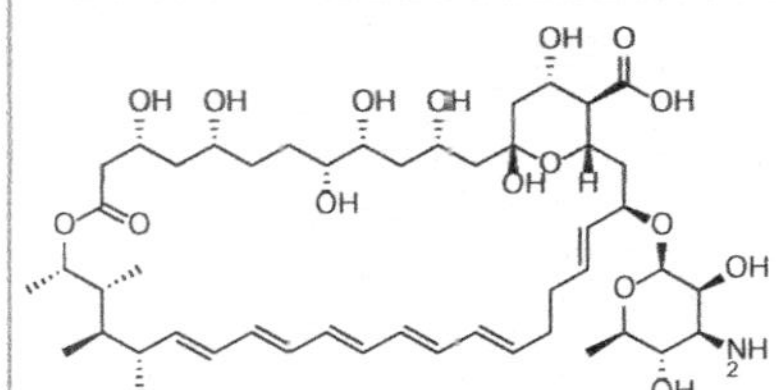	Cream, lotion, gels, ointments, Topical / Transdermal/subcutaneous	Fungal skin infections

both doxorubicin and a medicinally active transgene to HepG2 cells. The collective treatment enriches the cytotoxicity when compared to either of the two remedies alone. The increased potential of multi-drug therapies is further sustained recently by the observation that the therapeutic benefits of aerosol cisplatin can be improved by administration of a therapeutic transgene, using adenoviral-type 5(dE1/E3) (Cytomegalovirus promoter) as a vector, before cisplatin administration. Collectively, these point to the medicinal potential of multi-drug remedies. Regardless of this, the efficiency of multi-drug therapies may be fraught with if the co-delivered drugs are not well suited with each other. This is one of the foremost tasks to be addressed for multi-drug administration.

9 Conclusion

The significant headway in hydrogel study is shown to divulge a fast expansion of hydrogel-based systems during the last a few decades, from a simple crosslinking of macromolecular networks by chemical or physical process to further cutting-edge formulation systems for biomedical application. With particular focus on in vivo framework, this chapter has offered a concise picture of current progress in design and development of hydrogel nanoparticles for skin disease and has comprehensive approaches for change in the properties of the nanoparticles for drug delivery. With the improved knowledge in hydrogel chemistry, the practical application of hydrogel formulations has an extraordinary chance to be studied further. Transformation of hydrogel research into in vivo and therapeutic drug delivery applications is, consequently, expected to continue to advance at an astonishing rate. Taking this into consideration, what we anticipate in the hydrogel platform is the wide spread uses of technologies built on hydrogel-based formulations in the clinical setting for several therapeutic applications.

Acknowledgments DR is grateful to VIT-RGEMS for the financial support. We also thank DST-VIT-FIST for NMR, VIT-SIF for GC-MS and other instrumentation facilities. DR would also like to acknowledge the University of Central Florida, Orlando, USA for visiting professor program.

References

1. Gulrez SKH, Al-Assaf S, Phillips GO (2011) Hydrogels: methods of preparation, characterisation and applications. In: Program molecular environment bioengineering analysis modelling to technology application. InTech
2. Glavas-Dodov M, Fredro-Kumbaradzi E, Goracinova K, Calis S, Simonoska M, Hincal AA (2003) 5-Fluorouracil in topical liposome gels for anticancer treatment–formulation and evaluation. Acta Pharm 53:241–250
3. Lee KY, Mooney DJ (2001) Hydrogels for tissue engineering, 101

4. Siepmann J, Peppas NA (2012) Modeling of drug release from delivery systems based on hydroxypropyl methylcellulose (HPMC). Adv Drug Deliv Rev 64:163–174
5. Bettini R, Bonferoni MC, Colombo P, Zanelotti L, Caramella C (2014) Drug release kinetics and front movement in matrix tablets containing diltiazem or metoprolol/λ-carrageenan complexes. Biomed Res Int
6. Greenwald RB, Choe YH, McGuire J, Conover CD (2003) Effective drug delivery by PEGylated drug conjugates. Adv Drug Deliv Rev 55:217–250
7. Amsden B (1998) Solute diffusion within hydrogels. Mech Models Macromolec 31:8382–8395
8. Rice MA, Sanchez-Adams J, Anseth KS (2006) Exogenously triggered, enzymatic degradation of photopolymerized hydrogels with polycaprolactone subunits: experimental observation and modeling of mass loss behavior. Biomacromol 7:1968–1975
9. Khandare J, Minko T (2006) Polymer–drug conjugates: progress in polymeric prodrugs. Prog Polym Sci 31:359–397
10. Kumari K, Sara UV, Sachdeva M (2013) Formulation and evaluation of topical hydrogel of mometasone furoate using different polymers. Int J Pharm Chem Sci 2:89–100
11. Nnamani PO, Kenechukwu FC, Anugwolu CL, Attama AA (2014) Evaluation of hydrogels based on poloxamer 407 and polyacrylic acids for enhanced topical activity of gentamicin against susceptible infections. Trop J Pharm Res 13:1385–1391
12. Koehler J, Wallmeyer L, Hedtrich S, Brandl FP, Achim M, Koehler J, Brandl FP, Goepferich PAM (n.d.) Alkaline poly (ethylene glycol) -based hydrogels for a potential use as bioactive wound dressings
13. Minhas MU, Ahmad M, Ali L, Sohail M (2013) Synthesis of chemically cross-linked polyvinyl alcohol-co-poly (methacrylic acid) hydrogels by copolymerization; a potential graft-polymeric carrier for oral delivery of 5-fluorouracil. DARU J Pharm Sci 21:44
14. Rosiak JM (1999) Hydrogels Med Appl 151:56–64
15. Beynon T, Laverty D, Baxter A, Forsey P, Grocott P (2003) Lutrol gel: a potential role in wounds? J Pain Symptom Manage 26:776–780
16. Ranjha NM, Madni A, Bakar AA, Talib N, Ahmad S, Ahmad H (2014) Preparation and characterization of isosorbide mononitrate hydrogels obtained by free-radical polymerization for site-specific delivery. Trop J Pharm Res 13:1979–1985
17. Kaur LP, Guleri TK (2013) Topical gel: a recent approach for novel drug delivery. Asian J Biomed Pharm Sci 3
18. Kim SJ, Hahn SK, Kim MJ, Kim DH, Lee YP (2005) Development of a novel sustained release formulation of recombinant human growth hormone using sodium hyaluronate microparticles. J Control Release 104:323–335
19. Benamer S, Mahlous M, Boukrif A, Mansouri B, Youcef SL (2006) Synthesis and characterisation of hydrogels based on poly (vinyl pyrrolidone). Nucl Instrum Methods Phys Res Sect B Beam Interact Mater Atoms 248:284–290
20. Osmałek TZ, Froelich A, Jadach B (2018). Rheological investigation of high-acyl gellan gum hydrogel and its mixtures with simulated body fluids. https://doi.org/10.1177/0885328218762361
21. Kumar SV, Sasmal D, Pal SC (2008) Rheological characterization and drug release studies of gum exudates of *Terminalia catappa* Linn. Aaps Pharmscitech 9:885–890
22. Bashir S, Teo YY, Naeem S, Ramesh S, Ramesh K (2017) Correction: pH responsive N-succinyl chitosan/Poly (acrylamide-co-acrylic acid) hydrogels and in vitro release of 5-fluorouracil. PLoS ONE 12:e0185505
23. Grimaudo MA, Nicoli S, Santi P, Concheiro A, Alvarez-Lorenzo C (2018) Cyclosporine-loaded cross-linked inserts of sodium hyaluronan and hydroxypropyl-β-cyclodextrin for ocular administration. Carbohydr Polym 201:308–316
24. Peppas NA, Bures P, Leobandung W, Ichikawa H (2000) Hydrogels in pharmaceutical formulations. Eur J Pharm Biopharm 50:27–46
25. Chirani N, Gritsch L, Motta FL, Fare S (2015) History and applications of hydrogels. J Biomed Sci 4
26. Manju PJ, Fateh MV, Rao NGR (n.d.) World Journal Pharm Life Sci

27. Rowley JA, Madlambayan G, Mooney DJ (1999) Alginate hydrogels as synthetic extracellular matrix materials. Biomaterials 20:45–53
28. Ahmed EM (2015) Hydrogel: Preparation, characterization, and applications: a review. J Adv Res 6:105–121
29. Peppas NA (1991) Physiologically responsive hydrogels. J Bioact Compat Polym 6:241–246
30. Wichterle O, Lim D (1960) Hydrophilic gels for biological use. Nature 185:117
31. Dawson AL, Dellavalle RP, Elston DM (2012) Infectious skin diseases: a review and needs assessment. Dermatol Clin 30:141–151
32. Roberts MS (2007) Dermal absorption and toxicity assessment. CRC Press
33. Gupta M, Agrawal U, Vyas SP (2012) Nanocarrier-based topical drug delivery for the treatment of skin diseases. Expert Opin Drug Deliv 9:783–804
34. Pradhan SK (2011) Microsponges as the versatile tool for drug delivery system. Int J Res Pharm Chem 1:243–258
35. Jain NK (1997) Controlled and novel drug delivery. CBS Publishers & Distributors
36. Storm EJAN, Collier WS, Stewart FR, Bronaugh LR (1990) Metabolism of xenobiotics during percutaneous penetration: role of absorption rate and cutaneous enzyme activity. Toxicol Sci 15:132–141
37. Walters KA (1986) Percutaneous absorption and transdermal therapy. Pharm Tech 10:30–42
38. Yoshida R, Sakai K, Okano T, Sakurai Y (1993) Pulsatile drug delivery systems using hydrogels. Adv Drug Deliv Rev 11:85–108
39. Gong C, Qi T, Wei X, Qu Y, Wu Q, Luo F, Qian Z (2013) Thermosensitive polymeric hydrogels as drug delivery systems. Curr Med Chem 20:79–94
40. Vanbever R, Preat V (1999) In vivo efficacy and safety of skin electroporation. Adv Drug Deliv Rev 35:77–88
41. Cabral J, Moratti SC (2011) Hydrogels for biomedical applications. Fut Med Chem 3:1877–1888
42. Leipzig ND, Wylie RG, Kim H, Shoichet MS (2011) Differentiation of neural stem cells in three-dimensional growth factor-immobilized chitosan hydrogel scaffolds. Biomaterials 32:57–64
43. Gollnick H, Schramm M (1998) Topical drug treatment in acne. Dermatology 196:119–125
44. Hayati F, Ghamsari SM, Dehghan MM, Oryan A (2018) Effects of carbomer 940 hydrogel on burn wounds: an in vitro and in vivo study. J Dermatolog Treat 29:593–599
45. Kumar BK, Thiruvengada Rajan VS, Begum NT (2012) Analytical method development and validation of lidocaine in ointment formulation by U. V spectrophotometric method. Int J Pharm Pharm Sci 4:610–614
46. Ahuja N, Saini V, Bishnoi VK, Garg A, Hisoria M, Sharma J, Nepali K (2008) Formulation and evaluation of diclofenac sodium gel by using natural polymer. Rasayan J Chem 1:564–566
47. Samala ML, Sridevi G (2016) Role of polymers as gelling agents in the formulation of emulgels. Polym Sci 1:2
48. Proniuk S, Blanchard J (2002) Anhydrous Carbopol® polymer gels for the topical delivery of oxygen/water sensitive compounds. Pharm Dev Technol 7:249–255
49. Date AA, Naik B, Nagarsenker MS (2006) Novel drug delivery systems: potential in improving topical delivery of antiacne agents. Skin Pharmacol Physiol 19:2–16
50. Holland TA, Tabata Y, Mikos AG (2005) Dual growth factor delivery from degradable oligo (poly (ethylene glycol) fumarate) hydrogel scaffolds for cartilage tissue engineering. J Control Release 101:111–125
51. West JL, Hubbell JA (1995) Photopolymerized hydrogel materials for drug delivery applications. React Polym 25:139–147
52. Qiu Y, Park K (2001) Environment-sensitive hydrogels for drug delivery. Adv Drug Deliv Rev 53:321–339
53. Soppimath KS, Aminabhavi TM, Dave AM, Kumbar SG, Rudzinski WE (2002) Stimulus-responsive "smart" hydrogels as novel drug delivery systems. Drug Dev Ind Pharm 28:957–974
54. Fetih G (2010) Meloxicam formulations for transdermal delivery: hydrogels versus organogels. J Drug Deliv Sci Technol 20:451–456

55. Sahoo S, Pani NR, Sahoo SK (2014) Microemulsion based topical hydrogel of sertaconazole: formulation, characterization and evaluation. Colloids Surf B Biointerfaces 120:193–199
56. Chandra A, Sharma PK, Irchhiaya R (2014) Microemulsion-based hydrogel formulation for transdermal delivery of dexamethasone. Asian J Pharm Free Full Text Artic Asian J Pharm 3
57. Vashuk EV, Vorobieva EV, Basalyga II, Krutko NP (2001) Water-absorbing properties of hydrogels based on polymeric complexes. Mater Res Innov 4:350–352
58. Lee SJ, Kim SS, Lee YM (2000) Interpenetrating polymer network hydrogels based on poly (ethylene glycol) macromer and chitosan. Carbohydr Polym 41:197–205
59. Vishnubhakthula S, Elupula R, Durán-Lara EF (2017) Recent advances in hydrogel-based drug delivery for melanoma cancer therapy: a mini review. J Drug Deliv
60. Ta HT, Dass CR, Dunstan DE (2008) Injectable chitosan hydrogels for localised cancer therapy. J Control Release 126:205–216
61. Applications T (2018) Encapsulation of biological agents in hydrogels for, 1–30. https://doi.org/10.3390/gels4030061
62. Dimitrova N, Zamudio JR, Jong RM, Soukup D, Resnick R, Sarma K, Ward AJ, Raj A, Lee J, Sharp PA, Jacks T (2017) Public access NIH public access. PLoS ONE 32:736–740. https://doi.org/10.1371/journal.pone.0178059
63. Arias JL (2008) Novel strategies to improve the Anticancer action of 5-fluorouracil by using drug delivery systems, 2340–2369. https://doi.org/10.3390/molecules13102340
64. Parisi E, Garcia A, Marson D, Posocco P, Marchesan S (2019) Supramolecular tripeptide hydrogel assembly with 5-fluorouracil. Gels 5:5. https://doi.org/10.3390/gels5010005
65. Won H, Yeon D, Yeon D, Seon J, Mei L, Lee B, Ho J, Hyun B, Suk M (2013) Biomaterials Injectable intratumoral hydrogel as 5- fluorouracil drug depot. Biomaterials 34:2748–2757. https://doi.org/10.1016/j.biomaterials.2013.01.006
66. McCormick T, Ayala-Fontanez N, Soler D (2016) Current knowledge on psoriasis and autoimmune diseases. Psoriasis Targets Ther 7. https://doi.org/10.2147/ptt.s64950
67. De Gannes G, Huang C, Zhou Y (2005) Topical therapies for psoriasis 5:519–525
68. Lubrizol, Viscosity of Carbopol ® * polymers in aqueous systems-technical data sheet. Lubrizol Adv Mater (2010)
69. Di Tommaso C, Torriglia A, Furrer P, Behar-Cohen F, Gurny R, Möller M (2011) Ocular biocompatibility of novel cyclosporin A formulations based on methoxy poly(ethylene glycol)-hexylsubstituted poly(lactide) micelle carriers. Int J Pharm 416:515–524. https://doi.org/10.1016/j.ijpharm.2011.01.004
70. Luo J, Liu C, Wu J, Lin L, Fan H, Zhao D (2019) In situ injectable hyaluronic acid/gelatin hydrogel for hemorrhage control. Mater Sci Eng C 98:628–634
71. Schneider A, Garlick JA, Egles C (2008) Self-assembling peptide nanofiber scaffolds accelerate wound healing. PLoS ONE 3:e1410
72. Kawabata S, Kanda N, Hirasawa Y, Noda K, Matsuura Y, Suzuki S, Kawai K (2018) The utility of silk-elastin hydrogel as a new material for wound healing. Plast Reconstr Surg Glob Open 6

Chapter 11
Effect of Structural Properties of Hydrogel in Controlled Drug Delivery

Arjun Sabu, Priya Vijayaraghavan, Rugma Nair, and Fredi Francis Cheruvathoor

Abstract Hydrogels are extremely swollen, hydrophilic, three-dimensional polymer networks that are capable of absorbing vast amounts of body fluids or water. Hydrogels possess the ability to swell within their structure and hold a large fraction of water, but they may not dissolve in water. They have attracted tremendous attention as candidates for biomedical applications because of their ability to swell, under physiological conditions and their consequent biocompatibility. The ability of hydrogels to absorb large quantities of water is due to the presence of functional hydrophilic groups attached to their back bones or as lateral chains, whereas crosslinks between network chains result in their resistance to dissolution. Due to their specific physical properties, which make them promising materials for drug delivery, tissue engineering, and even in food and cosmetic manufacturing, they have attracted considerable attention in recent years. The interplay between their chemical–structure–property relationships and their interaction with the biological system, taking careful account of their physical, chemical, and biological properties, makes it possible to effectively design a hydrogel for biomedical applications. In this chapter, the structural parameters of polymer hydrogels and various drug release mechanisms of hydrogel drug delivery systems are discussed.

Keywords Hydrogels · Structural parameters · Structure property relations · Controlled release and mechanisms

A. Sabu (✉)
International and Inter University Centre for Nanoscience and Nanotechnology, Mahatma Gandhi University, PD Hills (PO), Kottayam, Kerala 686 560, India

P. Vijayaraghavan
Department of Biomedical Engineering and Environmental Sciences, National Tsing Hua University, Hsinchu, Taiwan (ROC)

F. F. Cheruvathoor
Department of Chemistry, National Tsing Hua University, Hsinchu, Taiwan (ROC)

R. Nair
College of Indigenous Food Technology, Pathanamthitta, Kerala, India

J. Jose et al. (eds.), *Nano Hydrogels*, Gels Horizons: From Science to Smart Materials,
https://doi.org/10.1007/978-981-15-7138-1_11

1 Structural Parameters

Swelling, porosity and permeation, stimuli responsiveness and mechanical stability are the most important properties of hydrogels which make them suitable for many applications. The significant structural factors which influence other hydrogel properties are the degree of swelling and mesh size. A hydrogel's mesh size ξ is a structural parameter that defines the average linear distance between neighboring crosslinks and the average molecular weight between the crosslinks is M_c. Using empirical evidence and theoretical models based on rheological, mechanical, thermogravimetric or size exclusion characterizations, mesh size is calculated. Hydrogel swelling is a physico-chemical parameter that can be measured directly via gravimetric techniques and is mathematically described as mass swelling (q) or volumetric swelling (Q).

$$q = \frac{m_s}{m_d}$$

$$Q = \frac{V_s}{V_d} = 1 + \frac{\rho_{HG}}{\rho_{sol}}(q - 1)$$

where $\boldsymbol{m}_s$ = swollen mass, $\boldsymbol{m}_d$ = dry mass, $\boldsymbol{V}_s$ = swollen volume, $\boldsymbol{V}_d$ = dry volume, $\boldsymbol{\rho}_{HG}$ = bulk density of the hydrogel polymer, and $\boldsymbol{\rho}_{sol}$ = swelling medium density [1].

Also, swelling ratio of hydrogels can be calculated by the following equation,

$$\text{Swelling}\ (\%) = \frac{W_s - W_d}{W_d} \times 100$$

where W_d = weight of dry hydrogel and W_s = weight of swollen hydrogel [2].

Hydrogels can be designed with stimuli responses which are controllable so as to shrink or swell with changes in external environmental condition like temperature, electric or magnetic field, light, pressure, sound, pH, solvent composition, ionic strength, oxidants and reductants, molecular species, protein, enzyme, sugars, etc. Hydrogel systems which can respond to changes in their environment are of special interest for biomedical applications due to the substantial changes occurring at several body locations as a result of a diseased state or during normal function.

In recent years, the use of potential pharmaceutical devices such as new drug delivery systems (DDS) has been of great interest as it proposes an effective means of delivering therapeutic agents on a site-specific and/or time-controlled basis. Different types of polymeric systems were used as containers for drugs or control barriers releasing rate, but among these, hydrogels are of primary interest. Therapeutically beneficial aspects of drug delivery can be harvested by hydrogel delivery systems and have attained a high impact in clinical use. Hydrogels serve as a basis for regulating the rate of release of various physiochemical interactions with the encapsulated drugs, which is possible because of their tunable physical properties, regulated degradability, and ability to avoid premature drug degradation before reaching the target location. Hydrogels provide the release of therapeutic agents, including cells, small and macro molecular drugs, with temporal and spatial controls.

The hydrogels' drug release kinetics mainly depend on their composition (polymer used, drug embedded, and additives used), geometry (shape and size), preparation method, and physiological conditions at the time of release of the drug [3]. The surface of the drug delivery system can often get wet with the releasing medium (water). This release medium can also penetrate (e.g., through pores) into the drug delivery system. Polymer or drug degradation can dramatically affect the kinetics of drug release. Drug release kinetics are often influenced by the diffusion, dissolution and/or precipitation of drugs and/or products from polymer degradation within the hydrogel matrix or in the fluid and micro-environmental pH shift inside the hydrogel matrix as a result of polymer degradation. Swelling of polymers and closing of pores caused by polymer swelling are another reasons. Creation or changes in acidic or basic microenvironments caused by degradation products in the dosage forms, physical drug-polymer interactions can also be a reason. A change in geometry and/or dimensions of the device for drug delivery caused by shearing forces has a clear effect on the same. All these phenomena concern the drug transport in the model system [4].

Various additional factors, such as enzymatic degradation, passive and active drug uptake into cells, protein binding, interactions with compounds in intra- and extra-cellular space, need to be taken into account to explain the drug transport process in the living body [5]. The mechanism of drug release consists of phenomena like exterior and interior diffusion [6], desorption, chemical reactions, etc. Other than these, shape changing processes (including heterogeneous and homogeneous erosion) and surface changing processes (desorption, reconstruction and reaction) may overlap with the factors listed above. Hydrogel matrix can also undergo a change in its shape during the drug release.

2 Chain Cleavage

The drug can be directly connected to the polymer or via a "spacer" group in hydrogel drug carriers. Polymers are eventually decomposed in the case of a biodegradable system and drugs are released, resulting in controlled drug release. If the drug is linked to the polymer through chemical crosslinks, different mechanisms can be used for the degradation of hydrogels. These mechanisms include cleavage of the crosslinker, pendant groups, or backbone chain (Fig. 1). Various covalent linkages were investigated such as highly stable amide bonds formed via carbodiimide chemistry, thiol-ene bonds and those formed via metal free click chemistry. Amide bonds have been used via an amine-hydroxysuccinimide reaction to conjugate TGFβ1 to a PEG hydrogel [7], while degradable click hydrogels have also been developed for regulated degradation and protein releases [8]. By combining PEG macromers that have been functionalized with various mercaptoacids and with maleimide functionalized PEG, hydrogels that degrade by either hydrolytic or hydrolytic and thiol

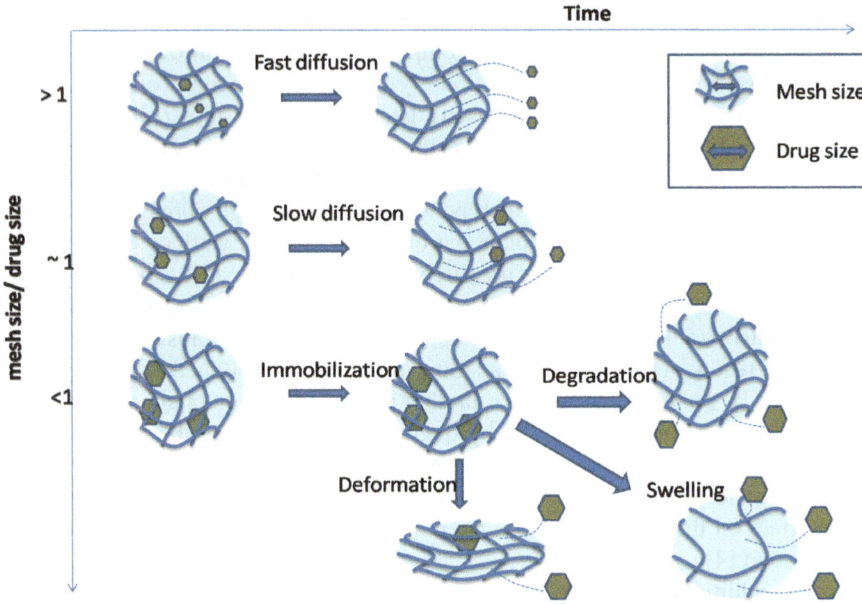

Fig. 1 Mediation of drug diffusion by mesh size. A smaller drug with $r_{mesh}/r_{drug} > 1$ results in a faster release of drug via diffusion. If both the drug and mesh are of comparable size ($r_{mesh}/r_{drug} \sim 1$), slow diffusion of drug takes place whereas when drug size exceeds the mesh size $r_{mesh}/r_{drug} < 1$ the drug cannot diffuse and the release happens via either degradation swelling or deformation

exchange mechanisms have been developed. For example, hydrolysis is accelerated through lowering the pH (Cancer tissues). UV light of considerable energy can trigger microgel degradation. Utilizing the conversion nanoparticles to combine two or more NIR photons into a UV photon, even using a low-energy near-infrared (NIR) light can activate hydrogel degradation. In a study, dexamethasone, a type of corticosteroid was attached to a photosensitive mono-acrylate PEG through a cleavable lactide bond. But, generally, the release of a drug which is covalently bound depends on the polymer—drug link's degradation rate. The majority of these interactions are hydrolytically degradable. As the network degrades, the mesh size increases, allowing drugs to disperse out of the hydrogel. This allows the drug release rate to be completely characterized by simple first-order kinetics (Fig. 1).

3 Hydrolytic Degradation

In hydrolytically degradable hydrogels, the degradation rate is affected by crosslinking density, local pH, and characteristics of the polymer network, including crystallinity, hydrophobicity, and polymer backbone molecular weight (Table 1). Synthetic hydrogels can be engineered in such a way to degrade via the hydrolysis

Table 1 Classes of hydrolysable bonds

Polymer class		Half life
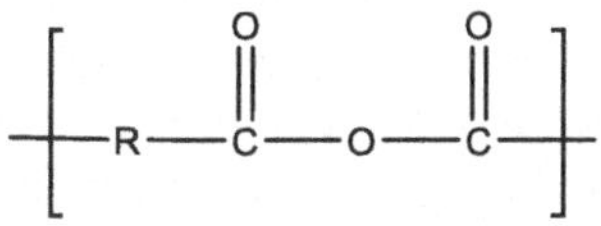	Poly(anhydrides)	0.1 h
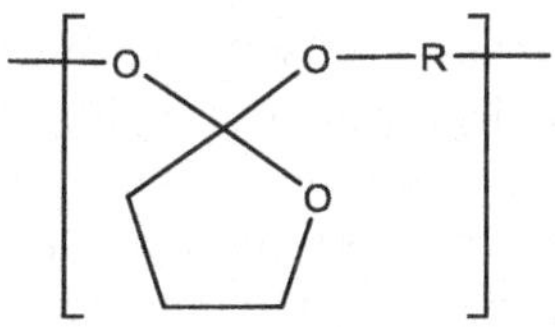	Poly(orthoesters)	4 h
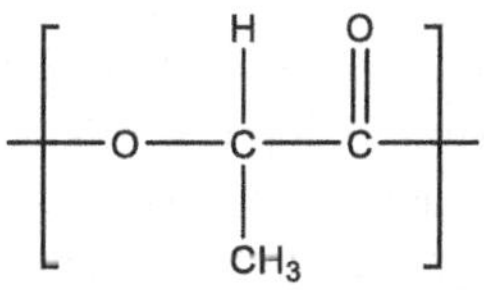	Poly(esters)	3.3 years
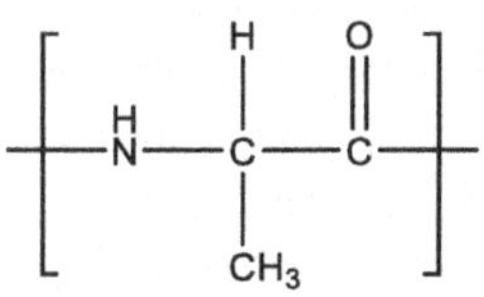	Poly(amides)	83,000 years

of ester linkages of the crosslinker or network backbone producing an alcohol and a carboxylic acid. Patenaude and Hoare reported the synthesis of thermo-responsive hydrogels which are hydrolytically degradable, using aldehyde and hydrazide functionalized PNIPAAM [9]. The hydrolysis rate of the hydrazone moieties in an acidic micro-environment was observed to be in the range of 2–6 h, finally resulting in the full cell-compatible hydrogels' degradation, and kinetic data extrapolation projected several months of degradation under physiological conditions. Zhang et al. devised the use of poly(e-caprolactone-colactide)-b-poly (ethylene glycol)-b-poly(e-caprolactone-co-lactide), a biodegradable tri-block copolymer hydrogel as an intestinal adhesion barrier for post-operative use [10]. The integrity of the hydrogel was preserved (in vivo) for almost 6 weeks and gradually degraded without significant cytotoxicity via ester hydrolysis.

4 Enzymatic Degradation

In the case of hydrogels made up of proteins, natural polymers or peptide linkages, degradation via cell-mediated enzymatic cleavage attracts special attention. In case of enzymatically degradable hydrogels, the enzyme concentration depends upon the types of tissues and cells. This enables drug release which is locally triggered. Enzymatic cleavage mediated by cells is of significant importance in case of this type of hydrogels. Enzymes responsible for the C–N, C–O, and C–C bonds hydrolysis belong to the family Hyaluronidase. It is known that the hyaluronidase concentration in various carcinomas is considerably higher. In such situations, as site-specific therapeutic delivery vehicles, enzymatically degradable HA-based hydrogels may be used. In the presence of hyaluronidase, HA-based hydrogels degrade. For protein delivery, an injectable hydrogel based on HA-tyramine is used for which the release of the cargo molecule partly depended on the degradation of hydrogel through hyaluronidase [11]. Approximately, 70% of the activity was retained in vitro by the released lysozyme, which was a model cargo protein. In theory, this approach can be used to prevent tumor growth by sustained, local therapeutic protein release [11].

In the above examples, the introduction of peptide- or protein-based linkages susceptible to proteases is also present which is a powerful tool for synthetic and in situ degradation control of hydrogels. Michael-type addition of thiols to maleimides is another reaction mechanism that can be utilized to synthesize enzyme-responsive PEG hydrogels. García et al. used thiol-maleimide crosslinking chemistry for the development of protease-responsive PEG hydrogels. MMP-cleavable hydrogels loaded with growth factor were administered to rats' infarcted myocardium and reported results demonstrated improved cardiac function [12]. Several examples of peptide-crosslinked hydrogel systems, which are MMP-cleavable, which include the systems prepared from Pluronic® triblock copolymer, silk and elastin, collagen, alginate, or heparin. Werner et al. documented the synthesis of star PEG-heparin hydrogel networks that are crosslinked with MMP-cleavable peptides that can be used for the controlled delivery of a variety of therapeutic molecules, via Michael-type addition [13].

5 Click Chemistry

Click chemistry is also a promising mechanism that can be used in synthesis of hydrogels. In recent years, due to its excellent selectivity, mild reaction conditions and high reactivity, for preparing hydrogels, click chemistry has emerged as the most promising strategy. One can also synthesize hydrogels with different patterns and dimensions.

The first report of hydrogel synthesis using "click chemistry" was in 2006 by Hilborn and co-workers [14]. Synthesis of poly(vinyl alcohols) (PVA) functionalized with either groups of acetylene or azides was reported. Immediately after the addition of $CuSO_4$/Sodium ascorbate, the hydrogel was formed.

Natural polymers based on hydrogels (also called natural hydrogels) have attracted a considerable interest attributable to their excellent biocompatibility and biodegradability for tissue engineering and drug delivery. Crescenzi et al. reported the synthesis of click hydrogels from azides- and alkyne-functionalized hyaluronic acid (HA) [15].

Studies of in vitro release have shown that the release of benzidamine and doxorubicin (DOX) from HA hydrogels ranges from hours to several weeks, depending on the densities of cross-linking. Drugs such as glucocorticoid dexamethasone (Dex) can be attached to an appropriate MMP-degradable peptide by conjugation to its *N*-terminus and then integrated into PEG gel scaffolds by thiol-norbornene reaction copolymerization to afford cell-mediated delivery of tiny bioactive molecules [16]. Covalently tethered dexamethasone from PEG hydrogels undergoing a controlled release can be facilitated by exploiting the dynamic nature of the DA reaction.

References

1. Goding J, Vallejo-Giraldo C, Syed O, Green R (2019) Considerations for hydrogel applications to neural bioelectronics. J Mater Chem B 7:1625–1636
2. Gupta S, Bit A (2018) 16-rapid prototyping for polymeric gels. In: Pal K, Banerjee IBT-PG (eds) Woodhead publishing series in biomaterials. Woodhead Publishing, pp 397–439. https://doi.org/10.1016/B978-0-08-102179-8.00016-8
3. Mauri E, Papa S, Masi M, Veglianese P, Rossi F (2017) Novel functionalization strategies to improve drug delivery from polymers. Exp Opin Drug Deliv 14:1305–1313
4. Kamaly N, Yameen B, Wu J, Farokhzad OC (2016) Degradable controlled-release polymers and polymeric nanoparticles: mechanisms of controlling drug release. Chem Rev 116:2602–2663
5. Grumezescu AM (2019) Nanomaterials for drug delivery and therapy. William Andrew
6. Zarzycki R, Modrzejewska Z, Nawrotek K (2010) Drug release from hydrogel matrices. Ecol Chem Eng S 17:117–136
7. Kim J et al (2015) TGF-β1 conjugated chitosan collagen hydrogels induce chondrogenic differentiation of human synovium-derived stem cells. J Biol Eng 9:1
8. Kharkar PM, Kloxin AM, Kiick KL (2014) Dually degradable click hydrogels for controlled degradation and protein release. J Mater Chem B 2:5511–5521
9. Patenaude M, Hoare T (2012) Injectable, degradable thermoresponsive poly(*N*-isopropylacrylamide) hydrogels. ACS Macro Lett 1:409–413
10. Zhang Z et al (2011) Biodegradable and thermoreversible PCLA-PEG-PCLA hydrogel as a barrier for prevention of post-operative adhesion. Biomaterials 32:4725–4736
11. Kharkar PM, Kiick KL, Kloxin AM (2013) Designing degradable hydrogels for orthogonal control of cell microenvironments. Chem Soc Rev 42:7335–7372
12. Phelps EA et al (2012) Maleimide cross-linked bioactive PEG hydrogel exhibits improved reaction kinetics and cross linking for cell encapsulation and in situ delivery. Adv Mater 24:64–70
13. Tsurkan MV, Levental KR, Freudenberg U, Werner C (2010) Enzymatically degradable heparin-polyethylene glycol gels with controlled mechanical properties. Chem Commun 46:1141–1143
14 Ossipov AD, Hilborn J (2006) Poly(vinyl alcohol)-based hydrogels formed by "click chemistry". Macromolecules 39:1709–1718
15. Crescenzi V, Cornelio L, Di Meo C, Nardecchia S, Lamanna R (2007) Novel hydrogels via click chemistry: synthesis and potential biomedical applications. Biomacromol 8:1844–1850
16. Yang C, Mariner PD, Nahreini JN, Anseth KS (2012) Cell-mediated delivery of glucocorticoids from thiol-ene hydrogels. J Control Release 162:612–618

Chapter 12
Elasticity, Strength, and Biocompatibility of Hydrogels

Arunima Reghunadhan, Athira Johnson, and A. R. Ajitha

Abstract Hydrogels have been a familiar term in the current biomedical research. Generally, hydrogels are swollen polymer networks with water. Biocompatibility and ease of preparation are the key properties which enable them to be used in a variety of biomedical applications. Hydrogels can be classified in a number of ways depending on a wide range of properties. The chapter discusses in detail about the general properties, classification, mechanical properties, and biocompatibility of hydrogels. The special emphasis is on the biocompatibility. The factors affecting the elasticity and mechanical strength will be discussed along with the characterization techniques.

Keywords Hydrogels · Elasticity · Biocompatibility · Mechanical properties

1 Introduction

Hydrogels are by definition, polymeric gel consisting of crosslinked molecules which are capable of holding large amounts of water. That means a three-dimensional system of polymers made from natural or synthetic materials with a high degree of flexibility owing to increased water content is called hydrogels. Hydrogels are like solids and also like liquids. Water fills the voids in the crosslinked three-dimensional networks. Particles can diffuse to these structures. They may be firm or dissociate or dissolve in water. Even though water molecules can diffuse or penetrate into the hydrogels, they are normally water-insoluble materials. The insolubility is a result

A. Reghunadhan (✉) · A. R. Ajitha
International and Interuniversity Centre for Nanoscience and Nanotechnology, Mahatma Gandhi University, P.D. Hills P.O., Kottayam, Kerala, India
e-mail: arunimarenjith02@gmail.com

A. Reghunadhan
Department of Chemistry, TKM College of Engineering, Karicode, Kollam-5, Kerala, India

A. Johnson
Department of Food Science, College of Life Science, National Taiwan Ocean University, Keelung, Taiwan

J. Jose et al. (eds.), *Nano Hydrogels*, Gels Horizons: From Science to Smart Materials,
https://doi.org/10.1007/978-981-15-7138-1_12

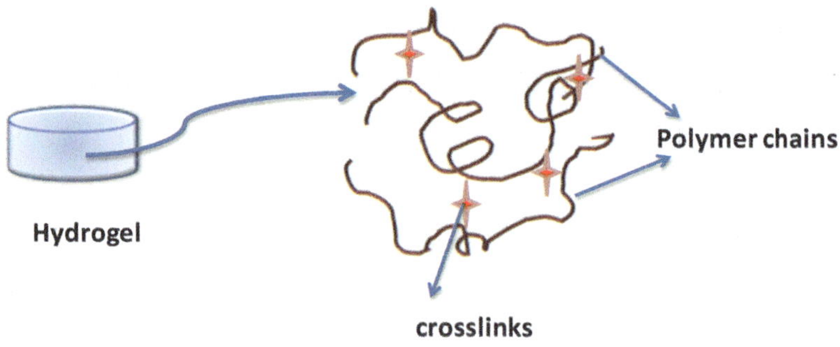

Fig. 1 Schematic representation of hydrogels

of the 3D crosslinks. At the molecular level, water in a hydrogel either binds to polar hydrophilic groups as bond water or fills the space between the network chains, pores, or voids as free water [1]. The presence of hydrophilic groups like $-NH_2$, $-COOH$, $-OH$, $-CONH_2$, $-CONH$, etc., is the reason behind the hydrophilicity (Fig. 1).

2 Classification of Hydrogels

Hydrogels can be classified in a variety of ways [2]. A large classification is possible in the case of these materials. The classification depends on many factors such as their physical properties, nature of swelling, methods of preparation, origin, charges, different sources, biodegradation, and nature of crosslinking.

Based on the origin or source, hydrogels can be divided into natural and synthetic.

The second division is based on the composition of the polymer involved. According the polymeric composition, hydrogels are classified into homopolymeric, co-polymeric, and multipolymeric IPNs.

1. Homopolymeric: These are polymer networks obtained from a single monomer species, a fundamental structural unit consisting of any polymer network. Homopolymers may have cross-linked skeletal structure based on the nature of the method of monomer and polymerization.
2. Copolymeric: They are comprised of two or more different monomer species with at least one hydrophilic component, arranged in a random, block or alternating configuration along the chain of the polymer network.
3. Multipolymer Interpenetrating polymeric: A significant class of hydrogels consists of two fully independent cross-linked synthetic and/or natural polymer components embedded in a network form. In semi-IPN hydrogel, one part is a cross-linked polymer and another part is a non-cross-linked polymer.

Next classification is based on crosslinking, and normally, two types exist: physical crosslinking and chemical crosslinking. Also based on configuration, they can be divided into crystalline, semi-crystalline and amorphous.

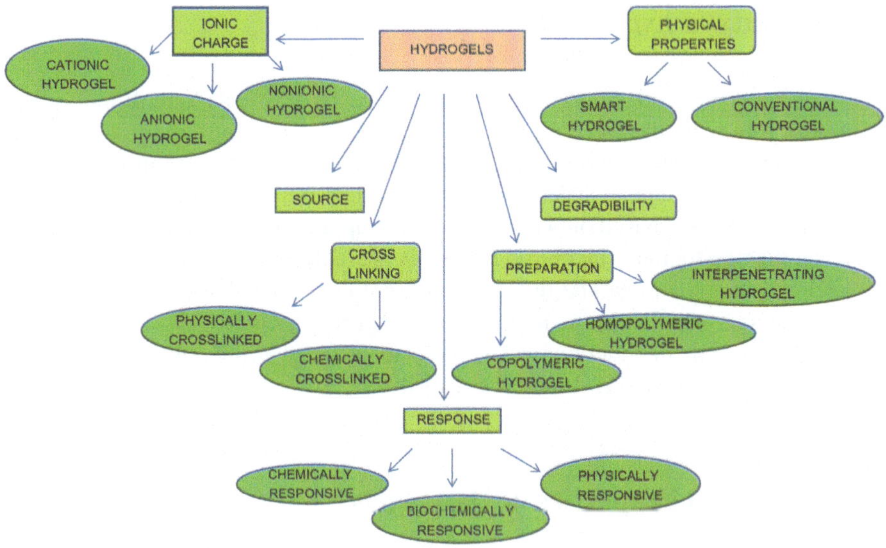

Fig. 2 Classification of hydrogels

Depending on appearance, they can be matrix, films, or microspheres. Based on the charge of the species, hydrogels may be grouped into four based on the presence or lack of electrical load situated on the crosslinked chains as nonionic (neutral), ionic (including cationic or anionic), amphoteric electrolyte (ampholytic) comprising acidic and basic groups and zwitter ionic comprising both anionic and cationic units in each structural repeating unit. Based on physical properties, they are subdivided into smart hydrogels and conventional hydrogels. A very important and broad classification is based on the response of the gels. Chemically responsive, biochemically responsive, and physically responsive hydrogels are there. Degradability is also considered as a measure to divide the hydrogels. Hydrogels can be biodegradable and non-biodegradable. All these classifications can be simply represented by a diagram as show in Fig. 2.

3 Properties of hydrogels

The general properties of hydrogels include the response, swelling, permeability, surface, optical, and mechanical properties. Rapid response to external stimuli is a crucial property in the view of applications. The swelling and mechanical properties depend on the degree of crosslinks in the polymeric material. All the properties of hydrogel materials depend on the environment too. Here, the detailed discussion will be for the elasticity, mechanical strength, and surface properties.

4 Elasticity of hydrogels

Elasticity is the physical entity of a substance by means of which it returns to its initial form after removing the force under which it deforms. The applied force is termed as stress, and the response is termed as strain. The stress-to-strain ratio is constant for a specified material and is defining mechanical property. The stresses and strains may be axial or shear based on whether the force applied is perpendicular or parallel to the supporting region. The elastic regime is characterized by a linear relationship between stress and strain. The theory of elasticity assumes that the strain reaction is instantaneous when stress is applied to the hydrogel. Hydrogels usually convey a non-purely elastic conduct owing to the viscoelasticity of the polymer chains and the poroelasticity caused by the presence of fluid.

5 Mechanical Properties of Hydrogels

As explained earlier, since the hydrogels are swollen with water, they have poor mechanical strength. There are a few explanations for the poor mechanical properties of hydrogel along with the random fiber arrangement and large water content inside the hydrogel. Monomer composition, crosslinking density, polymerization conditions, and degree of swelling play important role in determining the strength of gels. Crosslinks in the swollen structure are the main variable in evaluating strength. Mechanical properties are generally material dependent. The mechanical properties measured in the case of hydrogels are Young's modulus, Poisson's ratio, and viscoelastic properties. From the obtained Young's modulus, the crosslink density can also be measured [3]. The viscoelastic properties are better explained by Maxwell's model or theory. The relation between stress and deformation can be related as

$$\sigma(t) = \frac{\varepsilon_0}{t_1}\left[E_0 t_1 + \sum_{i=1}^{N} \eta_i \mathrm{e}^{-\frac{E_i}{\eta_i}\cdot t}\left(\mathrm{e}^{\frac{E_i}{\eta_i}\cdot t} - 1\right)\right]$$

where t is time, η_i an E_i represent the generalized Maxwell model parameters, N is the number of Maxwell elements considered (apart from the pure elastic element characterized by E_0), and t_1 is the time required to get the deformation ε_0.

Graci and coworkers used the above equation in order to relate the crosslink density and mechanical properties. They fitted the experimental data with the above theory and concluded that the Young's modulus and the crosslink density increased with increasing concentration of the polymer. From the mechanical properties, they calculated the network average mesh size [4].

Good mechanical strength is the utmost important property in biocompatible systems. As mentioned earlier, the hydrogels are poor in strength. Sometimes in order to increase the mechanical strength of hydrogels they are converted into composites with other materials having high strength. Such a modification was reported in the case of super porous hydrogel used for gastric retention devices. Chen and Park introduced a sol for making composite [5].

6 Analysis of Mechanical Properties

A good number of techniques are available for characterizing hydrogels in terms of their mechanical strength. Microindendation proved as the most successful technique to determine the tensile properties of hydrogels.

6.1 Compression Tests

Compression test is a common practice used to examine the mechanical characteristics of several distinct kinds of hydrogels. Suitability of this method is owed to the cylindrical shape of the hydrogels. In this test, a disk is compressed between two flat platens and can be expanded in the radial direction (sliding boundary conditions) [6]. As in this laboratory module, this test setup is usually conducted under displacement control. By considering the geometry of the disk sample (radius and thickness), the Young's modulus can be calculated. The pressure applied to the hydrogel's surface and the distance compressed by the hydrogel can be used to calculate the mechanical properties of the hydrogels using a theoretical model (Fig. 3).

6.2 Bulging Tests

The experiment includes deflating the hydrogel in the substratum across a window and measuring the corresponding displacement as a function of the stress applied. The displacement can be measured using either a camera or a laser. A finite element

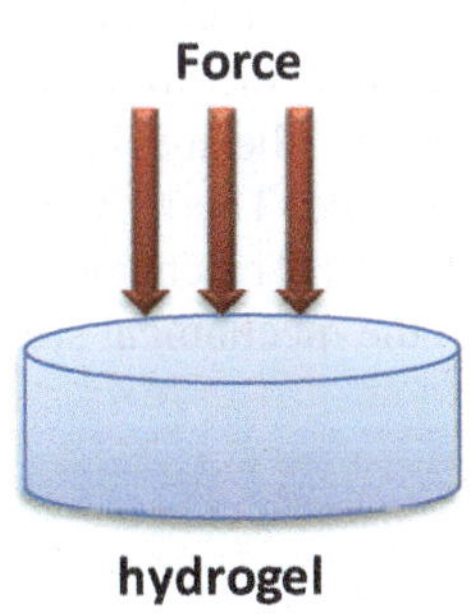

Fig. 3 Schematic representation of compression test

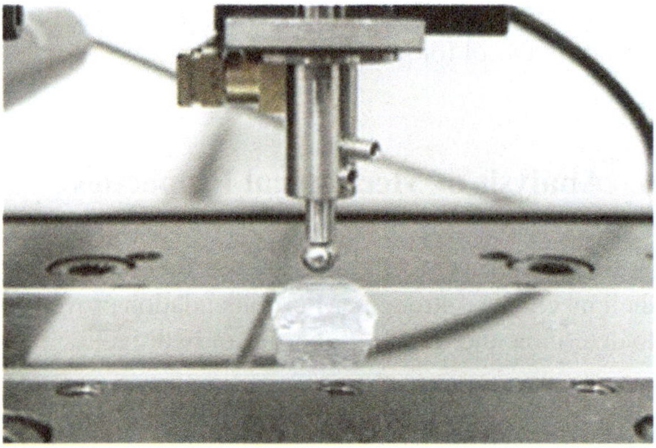

Fig. 4 Indentation on a hydrogel sample

template is then used to assess the information and compute values for the hydrogel's mechanical characteristics [7, 8].

6.3 Indentation

Indentation tests are the most favorable mechanical property analysis in the case of hydrogel and is the most successful technique [9–11]. This technique works by indenting a hydrogel at a single point to a predetermined displacement depth and measuring the reaction force required to cause the indentation. Indentation test are non-destructive approach in the field of mechanical characterization (Fig. 4).

6.4 Rheology

Rheological analysis is a common procedure to analyze the properties of polymer gels and viscous liquids. Rheology is generally considers as the study of the flow or it is considering the flow behaviour of substances. The rheological analysis can be done in different modes and all the modes generally deals with the shearing forces. The mechanical properties of hydrogels can be determined by rheological analysis. The hydrogels are subjected to shear force, and the response is measured (Fig. 5). The change in viscosity, storage and loss modulus are considered and related to the mechanical strength and processability.

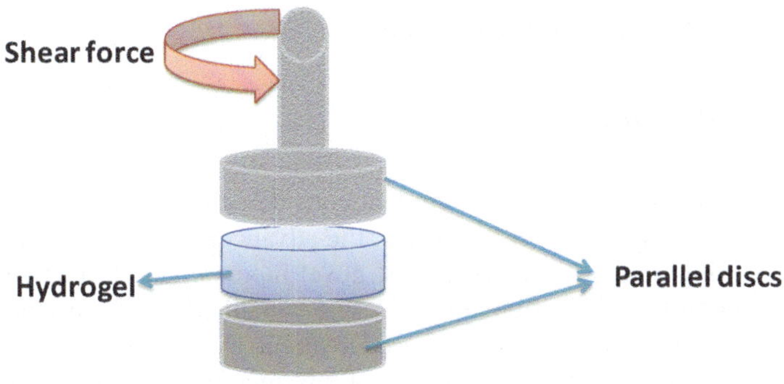

Fig. 5 Experimental setup for the rheological analysis of hydrogel

6.5 Particle Image Velocimetry

The method is based on the fact that small particles implemented in a fluid flow would move with the velocity of the local fluid. Basic measurements in particle image velocimetry (PIV) relate particle displacement over a period of time in such a manner that speed is measured as displacement proportion and time interval [12] (Fig. 6).

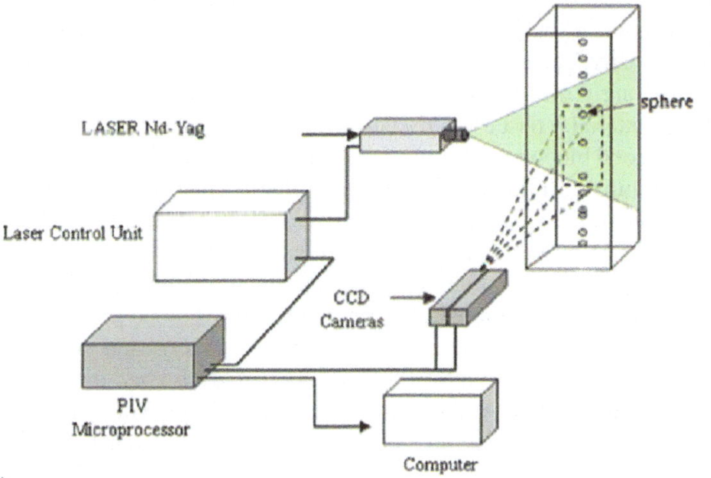

Fig. 6 Experimental setup of PIV

7 Biocompatibility of Hydrogels

7.1 Biocompatibility

"Biocompatibility" is an important term that considered during the preparation and execution of a biomaterial. In recent years, the advancement of biotechnology and tissue engineering facilitate the practice of novel biomaterials for clinical applications. According to the definition, a biomaterial is defined as "a substance that has been engineered to take a form which is used to direct, bycontrol of interactions with components of living systems, the course of any therapeutic or diagnostic procedure" [13]. The interaction between the biomaterial and living tissue is an important parameter because of the incompatibility. All of the biomaterials are considered as a foreign material when it will introduce into the body and that exerts certain immunological response known as foreign body responses (FBRs). Macrophages, dendritic cells, and adsorbed proteins are known as the key players that initiate the interaction between biomaterials and cells [14]. The need for non-toxic materials for therapeutic applications initiates the usage of term biocompatibility. It is defined as "the ability of the chosen material to achieve the best therapeutic performance in the target physiological environment, without adverse effects of the health of the host [15]." It creates significant challenges to the manufactures of the biomaterial in terms of the FBRs. Biocompatibility is also defined as the interdependent interaction mechanism between the biomaterial and living tissue, and it is categorized into interfacial (biological) and mechanical (bulk) biocompatibility [16]. A biocompatible material has an appropriate density, strength, rigidity, non-toxicity, and non-inflammatory response together with long-term storage capacity [17]. The biocompatibility is different from materials to materials, tissues to tissues, and cells to cells. So, the designing of a material with good biocompatibility is a challenge to researchers and manufacturers.

Biocompatibility is influenced by various biological pathways such as chemotaxis, neutrophil activation, and complement activation. The presence of foreign material (here: biomaterial) initiates neutrophil aggregation due to complement activation and leads to pulmonary dysfunction [18]. The incompatibility of the materials is marked by clotting and thrombosis. Host proteins such as blood proteins (fibronectin, fibrinogen, and vitronectin), opsonins(immunoglobin G), and the complement-activated fragment C3b were adsorbed onto the material when the material comes in contact with blood [19]. At the same time, frustrated phagocytosis occurred due to the large size of the biomaterial. As a result, leukocyte products (e.g., lysosomal proteases and oxygen-free radicals) are released to degrade the foreign material. After the neutrophil clearance, the chronic inflammation is arised due to the prolonged accumulation of monocytes, macrophages, and lymphocytes together with the proliferation of blood vessels and connective tissue [20]. This will initiate a foreign body response.

Both in vivo and in vitro methods are used to evaluate the biocompatibility of a material. The response of cells or tissues toward the biomaterials is roughly classified into (i) strong effects (cytotoxicity, genotoxicity), (ii) moderate to nearly negligible effects (complement activation, pharmacological effects), and (iii) the absence of measurable effects [21]. Cytotoxicity, sensitization, irritation or intracutaneous reactivity, mucous membrane irritation, systemic and subchronic toxicity, genotoxicity, reproductive or developmental toxicity, blood biocompatibility/complement activation, immune response, carcinogenicity, biodegradation, etc., are the some of the standards related to biocompatibility [21]. Final finished form of medical devices (ISO 10993–12), evaluation of the biological response due to device mechanical failure (specific to FDA), preparation of test article samples or test extracts (ISO 10993–12), evaluation of submicron or nanotechnology components (ISO 10993–22), testing of in situ polymerizing and/or absorbable materials (ISO/TR 37137), and the strategy for testing of extracts from multiple component devices (specific to FDA) are the major biocompatibility testing considerations [22]. The evaluation of the biocompatibility helps to predict whether the material is toxic or nontoxic to the living tissue. The hydrophilicity/hydrophobicity, wettability, surface energy, lubricity, chemical functions, smoothness, surface roughness, protein adsorption, swelling, and electrostatic effects are the important surface parameters of the biomaterials that are considered during the assessment of biocompatibility [23]. Both in vitro and in vivo tests are carried out to evaluate the cytotoxicity of the biomaterials. The prolonged exposure of biomaterials toward the target cell line is a widely accepted way to check the biocompatibility/toxicity of the material. 3-(4,5-Dimethylthiazol-2-yl)-2,5-diphenyltetrazolium bromide (MTT) assay, methylcellulose toxicity test, and nitro blue tetrazolium chloride (NBT) assay, etc., are some of the experiment that frequently used to evaluate the biocompatibility of the material in vitro. The subcutaneous implantation with histological and morphological evaluations are common in in vivo biocompatibility assessment [24].

7.2 Biocompatibility of the Hydrogel

Hydrogels are the network of polymer chains that swollen extensively in water. It is categorized according to cross-linking (physical and chemical crosslinking), physical state (solid, semisolid, and liquid), stimuli-responsive (pH-responsive, temperature, etc.), source (natural and synthetic), polymer composition (homopolymer, copolymer, and multipolymer), electric charge (nonionic, ionic, zwitterionic, and amphoteric), and configuration (amorphous, crystalline) [25–27]. The synthetic polymer-based hydrogels are considered to have low biocompatibility as compared to the natural one. The polymeric biomaterials are classified into biostable, bioabsorbable, and partially bioabsorbable based on their behavior in contact with the living tissue [23]. Hydrogel-related oral drug delivery has a wide application due to the strong pH variation from the mouth to the intestine and elimination from the body through feces. The degradation rate of the hydrogel is affected by the degree of crosslinking. An increase in the degree of crosslinking reduces the degradation rate of the material [28]. The physiochemical similarity to the extracellular matrix (ECM) and higher water content make the hydrogel become more biocompatible.

The polymers used to develop hydrogels are versatile in nature. They are capable of form hydrogels with good flexibility and softness. Like cells, the hydrogel maintains a hydrated nature and the elastic property that helps to reduce the irritation to the surrounding tissue. The negative immune response of the host cell is reduced by the low interfacial tension between the hydrogel surface and the body fluid. Furthermore, the mucoadhesive and bioadhesive characteristics of hydrogel enable the tissue permeability [29]. A biomaterial has the ability to perform desired functions without causing any toxicity to the cells/tissues. It must be immunocompatible and should not undergo significant functional changes during sterilization. The three-dimensional structure of the hydrogels is provided by cross-linking of the polymers. The mechanical properties also affect the cell migration, proliferation, and differentiation of the cells. Another important parameter is the degradation of the hydrogels. The hydrogels are mainly degraded via ester cleavage, enzymatic cleavage, photolytic cleavage or the combinations of this mechanism. The by-products formed after degradation must be non-toxic to the cells and the degradation kinetics is needed to be stable [18]. Alginate, dextran, hyaluronic acid, pectin, and xanthan are some of the natural polymers used for the preparation of hydrogels. The synthetic polymers such as acrylic acid (AA), poly(vinylalcohol), methacrylic acid (MAA), and poly(styrene) (PS) are used for the preparation of biocompatible hydrogels (Fig. 7).

A good hydrogel has the ability to control the specific molecular interaction such as receptor-ligand complexes, bound or soluble molecule interactions, and focal adhesion interactions at the cell-material interface. Poly(ethylene glycol) (PEG) hydrogel mimic collagenase substrates found in natural ECM proteins. Controlled resorption or dissolution is essential for the degradation of hydrogels [31]. At the macroscopic level, the physical texture of the hydrogels is altered by environmental parameters like temperature, pH, an electric signal, the presence of an enzyme or other ionic species. Biosafety and bio-functionality are the two elements of biocompatibility that

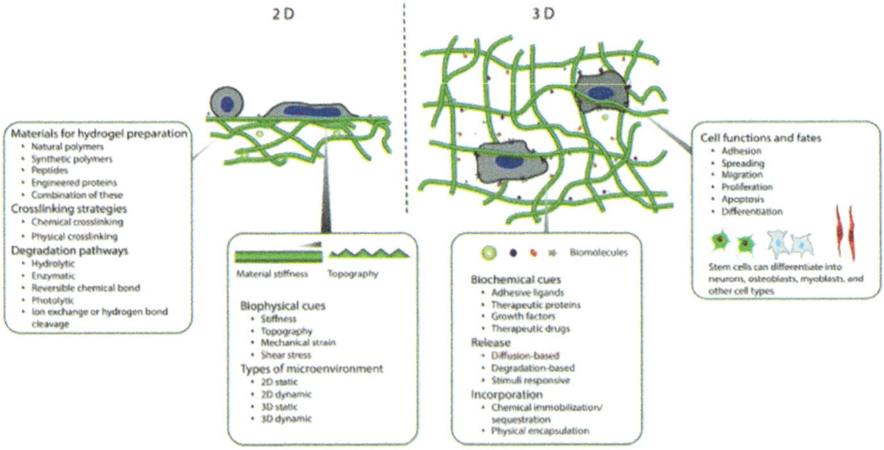

Fig. 7 Schematic illustration of parameters considered during hydrogel preparation [30]

ensure safe use and the ability to perform the desired task. In the case of hydrogels, the organic solvents, emulsifiers, initiators, crosslinkers, and unreacted monomers bring the toxicity toward cells. The purification of the hydrogels by dialysis or solvent washing reduces the toxicity of the hydrogel [32].

7.3 Biocompatibility of Natural Hydrogels

Natural polymers are known to have better interactions with the living tissues and promote them to exhibit high performance. Collagen, gelatin, agarose, alginate, chitosan, hyaluronic acid, etc., are widely used for biomaterial preparation. Alginate is a hydrophilic anionic polysaccharide obtained primarily from brown seaweed. It is composed of (1–4)-linked β-D-mannuronic acid (M) and α-L-guluronic acid (G)monomers. Due to the variations in the distribution of M and G residues and molecular mass in each algal source, the biocompatibility of the alginate is not guaranteed. So, the biocompatibility of alginate is depending on the purity, distribution of M and G residue, viscosity, and molecular weight [33]. Because of the gel-forming characteristics, alginate is generally used in the pharmaceutical field. The slower degradation rate of alginate is facilitated by the higher molecular weight. Because of the presence of the carboxyl group, alginate hydrogels are able to show a high swelling ratio at increasing pH values. Alginate-based hydrogels have a potential application in drug delivery and regenerative medicine. It was used for bone regeneration, wound healing, cartilage repairing, and drug delivery, etc. [34]. The hydrogel composed of N,O-carboxymethyl chitosan and oxidized alginate possesses good biocompatibility toward NH3T3 cells after 3-dayincubation [35]. In the case of calcium cross-linked alginate hydrogels, the stiffness and toughness improved with increasing cross-linking density [36]. Studies show that the high content of M contributes to the immune response by producing cytokines such as TNF-α, IL-1, and IL-6 [37]. Rapid release of the loaded drugs and low entrapment efficiency are the major disadvantages of alginate-based hydrogels.

Dextran is a bacterial polysaccharide consist of linear α-1,6-linked glucopyranose unit with some degree of 1,3 branching. Dextran has a molecular weight below than 100 kDa which is used as a plasma expander because of its relatively inert and nontoxic nature [38]. Different dextranases present in the liver, colon, and spleen have the capacity to metabolize the dextran. The reticuloendothelial system is able to degrade high molecular weight dextran [39]. Ferreira et al. showed that dextran-acrylate hydrogels have biocompatibility in both in vitro (human foreskin fibroblasts) and in vivo (subcutaneous and intramuscular implantation in Wistar rats for up to 40 days) [40]. It increases the longevity of therapeutic drugs and eliminates through the renal clearance (Mw < 40 kDa) [41].

Hyaluronic acid (HA) is a glycosaminogly can consist of repeating non-sulfated disaccharide units (α-1,4-D-glucuronic acid and β-1,3-*N*-acetyl-D-glucosamine) [42]. It is a major element in the ECM and involved in several biological functions such as regulation of cell adhesion, cell motility, and differentiation, etc. [43]. HA itself or association with other materials has been used to develop nanoparticles, hydrogels, microparticles, and other drug carriers [44]. Because of the high rate of elimination, modification of HA is needed for drug delivery. High structural analogy and poor interaction with blood facilitate the non-antigenic and nonimmunogenic effects [45]. Literature indicated that the HA is degraded by both reactive oxygen intermediates and hyaluronidases synthesized by endothelial cells, fibroblasts, and macrophages [46]. HA-based hydrogels are biologically inert, non-allergic, and non-carcinogenic during the degradation process. The non-toxicity of the HA hydrogels was confirmed by Kim et al. 2013 [47].

Pectin is an anionic polysaccharide found in the cell wall of the most plant and linked by 1,4-α-D-galacturonic acid residues [48]. It has a good gelling property and improves drug loading and releasing. The intermolecular interaction between pectin and tissues is determined by the presence of positive or negative charges on the pectin [49]. Pectin forms ionic interaction via calcium ions [50]. After the formation of hydrogels, these charges are partially or fully engaged. So that the further molecular interactions are reduced. Currently, pectin is used in tissue engineering, dentistry, and wound-healing applications, etc. [49].

Chitosan is a semi-synthetic polymer obtained from the deacetylation of chitin-whic is known as the analogous of the glycosaminoglycans (GAG) found in ECM of the cartilage [51]. It is approved by the FDA as a wound dressing material. This positively charged chitosan is known to stimulate the granulation and rebuilding of the tissues [52]. The positive charge of chitosan enables them to interact highly with the cells due to ionic interchanges between the intracellular and extracellular medium mediated by the $Na+$ /$K+$ pump [53]. Encapsulation of the drug within the chitosan carrier reduces the positive charge, thereby limiting the cellular uptake, and contribute toxicity [53]. The antibacterial and anticancer effect of chitosan is made then a suitable drug delivery system. In mammalian implantation model, the early migration of neutrophils was observed, and it was resolved with an increase in implantation time. The endotoxins were absent, and new blood vessels were formed [54].

8 Biocompatibility of Synthetic Hydrogels

Synthetic polymers do not occur in nature and made artificially through the process of polymerization. They got great acceptance because of its ease of modification. Generally, these kinds of polymers show less biocompatibility than natural polymers. Biocompatibility of some prominent synthetic polymers is given in Table 1. It gives an overall idea of the comparison between the biocompatibility of polymers based on tissue engineering applications [55]. Localized inflammation is observed during poly(lactic and glycolic) acid hydrogels, while polyethylene oxide and polyethylene glycol shows no inflammation during treatment. Polycaprolactone is degraded via hydrolysis, and it shows minimal inflammation to the tissues. Polyethylene glycol (PEG) is a synthetic polymer widely used for drug delivery applications. It was noted

Table 1 Biocompatibility nature of different types of synthetically manufactured hydrogels

Hydrogels from synthetic polymers	Biocompatibility nature	TE applications
Poly (lactic and glycolic) acid	Products degrade during metabolic pathway, lacalized inflammation	Bne, nerves, skin, ligament, tendon, vessels, cartilage, kindney, tumor, bladder, liver cells
Polyethyline oxide and plyethylene glycol	Hydrolysis, mild foreign in PEO and minimal foreign in PEG body reaction, no inflammation	Bone, skin, muscles, vessels, cartilage, nerves, cardiovascular, intraperitoneal, liver cells
Polycaprolactone	Hydrolysis, minimal inflammation	Sini, ligament, tendon, vessels, nerves, cartilage, bone, retina

that polyethylene glycol acts as a surface protector by reducing protein adsorption and cell adhesion [56]. It has been approved as a preservative additive by the U.S. Food and Drug Administration. Modification of nanoparticle with PEG helps them to escape from the recognition of the immune system and slowdown their removal. Apart from this, it was understood that PEG is able to inhibit the inflammatory response and will not accumulate in the body [57]. Covalent attachment of PEG to a molecule is called PEGylation. This kind of attachment will improve pharmacokinetics and biological functions [58] together with less protein adhesion. The coating with PEG limits protein adhesion, tissue damage, and antigenic activity [56]. The ability to resist protein adsorption is proportional to the polymer chain length and surface density. This is achieved by high mobility, steric hindrance effect, hydrophilicity, and large excluded volume [59].

Polyacrylic acid hydrogels are called superabsorbents because it has the capacity to absorba large amount of water [60]. Acrylic acid biomaterials are used widely in the pharmaceutical field and have been approved by the Food and Drug Administration (FDA). The hydrogels obtained by grafting the acrylic acid on cellulose was non-toxic to human embryonic kidney cells when cross-linked with ethylene glycol [61].

Polyvinyl alcohol is a water-soluble synthetic polymer widely used pharmaceutical field. Alexandre et al. reported that the PVA can be used as a vascular graft with good biocompatibility and hemocompatibility [62]. PVA-based artificial arteries, cartilage, muscle, etc., were reported. The strong hydrophilic nature of PVA-based gel contributes to bio-inert behavior [63]. It is a non-toxic material which has the ability to form films and exhibit emulsifying and cell adhesive properties. It is biodegradable, with high tensile strength and flexibility [64].

Poly(lactic-co-glycolic acid) (PLGA) is a biodegradable polymer which consists of polylactic acid and polyglycolic acid. It was approved by the FDA and currently used for various applications such as tissue engineering, drug delivery, and wound healing. During hydrolysis, the monomers are produced by the breaking of the ester bond and that can easily be metabolized by the Krebs cycle [65]. The biocompatibility is altered by initiating the inflammatory condition by lowering the pH value of the surrounding tissue. Hydration, initial degradation, constant degradation, and solubilization are the important steps involved in the degradation of the PLGA [66]. The biocompatibility of the PLGA was improved by incorporating various nanoparticle into it [67]. The previous study reported that the biocompatibility of PLGA with low concentration is satisfactory and the highest concentration of degradation product caused a toxic effect [68]. High lactide content of PLGA make them more hydrophobic and absorb less water. The crystallinity behavior of PLGA is directly linked to swelling behavior, mechanical strength, hydrolysis, and degradation property [69].

Polycaprolactone (PCL) is obtained by the ring opening polymerization of ε-caprolactone monomers. PCL is a biodegradable and biocompatible polymer widely used for biomedical applications. Under physiological condition, it will undergo degradation by hydrolytic mechanism and take more than 24 months for complete degradation [70]. The degradation of PCL is faster in the alkaline environment than acidic environment [71].

References

1. Okay (2010) General properties of hydrogels. In: Gerlach G, Arndt KF (eds) Hydrogel sensors and actuators, engineering and technology. Springer series on chemical sensors and biosensors. Springer, Berlin
2. Ahmed EM (2015) Hydrogel: preparation, characterization and applications. J Adv Res 6(2):105–121
3. Das N (2013) Preparation methods and properties of hydrogels: a review. Int J Pharm Pharm Sci 5(3):112–117
4. Grassi M, Sandolo C, Perin D, Coviello T, Lapasin R, Grassi G (2009) Molecules 14:3003–3017
5. Chen J, Park K (2000) J Control Rel 65(1–2):73–82
6. Svensson A, Nicklasson E, Harrah T, Panilaitis B, Kaplan DL, Brittberg M, Gatenholm P (2005) Bacterial cellulose as a potential scaffold for tissue engineering of cartilage. Biomaterials 26:419–431
7. Ranta-Eskola AJ (1979) Use of the hydraulic bulge test in biaxial tensile testing. Int J Mech Sci 21:457–465
8. Tsakalakos T (1981) The bulge test: a comparison of the theory and experiment for isotropic and anisotropic films. Thin Solid Films 75:293–305
9. Miller GJ, Morgan EF (2010) Osteoarthritis Cartilage 18(8):1051–1057
10. Simi R, Mathis CH, Spencer ND (2018) Polymer 137:276–282
11. Selby A, Maldonado-Codin C, Derby B (2014) J Mech Behav Biomed Mat 35:144–156
12. JohnsonJ B, BauerD M, NiedermaierW J, CroneD C, Beebe J (2004) Exp Mech 44:21
13. Williams DF (2014) There is no such thing as a biocompatible material. Biomaterials 35
14. Rahmati M, Mozafari M (2019) Biocompatibility of alumina-based biomaterials–a review. J Cell Physiol 234(4):3321–3335
15. Biesiekierski A et al (2018) Assessing the biocomptibility of biomaterials; A critical review of current in vitro toxicity assays, their advantages and limitations
16. Ikada Y (1993) Interfacial biocompatibility, in polymers of biological and biomedical significance. American Chemical Society, pp 35–48
17. Ahmed MH et al (2012) 1—Characteristics and applications of titanium oxide as a biomaterial for medical implants. In: Davim JP (ed) The design and manufacture of medical devices. Woodhead Publishing, pp 1–57
18. Remes A, Williams DF (1992) Immune response in biocompatibility. Biomaterials 13(11):731–743

19. Bryers JD, Giachelli CM, Ratner BD (2012) Engineering biomaterials to integrate and heal: The biocompatibility paradigm shifts. Biotechnol Bioeng 109(8):1898–1911
20. Johnston RB (1998) Monocytes and macrophages. N Engl J Med 318(12):747–752
21. Bruinink A, Luginbuehl R (2012) Evaluation of biocompatibility using in vitro methods: interpretation and limitations. In: Kasper C, Witte F, Pörtner R (eds) Tissue engineering III: cell–surface interactions for tissue culture. Springer, Berlin, pp 117–152
22. Baldrick P (2017) Biocompatibility assessments for medical devices—evolving regulatory considerations AU—Reeve, Lesley. Exp Rev Med Dev 14(2):161–167
23. Bernard M et al (2018) Biocompatibility of polymer-based biomaterials and medical devices—regulations, in vitro screening and risk-management. Biomater Sci 6(8):2025–2053
24. Draye J-P et al (1998) In vitro and in vivo biocompatibility of dextran dialdehyde cross-linked gelatin hydrogel films. Biomaterials 19(18):1677–1687
25. Ahmed EM (2015b) Hydrogel: preparation, characterization, and applications: a review. J Adv Res 6(2):105–121
26. Ullah F et al (2015) Classification, processing and application of hydrogels: a review. Mater Sci Eng C 57:414–433
27. Varaprasad K et al (2017) A mini review on hydrogels classification and recent developments in miscellaneous applications. Mater Sci Eng C 79:958–971
28. Sannino A, Madaghiele M (2008) and L. Biocompatibility and other properties of hydrogels in regenerative medicine, Ambrosio, pp 114–135
29. Parhi R (2017) Cross-linked hydrogel for pharmaceutical applications: a review. Adv Pharm Bull 7(4):515–530
30. Kharkar PM, Kiick KL, Kloxin AM (2013) Designing degradable hydrogels for orthogonal control of cell microenvironments. Chem Soc Rev 42(17):7335–7372
31. Seliktar D (2012) Designing cell-compatible hydrogels for biomedical applications. Science 336(6085):1124–1128
32. Das N (2013) Preparation methods and properties of hydrogel: a review, vol 5:112–117
33. Tam SK et al (2011) Factors influencing alginate gel biocompatibility, vol 98, pp 40–52
34. Sun J, Tan H (2013) Alginate-based biomaterials for regenerative medicine applications. Materials (Basel, Switzerland) 6(4):1285–1309
35. Li X et al (2012) Cytotoxicity and biocompatibility evaluation of N, O-carboxymethyl chitosan/oxidized alginate hydrogel for drug delivery application. Int J Biol Macromol 50(5):1299–1305
36. Schmidt JJ, Rowley J, Kong HJ (2008) Hydrogels used for cell-based drug delivery. J Biomed mater Res 87A(4):1113–1122
37. Orive G et al (2006) Biocompatibility of alginate–poly-l-lysine microcapsules for cell therapy. Biomaterials 27(20):3691–3700
38. De Groot CJ et al (2001) In vitro biocompatibility of biodegradable dextran-based hydrogels tested with human fibroblasts. Biomaterials 22(11):1197–1203
39. Van Tomme SR, Hennink WE (2007) Biodegradable dextran hydrogels for protein delivery applications. Expert Rev Med Dev 4(2):147–164
40. Ferreira L et al (2004) Biocompatibility of chemoenzymatically derived dextran-acrylate hydrogels. J Biomed Mater Res A 68A(3):584–596
41. Maia J et al (2014) Dextran-based materials for biomedical applications, pp 31–53
42. Ghosh K (2008) 28—Biocompatibility of hyaluronic acid: From cell recognition to therapeutic applications. In: Reis RL et al (2008) Natural-based polymers for biomedical applications. Woodhead Publishing. pp 716–737
43. Fakhari A, Berkland C (2013) Applications and emerging trends of hyaluronic acid in tissue engineering, as a dermal filler and in osteoarthritis treatment. Acta Biomater 9(7):7081–7092
44. Fallacara A et al (2018) Hyaluronic acid in the third millennium, vol 10, p 701
45. Necas J et al (2008) Hyaluronic acid (Hyaluronan): a review, vol. 53 (2008)
46. Choi S et al (2014) Purification and biocompatibility of fermented hyaluronic acid for its applications to biomaterials. Biomater Res 18(1):6

47. Kim J-T et al (2014) Biocompatibility of Hyaluronic Acid Hydrogels Prepared by Porous Hyaluronic Acid Microbeads. Metals Mater Int 20(3):555–563
48. Konovalova MV et al (2017) Preparation and biocompatibility evaluation of pectin and chitosan cryogels for biomedical application. J Biomed Mater Res A 105(2):547–556
49. Markov PA et al (2017) Mechanical properties, structure, bioadhesion, and biocompatibility of pectin hydrogels. J Biomed Mater Res A 105(9):2572–2581
50. Numata K et al (2014) Silk-pectin hydrogel with superior mechanical properties. Biodegradabil Biocompatibil 14(6):799–806
51. Akilbekova D et al (2018) Biocompatible scaffolds based on natural polymers for regenerative medicine. Int J Biol Macromol 114:324–333
52. Singh MR, Patel B, Singh D (2016) Chapter 9—Natural polymer-based hydrogels as scaffolds for tissue engineering. In: Grumezescu AM (ed) Nanobiomaterials in soft tissue engineering. William Andrew Publishing, pp 231–260
53. Rodrigues S et al (2012) Biocompatibility of chitosan carriers with application in drug delivery. J Funct Biomater 3(3):615–641
54. Porto I (2012) Polymer biocompatibility, pp 47–64
55. Saroia J et al (2018) A review on biocompatibility nature of hydrogels with 3D printing techniques, tissue engineering application and its future prospective. Bio-Des Manufact 1(4):265–279
56. Alcantar NA, Aydil ES, Israelachvili JN (2000) Polyethylene glycol–coated biocompatible surfaces. J Biomed Mater Res 51(3):343–351
57. Kong X-B et al (2017) Polyethylene glycol as a promising synthetic material for repair of spinal cord injury. Neural Regener Res 12(6):1003–1008
58. Hossain A (2015) Review on PEGylation (surface coating with polyethylene glycol) and potential use of PEGylated silica-based materials for biomedical applications. J Adhesion Soc Jpn 51(1):29–39
59. Chen J et al (2012) Biocompatibility studies of poly(ethylene glycol)–modified titanium for cardiovascular devices. J Bioact Compat Polym 27(6):565–584
60. Elliott JE et al (2004) Structure and swelling of poly(acrylic acid) hydrogels: effect of pH, ionic strength, and dilution on the crosslinked polymer structure. Polymer 45(5):1503–1510
61. Costa Milhomens G et al (2018) Biocompatibility and adsorption properties of hydrogels obtained by graft polymerization of acrylic acid on cellulose from rice hulls. Iranian Polym J 27
62. Alexandre N et al (2014) Biocompatibility and hemocompatibility of polyvinyl alcohol hydrogel used for vascular grafting—in vitro and in vivo studies. J Bioactive Compat Polym 102(12):4262–4275
63. Masanori K, Hyon SH (2010) Development and evaluation of polyvinyl alcohol-hydrogels as an artificial atrticular cartilage for orthopedic implants. Material 3
64. Desphande DS, Bajpai R, Bajpai AK (2013) Water sorption and biocompatibility evaluation of poly(vinyl alcohol—acrylonitrile) based hydrogels. Soft Mater 11(2):221–230
65. Chereddy KK, Vandermeulen G, Préat V (2016) PLGA based drug delivery systems: promising carriers for wound healing activity. Wound Repair and Regeneration 24(2):223–236
66. Gentile P et al (2014) An overview of poly(lactic-co-glycolic) acid (PLGA)-based biomaterials for bone tissue engineering. Int J Mol Sci 15(3):3640–3659
67. Ji W et al (2012) Biocompatibility and degradation characteristics of PLGA-based electrospun nanofibrous scaffolds with nanoapatite incorporation. Biomaterials 33(28):6604–6614
68. Ignatius AA, Claes LE (1996) In vitro biocompatibility of bioresorbable polymers: poly(L, DL-lactide) and poly(L-lactide-co-glycolide). Biomaterials 17(8):831–839
69. Makadia HK, Siegel SJ (2011) Poly lactic-co-glycolic acid (PLGA) as biodegradable controlled drug delivery carrier. Polymers 3(3):1377–1397
70. Thuaksuban N, Luntheng T, Monmaturapoj N (2016) Physical characteristics and biocompatibility of the polycaprolactone–biphasic calcium phosphate scaffolds fabricated using the modified melt stretching and multilayer deposition. J Biomater Appl 30(10):1460–1472

71. Malikmammadov E et al (2017) PCL and PCL-based materials in biomedical applications. J Biomater Sci Polym Ed 29:1–55

Chapter 13
An Overview of the Recent Developments in Hydrogels

K. S. Joshy, S. Snigdha, Sabu Thomas, and Tianduo Li

Abstract Hydrogels are extremely hydrophilic polymers that are physically or chemically cross-linked. They exist in many types varying according to their mechanical and structural characteristics, method of synthesis, or the nature present on the molecules. The present chapter presents an overview of hydrogels, and their properties and applications in the field of drug delivery. In the first part, relevant parameters defining hydrogel properties and the strategies for fine-tuning them are discussed. In the second part, the application of hydrogels in drug delivery, different modes of drug delivery, as well as an in-depth overview of the applications of hydrogels in current scenario is presented. From an application point of view, hydrogels can be used as an excellent drug delivery matrices and tissue engineering scaffolds.

1 Introduction

Hydrogels are hydrophilic three-dimensional network polymers capable of expanding up to thousand times of its dry weight when immersed in aqueous solutions. The interactions within the hydrogel network involve covalent bonds, physical cross-links, hydrogen bonds, strong van der Waals interactions, and crystallite associations. A hydrogel system consists of a combination of two or more associations of the aforementioned interactions. These are biocompatible and are extensively used for in vivo studies. Sol–gel transforming properties shown by hydrogel make them useful in different microenvironments present in the body with varying parameters such as pH, temperature, and enzymatic activities at the diseased sites. Physiological temperature (37 °C) and pH (7.4) are the common conditions which induce a

K. S. Joshy (✉) · T. Li
Shandong Provincial Key Laboratory of Molecular Engineering, School of Chemistry and Pharmaceutical Engineering, Qilu University of Technology (Shandong Academy of Sciences), Jinan 250353, China
e-mail: joshyk.s@gmail.com

S. Snigdha · S. Thomas
International and Inter University Centre for Nanoscience and Nanotechnology, Mahatma Gandhi University, Kottayam, Kerala 686560, India

J. Jose et al. (eds.), *Nano Hydrogels*, Gels Horizons: From Science to Smart Materials,
https://doi.org/10.1007/978-981-15-7138-1_13

hydrogel to transform from the sol-state to the gel state. Hydrogels are often used for the delivery of hydrophilic drugs due to the hydrophilic polymer matrix. However, hydrophobic drugs are generally incompatible with hydrogels. This is due to limited loading quantity of hydrophobic drugs and their homogeneity in hydrogel matrices. Therefore, hydrogel modification for delivery of hydrophobic compounds is essential. This is a major challenge as hydrophobic drugs are being increasing used in the current pharmaceutical treatment systems. It is estimated that ~40% of the marketed drugs and 60% of the compounds that are in the research and development state present poor water solubility.

The hydrogels' swelling properties and resistance to dissolution are dependent on the hydrophilic groups and degree of cross-linking in the structure. The water absorption capacity of the hydrogel is attributed to the hydrophilic groups in the polymer, and the dissolution resistance is primarily due to cross-linking within the polymer network. Water plays a key role in providing the peculiar characteristics of hydrogels. Numerous materials, including natural and synthetic, adhere to the above description of hydrogels. However, novel ideas are being innovated by researchers in order to enhance hydrogel properties such as mechanical properties, biocompatibility, and superporous nature. Various new generations of hydrogels such as grafted hydrogels, hybrid hydrogels, and genetically engineered triblock copolymers with high stability and fast response time imitating hydrogels promise a smart future for these useful materials.

2 Classification of Hydrogels

Hydrogels may exist in different physical forms. The classification and types of hydrogels can be done based on its properties like its origin (natural and synthetic), compositions (homopolymeric, copolymeric, multipolymeric interpenetrating hydrogels, etc.), configuration (crystalline, semicrystalline, and amorphous), and the interaction among polymer network (permanent/chemical gel and reversible/physical gel); besides these, some other categories are also possible. Hydrogels derived from only one type of monomeric species are known as homopolymeric hydrogels; however, when the hydrogel is comprised of two or more different types of monomeric units it is known as a copolymeric hydrogel. In copolymeric hydrogels, the monomeric units can be arranged in various fashions like random, alternating, or in block, along the chain of polymer network. The interaction between the polymer networks in the hydrogel is another category of hydrogels. When the interaction between networks is covalent, a chemical or permanent gel is obtained. Molecular entanglements and/or other types of secondary forces like hydrogen bonding, and hydrophobic and ionic interaction give rise to a reversible or physical type of hydrogel.

2.1 *Physical Hydrogels*

Thermosensitive hydrogels are known to undergo a sol–gel phase transition in response to temperature changes from room to physiological temperature. This sensitivity is particularly useful, since the temperature control is easy. Thermosensitive hydrogels are generally triblock polymers constituting poly(ethylene glycol) (PEG) linked to hydrophobic polymer blocks. The triblock consists of A blocks and B blocks organized as ABA or BAB, where PEG (A block) is well established in hydrogel formulation due to its high water solubility, biocompatibility, and low immunogenicity. The B blocks increase the hydrophobicity of the hydrogel and thereby the drug loading capacity of hydrophobic drugs through micellization. Usually, thermosensitive hydrogels have a gelation transition temperature of 37 °C, which causes hindrances during syringe/needle administration. The patient's body at 37 °C induces rapid gelation of the hydrogel which blocks the needle. To overcome this barrier, researchers introduced pH-sensitive moieties to thermosensitive copolymers, so that a second condition must be fulfilled in order for gelation to begin.

2.2 *Covalent Hydrogels*

Another technique to confer hydrophobic domains in a conventional hydrogel network could be the cross-linking of hydrophobic chains/monomers with hydrophilic ones. A similar end result can be achieved with hydrophobic cross-linkers. Such hydrogels are referred to as amphiphilic hydrogels. Several strategies have been used to synthesize such hydrogels. Condensation between anhydrides and alcohols could lead to formation of such hydrogels by a simple synthetic process. For example, pyromellitic anhydride, a hydrophobic cross-linker with anhydride groups, can react with OH groups in other polymer chains. This strategy is advantageous over the others, due to the absence of initiators, coupling agents, or additives that could limit the biomedical applications of the hydrogels due to toxicity issues.

2.3 *Nanoparticle-Containing Hydrogels*

The nanoparticles can effectively introduce hydrophobic moieties in the hydrogel. Covalent linkage or absorption can be employed to introduce the nanoparticle into the hydrogel system. Nanoparticles can be covalently linked if they possess polymerizable groups on their surface that can be copolymerized with hydrophilic monomers. In addition, multifunctional particles can be used as cross-linkers for the hydrogel matrix. This approach could prevent loss of nanoparticles due to diffusion during the swelling process. Usually, the nanoparticles are incorporated before the cross-linking (physical or chemical) occurs; in this case, the particles are prepared in advance and introduced into the reaction mixture. This technique enables easy incorporation of the nanoparticles, but they have the tendency to diffuse out of the matrix during swelling as they are not covalently attached to it.

2.4 *Hydrogels Containing Cyclodextrins*

Cyclodextrins (CDs) have been in great demand to produce hydrogels that form inclusion complexes with hydrophobic drugs. CDs are cyclic oligosaccharides formed from dextrose units bound by 1–4 carbon bonds. There are three classes: α (6 units), β (7 units), and γ-CD (8 units). Their structure is a truncated cone of hydrophilic outer surface enclosing a hydrophobic cavity. The hydrophobic cavity encourages the formation of inclusion complexes with hydrophobic molecules. The CDs are used in combination with chemical cross-linkers such as epichlorohydrin (EP), triazine, or diisocyanates. The CD molecules contain multiple OH which can readily react with the cross-linkers to yield hydrogels [1].

3 Hydrogel Network Properties

The bulk structure of hydrogels defines their suitability as biomedical materials and their performance in a particular application. The important parameters for characterizing the network structure of hydrogels include: (1) the molecular weight of the polymer chains between two neighboring cross-links (Mc), (2) the corresponding mesh size (ξ), and (3) the effective network density (ve). These parameters are interrelated and can be determined by applying the equilibrium-swelling theory and the rubber elasticity theory. Recently, an alternative method for characterization of cross-linked hydrogel networks was presented. High-resolution magic angle spinning (HR-MAS) NMR spectroscopy enables characterization and quantification of any unreacted cross-linkable moieties that occur in a chemically cross-linked, swollen hydrogel network. This methodology was first applied to quantify unreacted methacrylic amide residues in chemically cross-linked gelatin hydrogel. Since HR-MAS NMR spectroscopy is a fast, accurate, straightforward, and nondestructive technique, it may be applied more frequently in the future studies involving hydrogel network properties.

3.1 *Temperature-Induced Hydrogel Formation*

A large number of hydrogels tend to self-structure upon temperature variation. Temperature-sensitive materials are of two types: upper critical solution temperature (UCST) and lower critical solution temperature (LCST) materials. Both these systems have great demand for biomedical applications that require the materials to gel or dissolve in situ depending on the exact UCST or LCST behaviors.

3.1.1 Upper Critical Solution Temperature

Reversible gelation through intermolecular hydrogen bonds of many biopolymers can be induced by the temperature. This thermoreversible process is characteristic behavior shown by gelatin (i.e., partially hydrolyzed collagen) and certain polysaccharides such as agarose, amylose, amylopectin, and carrageenan. The nucleation and growth of the helical aggregates are by the formation of double (for polysaccharides) or triple helices (for gelatin). Many synthetic polymers also form physical hydrogels via hydrogen bonding.

3.1.2 Lower Critical Solution Temperature

Another class of temperature-sensitive materials is the LCST systems, in which a homogeneous solution is obtained at low temperatures. On heating, aggregation of the hydrophobic moieties starts which induces phase separation and hydrogel formation. This endothermal gelation is driven by an entropy change, where the entropy increases during the hydrogel formation, even though there is an increase in order due to hydrophobic segments aggregating. This occurs due to the release of large quantity of water by the hydrophobic region of the polymer.

3.2 Cryo-Induced Hydrogel Formation

In addition to ambient temperature hydrogel formation, hydrogels can also be synthesized using cryogenic treatment. Cryogelation typically decreases both the critical monomer/polymer concentration and the reaction time required for gelation. Cryotropic gelation (aka cryogelation) is a specific type of gelation that takes place when gel-forming systems are cryogenically treated.

The primary requisite for cryogel formation is the bulk crystallization of the low-molecular-weight liquid present in the initial system. The crystallization of the pure solvent results in the total volume of the nonfrozen liquid microphase (NFLMP) being lower than the initial reaction volume. Consequently, the concentration of polymer/monomer in the NFLMP is significantly higher than the initial concentration. The polymer gel phase can be formed during one of the stages of cryogenic treatment: during freezing of the initial system, during storage of the samples in the frozen state, or during thawing of the frozen specimens. The aforementioned process results in the formation of a cryogel which is the porous scaffold of the hydrogel starting material.

4 Biopolymer-Based Hydrogel Systems

The polysaccharides and proteins frequently used for hydrogel preparation in regenerative medicine are as follows.

4.1 Polysaccharide Hydrogels

4.1.1 Chondroitin Sulfate

Chondroitin sulfate (CS) is a glycosaminoglycan composed of alternating units of N-acetyl-D-galactosamine and D-glucuronic acid. It possesses excellent bio-characteristics including the binding and modulation of certain growth factors. Because natural CS is readily water-soluble, chemical cross-linking of CS is required for in vitro or in vivo hydrogel application.

A variety of methods was described for cross-linking CS. A biocompatible hydrogel film was prepared using the adipic dihydrazide derivative of chondroitin sulfate (CS-ADH), in which a pendant hydrazide functionality generated a gel using a small molecule or a macromolecular cross-linker. The most frequently applied cross-linking reagents include a combination of 1-ethyl-3-(3-dimethylaminopropyl)carbodiimide (EDC) and N-hydroxysuccinimide (NHS). The cross-linking reaction has often been performed in the presence of collagen or other amine-containing reagents (e.g., 1,12-diaminododecane). However, cross-linking using EDC often resulted in (partial) matrix collapse in aqueous media.

CS-based hydrogels have previously found widespread application in the field of tissue engineering. Hydrogels composed of gelatin and CS were applied as controlled release systems for antibacterial proteins. Incorporation of CS in cross-linked gelatin gels significantly increased the protein loading capacity of the gels and extended the release time. Alternatively, gelatin-CS-hyaluronantric copolymer scaffolds were selected to mimic natural cartilage. It was observed that the presence of CS promoted the secretion of proteoglycan and type II collagen. Bilayer gelatin-CS-hyaluronan biomatrices have also been studied for wound treatment. The results showed that in addition to a permanent coverage with histologically normal and adequately differentiated epithelial tissue, a well-defined dermal–epidermal junction and a collagen network in the dermis were present. As a result, the skin substitute had a positive effect on the promotion of the wound healing process and could be used to assist the regeneration of full-thickness skin defects. Another application of the tri-copolymer scaffold included the regeneration of the human nucleus pulposus. Furthermore, both microcarriers and membranes, composed of CS and gelatin, were prepared in view of different therapeutic strategies.

4.1.2 Hyaluronic Acid

Hyaluronic acid (i.e., hyaluronan, HA) is a non-sulfated glycosaminoglycan, composed of alternating units of D-glucuronic acid and D-N-acetylglucosamine, linked together via alternating β-1,4 and β-1,3 glycosidic bonds. HA is one of the major components of the extracellular matrix of skin, cartilage, and the vitreous humor. The first hyaluronan-based biomedical product (Healon) was developed in the 1970s and is FDA approved for the use in eye surgery (e.g., corneal transplantation). At present, the most often used commercially available HA-based product is HYAFF (i.e., benzyl ester of HA). The product exists with varying esterification degrees, and various research groups have already reported on their differences in mechanical properties and biological response. HA has also been combined with alginate and poly-L-lysine to develop scaffolds for a variety of tissue engineering applications including nerve regeneration. More recently, composite scaffolds were also prepared starting from complementary chemical functionalities.

4.1.3 Chitosan

Chitosan is the partial deacetylated derivative of chitin, which is obtained from the shells of crabs and shrimp. This biocompatible, cationic polymer dissolves in water up to a pH of 6.2. An increased basicity results in a gel-like precipitation of the hydrated polymer by neutralization of the amine groups. The pH responsiveness can be extended to a pH-dependent, thermoresponsive system (i.e., LCST-characterized system) by adding polyol salts including β-glycerophosphate (GP). These formulations dissolve at neutral pH and ambient temperature. Upon heating to body temperature, gelation occurs. It was observed that both the stability at room temperature and the gelation time increase with decreasing deacetylation degree. The solubility at ambient temperature and pH 7 is induced by the hydration of the chitosan chain, promoted by the GP. Upon heating to body temperature, the bound water is partially released inducing chain interactions and subsequent gelation [2].

5 Methods for Preparation of Hydrogel

Cross-linking of polymer chain is the main principle behind hydrogel preparation. This can be done by either using inherent ability of the polymer to cross-link, external cross-linking agent, chemical modification, temperature variations or exposure to high-energy radiation. The hydrogel preparation can be broadly classified into two categories, i.e., physical and chemical cross-linking techniques. Chemical techniques involve the formation of new covalent bonds between polymer chains in the hydrogel, while physical interactions exist between polymer chains in physically cross-linked hydrogel. Both physical and chemical techniques have their own benefit and drawbacks.

5.1 Physical Cross-Linking Methods

Physical cross-linking involves various physical interactions among polymer chains like ionic interaction, hydrophobic interaction, stereocomplex formation, hydrogen bonding, and protein–polysaccharide interaction resulting in hydrogel formation. Physical cross-linking techniques are being evolved as an important tool due to the absence of external cross-linker and its associated side effects. Physical cross-linking provides reversible hydrogel, and they are subject to structural imperfections or in homogeneities due to the presence of free chain ends.

5.2 Ionic Cross-Linking or Ionic Interaction

Ionic polysaccharides like sodium alginate can be cross-linked by the addition of counter ions (like calcium ions). The hydrogel can be cross-linked under mild conditions, at physiological pH and temperature. However, the gelation rate is hard to control and non-uniformity in the structure is an additional issue. The gelation rate increases at low concentrations of alginate and increases with increasing concentration of counter ions and temperature. Slow gelation was found to yield mechanically robust gels with uniform structure.

5.3 Hydrophobic Interaction

Polymers with hydrophobic domains are known to cross-link in aqueous atmosphere via reverse thermal gelation or "sol–gel" chemistry. Hydrophobic interaction occurs in amphiphilic polymer solution at elevated temperature. Though such polymers are soluble at low temperatures, when the temperature increases, aggregation of the hydrophobic domains takes place, in order to minimize the contact with water molecule. This process maximizes the solvent entropy in the solution. The larger hydrophobic segment contributes more toward solvent entropy, driving more hydrophobic interaction and lowering the gelation temperature.

5.4 Thermoreversible Gelation

Polysaccharides like carrageenan or gelatin undergo physical cross-linking upon cooling forming a hydrogel. The gel formation is due to helix formation, helix association, and formation of junction zones. Carrageenans exist as random coils above their transition temperature, which upon cooling turns to rigid helical rods. Stable gels form in aggregates in the presence of ions (Na^+, K^+, etc.) due to repulsion of sulfonic group (SO^{3-}).

5.5 *Complex Coacervation*

The mixing of poly-cationic and poly-anionic polymer results in a complex coacervate gel. This technique is driven by the principle of oppositely charged polymers aggregating together to form complexes that are highly dependent on pH and concentration of the solution. The mechanical properties of the hydrogel change from fragile (at pH close to pKa of chitosan, amine groups) to stretchable and strong (at pH close to pKa of hyaluronic acid, carboxylic groups). Similarly, proteins below their isoelectric point are positively charged and they tend to associate with anionic polysaccharides to form coacervate complex hydrogels.

5.6 *Hydrogen Bonding*

Hydrogen-bonded hydrogel can be produced by lowering the pH of the solution containing carboxyl functionalized polymer. For the synthesis of carboxymethylcellulose (CMC)-based hydrogel, the CMC is first dispersing in 0.1 M HCl solution. In acidic solution, sodium ions were replaced by hydrogen promoting hydrogen bonding and thereby decreasing the solubility of CMC, resulting in an elastic hydrogel. Polyacrylic and polymethacrylic acid forms a hydrogel with polyethylene glycol at low pH, due to the H-bonding interaction between the acidic group (−COOH) of acrylate and the hydroxyl groups (−OH) of PEG.

5.7 *Freeze–Thaw*

The freeze–thaw technique is one of the most promising techniques for hydrogel synthesis, especially for polysaccharide-based gels due to their biocompatibility and nontoxicity. Freeze–thaw usually involves freezing of polymer solution to a relatively low temperature (−20 to −80 °C) followed by thawing at room temperature. The hydrogel properties can be controlled by monitoring the pH, freezing duration, temperature, rate of thawing, and number of thawing cycles.

5.8 *Chemical Cross-Linking Methods*

Though physically cross-linked hydrogels have the advantage of developing without any cross-linking agents or chemical modification, they are limited by their poor mechanical performance. This in turn affects various other properties directly. However, chemically cross-linked hydrogels are mechanically robust, resist dilution of hydrogel matrix, and prevent diffusion of hydrogel. Chemical cross-linking involves chemical modification of polymer chains or use of additional cross-linking agent to bind polymer chains. Different chemical cross-linking techniques have been reported in the literature, and two important chemical techniques are discussed below.

5.8.1 Grafting

The grafting technique involves the polymerization or addition of a monomer on the backbone of a preformed polymer, like polysaccharides. The activation of polymer chains is carried out by the action of chemical reagents or by treatment with high-energy radiation. Thus, the grafting of functional monomer on activated polymer chains results in branching, and this is followed by cross-linking. The chemical modification of edible polymers via grafting constitutes an important method to improve their properties and expand the range of its application. Starch grafted with hydrophilic monomers like acrylic acid, acrylamide, and acrylonitrile has been used as a super-absorbent hydrogel. Such hydrophilic monomer-grafted polysaccharide exhibits higher water absorption capacity. The grafting technique can be chemical or radiation grafting, depending on the source of activation. Chemical grafting uses chemical initiators (like potassium persulfate, benzoyl peroxide, etc.) for the activation of polymer chains, while radiation grafting involves the use of high-energy radiation (like γ-radiation) as a source of initiators.

5.8.2 Cross-Linking

The use of a chemical cross-linker, such as glutaraldehyde, epichlorohydrin, glyoxal, PEG, in situ generated cross-linker, etc., in hydrogel formation has being practiced with both synthetic and natural polymers. This type of cross-linking involves the insertion of a new molecule with reactive functionality between the polymeric chains. However, this cross-linker (like glutaraldehyde) increases the toxicity of hydrogel which limits their application potential. In order to counter such problems, polysaccharide-derived novel biocompatible cross-linkers that are generated in situ were applied as a superior alternative for chemical cross-linker. Such biocompatible hydrogels find wider applications in biomedical, agriculture, and food-related applications. Periodate oxidation of polysaccharide to generate dialdehyde groups was reported as a safe and efficient biocompatible cross-linker. The degree of cross-linking can be controlled by monitoring the extent of oxidation.

6 Edible Polymer-Based Hydrogels

Hydrogel preparation is carried out using both synthetic and natural polymers. However, some synthetic hydrogels may be non-biodegradable, may elicit inflammatory responses, and may have toxic side effects. Although synthetic polymers have precisely controlled chemical structures which are suitable for hydrogel designing at the molecular level, natural polymers have also shown favorable properties for forming hydrogels. Thus, natural polymers can act as an alternative sources to traditional synthetic polymers with increased perks of good biodegradability and biocompatibility properties as well as minimal waste and pollution. Many natural hydrogel-forming polymers have been found to be edible; however, the mechanical properties of these edible polymers have been a subject of concern. Although it can be improved by using suitable bio-cross-linker or plasticizer, the toxicity of the cross-linkers remains to be tackled. The properties of the hydrogels are greatly influenced by the nature of the polymers. Linear polysaccharide associated with proteins has a stiff and rigid nature and is found in membrane, sheets, and coatings, while flexible and globular polysaccharides form film-type hydrogels. To date, numerous types of edible natural polymer-based hydrogels have been synthesized and utilized for different applications such as coating, drug delivery and packaging. The subsequent section concisely describes different types of edible polymer-based hydrogels [3].

7 Applications of Hydrogel

7.1 Drug Delivery

The fascinating physical properties of hydrogels, especially their porosity, offer tremendous edge in drug delivery applications. A local concentration of active pharmaceutical ingredient can be retained over a long period of time through release mechanism that can be controlled by diffusion, swelling, chemical or on environmental stimuli. Hydrogels that deliver drugs via diffusion control make use of reservoir or matrix devices that release drugs by diffusion through a hydrogel mesh or pores filled with water. The reservoir delivery system is composed of a hydrogel membrane coated on a drug-containing core. The cargo can be in the form of capsules, spheres, or slabs with high drug concentration in center of the system that ensures a constant drug release rate. While the reservoir delivery system produces time-independent and constant drug release, the matrix system works via the macromolecular pores or mesh. In this type of time-dependent drug release, the initial release rate is proportional to the square root of time, rather than being constant.

The hydrogels showing swelling-controlled drug release make use of drugs dispersed in a glassy polymer which starts swelling upon associating with bio-fluid. The expansion of the polymer during the swelling process facilitates drug diffusion and polymer chain relaxation. This process termed Case II transport supports time-independent, constant drug release kinetics. In addition, the gradient between the dispersed drug in the hydrogel and its surrounding environment facilitates the active diffusion of the drug from a region of higher concentration (hydrogel matrix) to a lower one, and this phenomenon is referred to as anomalous transport since the processes of diffusion and swelling that facilitate drug release are combined. Ocular drug delivery carriers make use of covalently cross-linked hydrogels. These soft, biodegradable hydrogels that have high swelling capacity remain in situ in the lacrimal.

Poly(ethylene glycol) hydrogels are commonly used for producing ophthalmic drug delivery systems. Drug release on exposure to environmental stimuli would be ideal for a delivery system as the release is controlled. The non-specific side effects associated with nontarget sites can also be prevented. Therefore, stimuli-responsive drug delivery vehicles that respond to changes in pH, temperature, ionic strength, or glucose concentration are being preferred for treatment of diseases such as cancer and diabetes, which are characterized by physiologically different microenvironments that are specific to various disease stages. The polymer composition of such hydrogels is manipulated in order to induce responsiveness to the environment [4].

Hydrogels enhance therapeutic outcome of drug delivery, and therefore they have found enormous clinical application. Hydrogels have greatly enhanced the temporal and spatial delivery of macromolecular drugs, small molecules, and cells. Hydrogel-mediated drug delivery has its share of challenges and requires constant improvements for being best suited for specific drug delivery purposes.

7.1.1 Ocular Delivery

Hydrogels containing hydrophobic moieties have been used for the delivery of hydrophobic drugs. However, ocular delivery of hydrophobic drugs using hydrogels has not been extensively explored. The two routes for ocular administration are implantable systems or drug-loaded contact lenses. For example, a PEG/silica hydrogel matrix has the potential to deliver hydrophilic and hydrophobic drugs. This system was to be injected directly into the eye for the sustained delivery of dexamethasone. In the study, multiarm poly(ethylene glycol) (PEG)/silica hydrogels were synthesized using the sol–gel method by hydrolysis and condensation of poly(4-arm PEG silicate). Similarly, thermosensitive injectable hydrogel using poly(trimethylene carbonate) and Pluronic F127 for mitomycin C delivery has also reported. The hydrogel system released all the drug within 25 days.

7.1.2 Transdermal Delivery

The transdermal route could be a good alternative to oral drug delivery. It can be self-administered painlessly. Moreover, transdermally administered drugs can avoid the harsh conditions of the GI tract. However, the transdermal route of administration is limited by the fact that only a few drugs have the physicochemical requirements to permeate passively through the skin. pH-sensitive hydrogels capable of loading hydrophobic drugs are used to treat different skin conditions. A pH imbalance leads to skin inflammation and acne. Under normal conditions, the surface of the skin has pH ranging between 5 and 6. Changes in the skin pH can compromise the barrier function of the stratum corneum. A novel hydrogel system consisting of hyaluronic acid and cellulose was reported as the hydrophobic molecule, to deliver an antimicrobial drug (isoliquiritigenin) to inhibit acne growth. This hydrogel system showed pH sensitivity and released maximum drugs at around pH 7. The colony formation of acne presents the peak of activity at this pH. The drug was able to permeate the skin barrier via the follicular pathway as the hydrogel aided in swelling of the skin.

Injectable hydrogels are greatly sort out in drug delivery and tissue engineering. Though hydrogel applications for brain disorders are restricted to preclinical investigations, hydrogels are being projected as effective tools in the treatment of neurodegenerative diseases and cerebrovascular disorders in forthcoming years. The minimally invasive implantation and unique mechanical properties relatable to soft tissues required for the brain and spinal cord can be achieved using hydrogels. They have been known to facilitate cell transplantation survival and stabilize the short half-life of drugs. Furthermore, polymer-based hydrogels can be used for local delivery of pharmacological moieties directly to the host tissue, thereby reducing systemic side effects.

7.2 Hydrogel-Based Targeted Drug Delivery

7.2.1 Supramolecular Hydrogels

The supramolecular hydrogel system is composed of two or more molecular entities held together by non-covalent intermolecular interactions. The non-covalent cross-linking helps resolve the issues of limited drug loading potential and drug incorporation in implantables. This non-covalent cross-linking provides physical stability as well as simultaneous drug loading and gelation in an aqueous environment without the need for a covalent cross-linking. Recently, supramolecular hydrogels prepared using self-assembled inclusion complexes of cyclodextrins and biodegradable block copolymers have exhibited sustained and controlled release of macromolecular drugs.

8 DNA Hydrogels

Hybrid bio-nanomaterials could be developed using DNA as the building block. Predictable two- or three-dimensional structures are formed from DNA molecules. Highly structured networks are formed by hybridizing complementary DNA molecules, and the resultant hydrogel structures expand upon encounter with an aqueous environment. These materials tend to append to other type of nucleic acid molecules (such as siRNA and miRNA) and are also capable of loading DNA binding drugs. Such hydrogels possess high solubility, biocompatibility, versatility, and responsiveness. They can also be fluorescently tagged for tracking in in vitro biological experiments. There has been great improvement in hydrogel modifications in order to enhance shape (e.g., external stimuli such as temperature). This stress responsivity behavior is an example of the construction of supramolecular hydrogel with tunable mechanical properties and multi-shape-memory effects. These hydrogels make use of physically cross-linked agar and a supramolecular network that is cross-linked by suitable chemical bonds that fix shapes temporarily and produce a multi-shape-memory effect. The supramolecular hydrogels are biocompatible and biodegradable and rely on non-covalent interactions to promote self-assembly of small molecules in water. The structures thus formed have supramolecular architectures and encapsulate water.

A programmed temporary shape can turn into the memorized original shape when placed in an appropriate environment or exposed to a trigger. Such shape-memory hybrid hydrogels could also be synthesized using DNA cross-linkers. These hydrogels not only undergo phase transitions in the trigger of the stimulus, but also possess memory code to recover to the original matrix shape.

9 Bio-Inspired Hydrogels

A newer variety of drug delivery hydrogels used for biomedical applications are the bio-inspired hydrogels. These 3D materials replicate biological microenvironment pertaining to the disease condition and support studies on how the targeted drug delivery process could be optimized, how the therapy behaved in vivo, how the disease progressed, and so on. These are particularly useful in cancer therapy as the disease is particularly complex and associated with intricate cellular and physiological changes that require monitoring. Engineering such microenvironments would thus be a very useful approach to promote research and study the disease condition and therapeutic process better. The stiffness of the 3D model used for studying liver cancer is a critical attribute to regulate molecular diffusivity and malignancy. The elastic moduli of the collagen gels were increased by stiffening interconnected collagen fibers with varied amounts of poly(ethylene glycol) di(succinic acid N-hydroxysuccinimidyl ester). The softer gels produced malignant cancer spheroids, while the stiffer ones showed suppressed malignancy. The model provided better understanding and regulation of the emergent behaviors of cancer cells.

10 Translation to the Clinic

With enormous potential for therapeutic applications, several hydrogel formulations have crossed the barriers of in vitro/preclinical studies into the market. Some of them are still in the clinical study phases. Hydrogels have evolved over time to one of the best and the most versatile drug delivery platforms [4].

11 Conclusions

Hydrogels offer a versatile platform for the therapy of several diseases including cancer and diabetes. The water-loving nature of hydrogels and the ability to shrink and swell depending according to environmental cues or the presence of water are appealing for drug delivery applications. They have a high degree of porosity, and the polymers building blocks could be cross-linked to varying degrees by adjusting their densities. The ability to modify the physical structure in several ways and the hydrogel applications can be extended beyond targeted drug delivery. They can be used for hygiene products, wound dressings, contact lenses, and tissue engineering. The recent developments of hydrogels for targeted drug delivery include modification with targeting ligands and diverse polymer types. Ophthalmic drug delivery is receiving significant attention in therapy from hydrogels. From comfortable contact lenses to biodegradable drug delivery, the applications in eye care have been enormous. They are 90% water and provide sustained drug release over a period of days or months. They are capable of delivering small molecules or large proteins and are fully absorbed in delivery, and they may remain visible during monitoring. The application of pH-responsive hydrogels for cancer therapy and glucose-responsive hydrogels for diabetes are noteworthy developments. The use of modified stem cell membranes for targeted delivery is a very recent and attractive strategy for drug delivery. These membranes coated on hydrogels (nanogels) loaded with drugs are highly specific to the disease site in cancer and are highly biocompatible. Though the hydrogel-based drug delivery was originally influenced by the hydrophobicity of the drugs, several improvements have been made recently including development of cyclodextrins modified to accommodate the hydrophobic drug. Adhesive and conductive patches developed using hydrogels have been useful in cardiac repair and vascularization. Remotely controlled motility of hydrogel (mimicking motion of a magbot) and the DNA hydrogels are novel ideas to facilitate targeted drug delivery. There are several hydrogel formulations in clinical use, and there is always scope for improvement and modification of hydrogels to enhance their applications. With subtle modifications to the existing ones, the hydrogels could become superlative drug delivery vehicles. Such hydrogel systems could outperform several conventional delivery forms and provide promising therapy of several illnesses.

References

1. Larrañeta E et al (2018) Hydrogels for hydrophobic drug delivery. Classification, synthesis and applications. J Funct Biomater 9(1):13
2. Van Vlierberghe S, Dubruel P, Schacht E (2011) Biopolymer-based hydrogels as scaffolds for tissue engineering applications: a review. Biomacromolecules 12(5):1387–1408
3. Ali A, Ahmed S (2018) Recent advances in edible polymer based hydrogels as a sustainable alternative to conventional polymers. J Agric Food Chem 66(27):6940–6967
4. Narayanaswamy R, Torchilin VP (2019) Hydrogels and their applications in targeted drug delivery. Molecules 24(3):603

Chapter 14
Self-assembled Hydrogels: An Overview

Athira Anil and Jiya Jose

Abstract Self-assembled hydrogels are a three-dimensional network of polymeric materials that are self-assembled either by physical or chemical crosslinking. Excellent biocompatibility, biodegradability, and sensitivity towards physiological stimulus make these materials as the best candidate for tissue culture, drug delivery, and development of sensors that can be. implanted on the human body. Whereas, versatile bonding that exists between the polymeric chain and water molecules and its ability to chelate metal ions extends its applications to photovoltaics and optics. This chapter focusses on the classification of self-assembled hydrogels based on their source and the nature of crosslinking force. The hydrogels formed by the self-assembly of biomolecules and the various factors governing their self-assembly like coiled-coil motifs, beta sheets, and beta-hairpin were discussed in the part, which was followed by a discussion synthetic hydrogels and their three different categories based on their nature of crosslinking force. Self-assembled hybrid hydrogels that are developed by the two distinct types of molecules are also evaluated.

1 Introduction

Solids, liquids, and gases constitute the three different phases of matter. Depending upon the temperature and pressure, we can govern the phase transitions among these. If we mix a pinch of gelatin powder with boiling water, the resultant product is neither solid nor water but has both the properties of solids and water. Like solids, they would not flow, and like liquid, they diffuse. These materials are called hydrogels. Hydrogels are three-dimensional polymeric materials that can possess a remarkable amount of water without dissolving in water [1]. This exceptional behaviour of swelling without dissolution in aqueous medium was originated from its structural peculiarities. Hydrogel structure consists of a hydrophilic head supported in a polymeric backbone, which is cross-linked together to form a three-dimensional

A. Anil · J. Jose (✉)
Department of Materials and Environmental Chemistry, Stockholm University, Stockholm SE-10691, Sweden
e-mail: jiyajose@gmail.com

J. Jose et al. (eds.), *Nano Hydrogels*, Gels Horizons: From Science to Smart Materials,
https://doi.org/10.1007/978-981-15-7138-1_14

network [2]. The three-dimensional network of polymer chains resist the hydrogels from dissolution, whereas the hydrophilic head with polymeric backbone significantly contributes to its ability to retain water. Based on various parameters like cross-linking, source, degradability, ionic charge, physical properties, etc., hydrogels can be classified into various categories [1]. One of the major classifications is based on the strength of cross-linking force. Depending on this, hydrogels can be categorized as physical hydrogels and chemical hydrogels [3]. If the non-covalent interactions such as electrostatic forces, hydrogen bonds, chain entanglements, and hydrophobic interactions result in the cross-linking, then they are physical hydrogels, and in turn if strong covalent bonds bind them together, they are chemical hydrogels.

When the hydrogels are formed by the spontaneous association of polymeric chains that are held together by noncovalent interactions without the presence of an external agent, such type of physical hydrogels are called self-assembled hydrogels. The scale of self-assembly can be tailored from nanometers to micrometres, thus opening a vast window of application to self-assembled hydrogels [3–5]. Ordered structure and the presence of water content have an inverse relation, and hence, it is a major challenge to produce self-assembled hydrogels with ordered manner. Liquid crystalline molecules [6], block polymers [7], and amphiphile [8] are the typical synthetic molecules that are capable of forming a perfectly ordered structure in an aqueous medium. Like synthetic copolymers, numerous biomaterials [9, 10] or genetically modified proteins [11, 12] also have the property to self assemble to form hydrogels. Hybrid hydrogels are another distinct class of hydrogels where two different types of macromolecules are cross-linked and self-assembled to form hydrogels [5, 13, 14]. For example, these class of molecules can have both synthetic as well as biomaterials cross-linked together non-covalently, and self-assembled to form a new type of hydrogels. These gels formed by the cooperation of two different types of molecules not only possess perfectly order structure but also they are packed with a huge amount of novel properties [4, 15]. In this chapter, we discuss the different varieties of self-assembled hydrogels and their properties.

2 Hydrogels Formed by the Self-assembly of Biomolecules

The presence of electrostatic interactions, hydrogen bonds, pi stacking, and van der Waals interactions that present in biomacromolecules makes them as better building blocks for the synthesis of self-assembled hydrogels. Many of these building blocks can form fibres, which in turn entangles to form networks of hydrogels [16]. Peptides like collagen, filamentous actin, and gelatin can be triggered by various external factors like temperature, pH, and charge to undergo self-assembly [16, 17]. Collagen is a structural protein having amino acid groups that are winded together to form a triple helical structure. Upon high salt concentration or at high temperatures, these self-assembled semi-crystalline collagen hydrogels change their conformation to form amorphous and compact coils [18, 19].

There are various factors that govern the self-assembly of biomaterials like peptides, which are discussed below.

3 Coiled-Coil Motif

Coiled-coil is the basic folding pattern of most of the peptides that consist of a single left-handed superhelix formed by the winding of two right-handed alpha helixes [20, 21]. The primary structure of the coiled-coil motif includes a sequence of seven repeating units where the 2–7 alpha helixes are coiled together [21]. The seven repeating units or the heptads can be designated as (a, b, c, d, e, f, g) with each having its prime significance: a and d are hydrophobic, whereas all the remaining are polar [21, 22]. Hydrophobic units help in the winding or association of the two different helices, thus making the polar b, c, and f to face outside. E and g govern the stability of the helices with its strong electrostatic interactions offered by its polar nature. As the heptads are coiled together to form like strands in a rope, on undergoing self-assembly, they can quickly form hydrogels with ordered fibrous structures. The presence of proper spatial recognition and arrangement present for the association and dissociation of helices makes it as the best building block for the synthesis of order macromolecules including hydrogels because we can predict the properties of the ordered hydrogels based on the primary sequence. The presence of hydrophilicity also offers the possibility to attach functional moieties in the primary structures, which can impart various types of self-assembly mechanism for these materials. These motifs are now widely exploited for the synthesis of hydrogels for cell culture (Fig. 1).

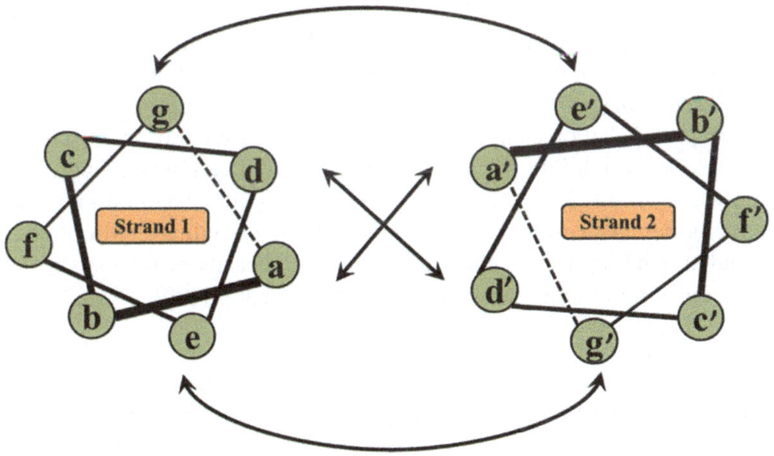

Fig. 1 Helical wheel diagram of a two stranded coiled-coil motif

4 Beta Sheets

Beta sheets are the most significant structural motif that contributes to the secondary structure of peptides. These sheets consist of multiple peptide chains with an extended backbone that is laterally aligned to form hydrogen bonds between the carbonyl oxygen of amino acid of one strand to the second amino acid in another strand, together resulting in a pleated structure [14, 23]. The strength of the hydrogen bond interactions governs the stability of beta sheets. Based on the orientation of beta sheets, we can classify it as parallel or antiparallel. If all the C terminals are at one end of the structure, they are called parallel or if the N terminal and C terminal alternate, they are called antiparallel. The interaction between enantiomeric beta sheets can be homochiral and heterochiral. Various studies have proved that the beta sheets with homochiral interactions self-assemble to form amyloid-type nanofibrils, which further assemble to form scaffold hydrogels by the changes in temperature, and pH whereas the heterochiral interactions operate between the beta sheets, and it results in its agglomeration [24, 25]. Various studies and discussions have done on the self-assembly of beta sheets, as it has high biological importance. For example, Scherman et al. have discussed the tunability in the pentapeptide self-assembly of beta sheets [26]. By altering the charge and concentration of the pentapeptide, they have tuned the stiffness of the hydrogels to a magnitude of two orders, which has a high impact in tissue engineering and three-dimensional printing applications [26].

5 Beta-Hairpins

One of the alternatives to beta sheets is beta hairpins. Beta hairpins consist of two beta sheets that are arranged in two antiparallel directions and linked together by a loop of 3–5 amino acids to form a hairpin-type structure [27]. Beta hairpins can self-assemble to form hydrogels or can undergo beta sheet transition or random coil(or vice versa) with the presence of external stimuli like pH, the concentration of sequence, and temperature [28, 29]. For example, MAX 1 beta hairpin self-assembles to form fibrillar networks which intern lead to the formation of responsive hydrogels [30]. The beta sheet assembly is mostly driven by intermolecular and intramolecular interactions, including electrostatic interactions, hydrogen bonding, hydrophobic interactions, and pi bonding. Hence, the self-assembly can easily be tuned using changes in the pH, concentration, temperature, and solvent medium [29].

6 Hydrogels from Self-assembly of Synthetic Molecules

Inspiring from the natural hydrogels made up from protein molecules, and so on, researchers have been working in macromolecules that are tailored by functional groups which can act like pre-programmed materials that can immediately self-assemble to form hydrogels. Amphiphiles, block copolymers, and liquid crystals are three different types of materials that form self-assembly in aqueous solutions [7].

7 Supramolecular Hydrogels

Noncovalent crosslinking like hydrogen bonds, metal–ligand coordination, electrostatic interactions generate supramolecular hydrogels [31, 32]. As the mode of interaction is purely physical, these hydrogels will not only moderate in their mechanical properties but also shows high gel to sol transition [33] behaviour in the presence of biological stimuli like pH, temperature, reducing and oxidizing agents, enzymes, etc. [34, 35]. High mass transfer rate, structure control, nontoxic preparation condition with strong biocompatibility and biodegradability make supramolecular hydrogels as a potent candidate for drug delivery in biological systems [36, 37].

Thermal reversibility is considered as one of the major features of supramolecular hydrogels as the hydrogen bonds and hydrophobic interactions are temperature dependent. Other than temperature, ultrasounds also act as a physical stimulus for the synthesis of supramolecular hydrogels [38, 39]. The weak interactions like intramolecular hydrogen bonding and pi-pi stacking forces can be spontaneously triggered and rearranged to form intermolecular interactions along with the water molecules and thereby enhancing the speed of gel formation [32], whereas pH holds the tag of the simplest and most effective method for triggering the supramolecular hydrogel formation as any changes in the pH can be easily identified using the pH papers and pH metres. By changing the pH of the precursor, solutions affect the protonation and deprotonations of the functionalities present in the hydrogelator, and thereby, it changes the strength and intensity of hydrogen bonding which operates between the hydrogelators and water molecules. One of the major examples is peptides. Peptides are chains of amino acids containing both amino and carboxylic groups. Based on different pH, peptides can self-assemble in a various manner, and thus, they can be classified into different categories. Self-assembly of N terminal blocked peptides forms hydrogels that are stable at lower pH [40]. Supramolecular hydrogels that are constituted by amphiphile belongs to the category of Hydrogels that can be stabilized in physiological pH [41]. Here, the hydrophilic ends support the solubility, and the hydrophobic body helps in its aggregation in the solvent resulting in the formation of 3D network structure [32]. As they are can be formed and stabilized in physiological pH, they are very promising for biological applications.Peptides having highly hydrophobic groups with primary amines stabilize such peptide self-assemblies in higher pH [42].

Although many monomers with carboxylic acid groups self-assemble by itself, various reports have shown the possibility of incorporating both transition metal ions and alkali metal ions into it during the self-assembly [43]. The incorporation of inorganic salts not only fastens the gelation of supramolecular hydrogels at a lower concentration of gelators but also enhances the mechanical strength of it. Enzyme induces self-assembly is an enzyme-catalyzed process where the enzyme converts the precursor molecule which can easily undergoes self-assembly [44]. This opens a wide set of opportunities to the biomedical applications like the intracellular formation of self-assemblies in physiological condition. Recent researchers have developed supramolecular hydrogels which can form instantly in intracellular matrixes rather than the outer cellular region that can determine the fate of the cell. The endogenous esterases that are present in mammalian cells can convert Fig. 2a into Fig. 2b which can undergo rapid self-assembly to form nanofibres when the threshold concentration is reached [32, 45]. The as-formed hydrogels change the viscosity of the cytoplasm and ultimately leads to cell death. Unlike endoenzymes, ectoenzymes stay in the surface of the cell with catalytical domains in the cytoplasm [46]. Such enzymes can help in the self-assembly of nanofibers in pericellular spaces which can selectively inhibit the growth of targeted cells without harming the normal cells [32, 47].

High tunability, feasibility, and efficiency make enzyme instructed self-assembly (EISA) as a novel technique for the supramolecular hydrogel assemblies which have wide biomedical applications. Light harvesting supramolecular assemblies were synthesized spontaneously by the electrostatic and van der Waals cross-linking of L-glutamate derivatives and anionic fluorescent dyes [48]. Phosphatase is an abundant enzyme, and Wang and his coworkers have reported the formation of supramolecular assembly of leaf-like structures ion ultra-low gelation concentration of 0.01 wt%

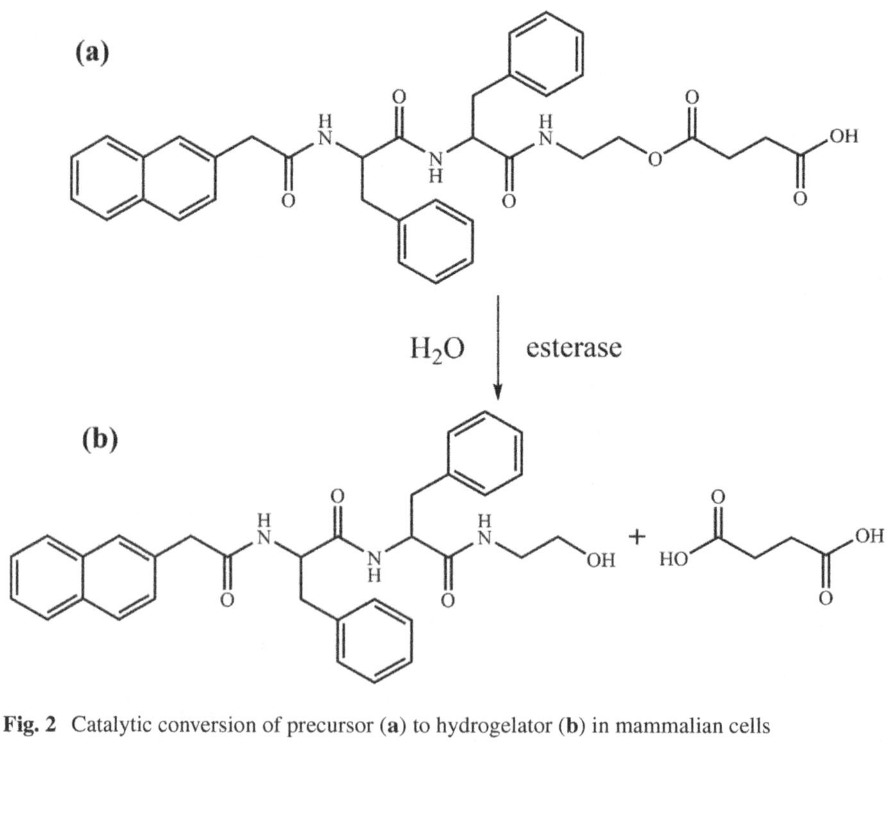

Fig. 2 Catalytic conversion of precursor (**a**) to hydrogelator (**b**) in mammalian cells

[49]. The very low level of toxicity, high biocompatibility of these materials with ultra-low gel concentrations, increases its further scope in tissue engineering, cell culture, and drug delivery.

8 Self-assembled Block Copolymers

The polymerization of more than one type of monomer units leads to the formation of copolymers. When the two monomer units of copolymer clustered together to form blocks of repeating units, such copolymers are called block copolymers. For example, a polymer made up of monomer units A and B, formed like -A-A-A-A-A-A-A-A-B-B-B-B-B-B-B-B-A-A-A-A-A-A-A-A-B-B-B-B-B-B-B-B-, where A-A-A-A-A-A-A-A and B-B-B-B-B-B-B-B-B are the blocks [50]. Synthetic copolymer-based hydrogels are of atmost interest due to their reversible sol–gel mechanism towards external stimuli sensitivity towards pH, temperature, ionic strength, electric field, light, etc. Among these, hydrogels that are made from temperature-responsive polymers are of wide interest, as they can undergo a volume phase transitions at their critical temperatures. Upon increasing temperature, LCST polymer hydrogels exhibit soluble to insoluble transition in aqueous media whereas UCST exhibits insoluble to soluble transition [51]. The competition between hydrophobic interaction, intermolecular hydrogen bonding, intramolecular hydrogen bonding, and the weak van der Waals forces governs the collapse of these hydrogel structures. polymerizing hydrophilic polyethylene glycol with biodegradable and thermosensitive polyesters like polylactide, polyglycolide result in the formation of biodegradable thermoresponsive block copolymer hydrogels. One of the first biodegradable thermoresponsive block copolymers was developed by Jeong B using polyethylene glycol (PEG) and poly (L lactide) (PLLA) [52]. The diblock and triblock copolymers, PEG-PLLA, PEG-PLLA-PEG show gel to sol transitions in higher temperature. Hydrophobicity and crystallinity of the polyesters can tune the critical gel concentration and gel to sol transition [53]. For example, longer the polyester bonds (more the hydrophobicity) and shorter PEG imparts, lower critical gel concentration has a higher gel to the sol transition temperature. Figure 3 shows the structure of PEG-PLA-PEG copolymer.

In an aqueous medium, the hydrophobic PLA molecules self-assembles to form micellar cores, whereas the hydrophilic PEG groups bridge between the micellar cores [54]. Temperature responsive of PCL-PEG-PCL copolymer shows a clear sol

Fig. 3 PEG-PLA-PEG copolymer

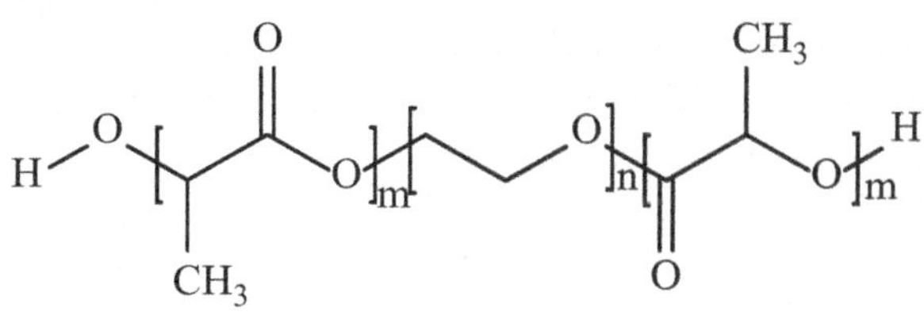

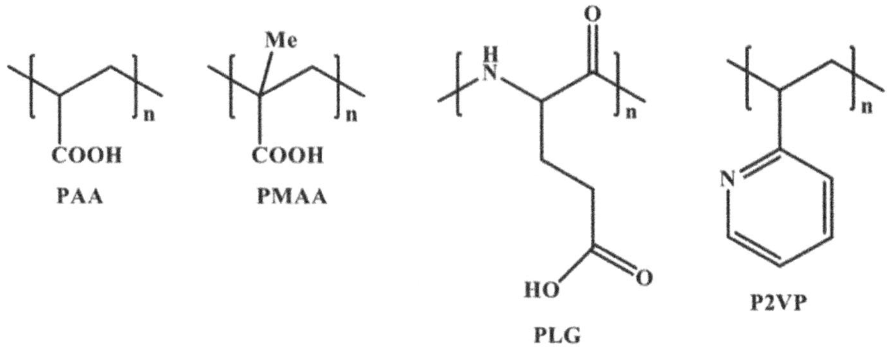

Fig. 4 Polyacidic electrolytes like PAA, PMMA, PLG, and polybasic electrolytes like P2VP

to gel to turbid sol transition in increasing temperatures [55]. The sol to gel transitions indicates the formation of micellar phases, whereas the gel to turbid sol transitions is due to the disintegrations of micellar phases. pH is another external stimulus that governs the gelation behaviour of block copolymer hydrogels. Since the stomach, intestine, and many other organs are pH sensitive, pH-responsive hydrogels have a vast biological application in tissue culture and drug delivery. The ionizable groups present in these materials help in its drastic changes in morphologies at varying pH. Chemical structure of polyacidic electrolytes like PAA, PMMA, PLG, and polybasic electrolytes like P2VP are shown in Fig. 4. pH-thermoresponsive hydrogels are the new class of block polymer hydrogels with vast biological applications due to their duel behaviour.

9 Liquid Crystalline Hydrogels

Even though block copolymer hydrogels and supramolecular hydrogels are excellent in its biocompatibility and wide biological applications, the poor mechanical strength limits their applications in chemomechanical systems [7]. Liquid crystalline gels consist of liquid crystals and aggregates of molecules that are called gelatos. They are macroscopically smooth and soft materials with enhanced electrical, magnetic, photoinduced properties along with the high mechanical strength [56]. Liquid crystalline gels show a versatile amount of properties of both liquid crystals and gels, thus making them more unique than other hydrogels. Due to their excellent mechanical strength and electrical properties, they were even used as dopants in other physical hydrogels and also widely exploited for the development of mechano-optical sensors [57].

Liquid crystal hydrogels also show multiphase behaviour with various water concentrations. For example, Oswada and his coworkers investigated this multiphase behaviour [6, 58]. Liquid crystalline hydrogels were prepared by the copolymerizationof hydrophobic 11-(4′-cyanobiphenyloxy) undecylacrylate (11CBA) with the hydrophilic acrylic acid monomers. At lower concentrations of molefractions of copolymers, for molefraction, $F < 0.18$, the copolymers tends to dissolve completely in water, whereas in the concentrations higher than 0.26, the hydrophobic interactions that operated between the side chains lead to the formation of hydrogels; i.e., at higher molar concentrations, these are forming liquid crystalline structures in the dry state, whereas copolymers of $F < 0.18$ form the amorphous structure. This synthesized liquid crystal hydrogels showed various phases at varying water concentrations. At lower water concentration with $F > 0.26$, hydrogels showed Smetic A structure (bilayers are formed by the side chains that aligns perpendicular to the main chainaxis), whereas at higher water contents, the liquid crystalline phases transform into the amorphous structure. They have also investigated with higher molefractions $F > 0.29$ and lower water contents, where the Smetic I (side chains normal to the main chain axis) structures are formed. The Smetic I to smetic A transitions were also observed by the application of mechanical stress [59]. By the application of magnetic, electric, and shear stress, the liquid crystalline hydrogels can be formed with high anisotropy ranging from the sub-micrometre to the macroscopic scale [60]. Several researchers have developed the hydrogel with macroscopic lamellar or micellar structured by applying a shear flow to the precursor solution before polymerization [61]. Centimetre scale liquid crystalline hydrogels can be also prepared by the self-assembly of polyion complexes that are semi-rigid [62]. For example, PBDT is a water-soluble semi-rigid polyanion with high molecular weight and negative charge similar to that of many natural biomacromolecules like DNA and fibrous actin. Dialysis of negatively charged PBDT solutions with $CaCl_2$ can lead to the electrostatic complexation of PBDT with Ca^{2+} and thereby self-assembling to form hydrogels with anisotropy or long-range order in centimetre scale, showing strong birefringence [63, 64]. Introducing liquid crystals as a dopant to chemical hydrogels leads to the tremendous rise in new properties in these hydrogels. Several reports show the usage of PBDT as a dopant in the photoinduced copolymerization of cationic monomer N-[3-(N,N-dimethylamino)propyl] acrylamide methyl chloride quaternary (DMAPAA-Q) [65, 66]. The as-synthesized transparent hydrogels showed high ordering in millimetres scale and strong birefringence which can be resulted from the molecular orientation ordering due to electrostatic interaction between cationic DMAPAA-Q and anionic PBDT.

10 Hybrid Hydrogels

Hybrid hydrogels are a type of hydrogels that are formed by the crosslinking of at least two different macromolecules or polymers (either synthetic or biological) systems covalently or non-covalently. Inter-wining the properties of synthetic molecules with natural copolymers can lead to the generation of hybrid hydrogels with magnificent properties. The high homogeneity, well-defined order and structure, stable mechanical strength, and folding-unfolding patterns are the major advantages and characteristics of protein motifs, whereas synthetic copolymers can easily synthesize in large quantities with controlled molecular weight, morphologies, and functional groups. Readily accessible functional groups can be added to the defined areas more precisely in synthetic polymers. This can help in the well-defined cross-linking between the synthetic polymers with the natural copolymers. Attaching the synthetic molecules to the protein motif improves not only the thermal stability of the hydrogel but also its conductivity [67]. Various studies have shown the improvement of thermal stability of the hybrid hydrogels formed by attaching polyethylene glycol (PEG) molecules into coiled-coil motif forming peptides [68, 69].

Self-assembling of alpha-helical motif with the HMPA polymer is one of the earliest and successful hybrid hydrogel self-assemblies [70, 71]. Several researchers were able to superimpose the properties of the coiled-coil helical motif in the whole hydrogel. Even the melting temperature of the protein motif and the phase transition temperature of the hybrid hydrogels are similar. This results in the creation of hydrogels with tremendous collapse and phase transition in particular temperatures. This technique has recognized wide attention as they were able to create various hydrogels with various phase transition temperatures by just replacing the coiled-coil motif with another coiled-coil motif which can melt at different temperature.

Human cardiac protein, also known as cardiac titin, is a giant protein that functions as a molecular spring which governs the passive elasticity of cardiac muscles. Titin comprises of two different modules, first the fibronectin type of domains and second the immunoglobulin domains. Immunoglobulin domains comprise of two anti-parallel beta sheets that unfolds at the temperature of 58 C. Self-assembling the immunoglobulin domains of cardiac titin with the acrylamide copolymers can result in the formation of temperature-sensitive hydrogels. Since the beta sheets unfold at 58 C, the hydrogels swell above its melting temperature. Thus, self-assembling cardiac titin with acrylamide can result in the creation of highly temperature-sensitive and responsive hydrogel.

Protein PEG graft hydrogels are another class of hybrid hydrogels that can mimic the extracellular matrix of a cell. Photopolymerized self-assembly of polyethylene glycol diacrylate along with genetically synthesized protein forms protein PEG graft hydrogels. The as-synthesized hydrogels permit the cell attachment and also help in proteolytic penetration. Concanavalin A is a naturally occurring glucose-binding protein. Physical crosslinking and self-assembly of concanavalin A with poly(acrylamide-co-allyl glucose) leads to the formation of a glucose-sensitive hydrogel. Competition of free glucose for the concanavalin A glucose-binding sites not only disturbs the physical crosslinking networks but also leads to the swelling of hydrogel.

11 Applications

The high biocompatibility and the biodegradability of self-assembled hydrogels make them as a potent candidate for drug delivery and tissue engineerings. Not only on biological applications but also these materials share vast electronic applications. Wang et al. recently reported the synthesis of fluorescent hydrogels with the self-assembly of peptides and transition metals [72]. The metal ions are chelated by the ligands present in the peptide motifs, thus stabilizing the hydrogels and preventing the organometallic chromophore aggregation. They have demonstrated the usage of this highly stable white light fluorescent material for 3D printing, thereby opening a vast window of its applications in the field of soft electronics. Conductive polymer hydrogels are another class, which is widely used in the electronic implanting device due to their high conductivity, toughness, and easy in patterning [15, 73]. One such example is the hybrid hydrogel synthesized by the self-assembly of polyion complex and polyaniline molecules [15]. These hybrid hydrogels show remarkable self-recovery behaviour and thereby used as strain sensors to detect the human motion [15, 74].

Extensive reports have proved the application of using self-assembled hydrogels as the promising candidate for drug delivery system, regenerative medicine, etc., as they are highly sensitive to changes in temperature, pH, electric field, light, and other external stimuli [75]. One of the best examples of regenerative medicine is the self-assembled peptide nanofibril that consists of amphiphilic oligopeptides. These amphiphilic oligopeptides consist of alternating repeating units of positively charged aminoacids like lysine or arginine and negatively charged aminoacids like asparagine which are separated by highly hydrophobic amino acid, alanine. These amphiphilic oligopeptides can form self-assemblies in physiological environmental like cerebral spinal fluid. The further scope of this work was investigated by Ellis-Behnke et al. [76]. They have developed a peptide solution with Ala-Asp-Ala repeating units, whose 1% injection on brain spontaneously undergoes self-assembly that can enable the reconnection of nerve tissue. Rather than biological applications, self-assembled hydrogels serve a vast optical and electronic applications also. For example, azobenzene units were incorporated along with the cholesterol or maltose-based hydrogelator brought up a hydrogel with very high photoresponse [32]. Similarly by combining the coordination chemistry along with self-assembly can also pave the way for the generation of photoresponsive hydrogels. Chelation of metal ions with the gelators forms the highly stable triplet excited state which emits lights strongly in the visible region [77]. This property of the metallogels can be widely used in photovoltaics, photocatalysis, and phosphorescence or luminescence-based cells and other technologies. By replacing one metal ion with another the phosphorescence wavelength can be tuned. For example doping and undoping of trinuclear gold (1) pyrazolatemetallogel with silver induces a reversible red–green–blue luminescence which was further explored for the creation of security inks for the rewritable fluorescent paper [78]. Highly catalytically active palladium and platinum can also undergo self-assembly with the gelators forming the catalytically active gels. For example, several palladium gels are used for the catalysis of benzyl alcohol to benzaldehyde [79].

12 Conclusions

Self-assembled hydrogels are the newly emerging class of materials with numerous applications. Their highly biocompatibility and sensitivity towards the stimuli like pH, temperature, salt concentration give rise to their wide applications in the biological field like tissue engineering, drug delivery, biosensors, and so on. Based on the source, we have categorized the self-assembled hydrogels into three categories, hydrogels with self-assembled biomacromolecules, hydrogels with self-assembled synthetic molecules, and hybrid hydrogels. Physical crosslinking imparts stimuli-sensitive behaviour to the hydrogels, whereas chemical covalent bonds improve the mechanical strength of these materials. In general, self-assembled supramolecular hydrogels and block copolymer hydrogels belonged to the category of physically crosslinked synthetic hydrogels, whereas liquid crystalline hydrogels belong to the category of chemical hydrogels. Incorporating one type of hydrogel with other hydrogels results in the formation of hybrid hydrogels with unique properties.

References

1. Ahmed EM (2015) Hydrogel: preparation, characterization, and applications: a review. J Adv Res 6:105–121
2. Chen X et al (2018) Supramolecular hydrogels cross-linked by preassembled host–guest PEG cross-linkers resist excessive, ultrafast, and non-resting cyclic compression. NPG Asia Mater 10:788–799
3. Kopeček J, Yang J (2009) Peptide-directed self-assembly of hydrogels. Acta Biomater 5:805–816
4. Kopeček J (2007) Hydrogel biomaterials: a smart future? Biomaterials 28:5185–5192
5. Xu C, Kopeček J (2007) Self-assembling hydrogels. Polym Bull 58:53–63
6. Kaneko T, Yamaoka K, Gong JP, Osada Y (2000) Liquid crystalline hydrogels. 2. Effects of water on the structural ordering. Macromolecules 33:4422–4426
7. Wu ZL, Gong JP (2011) Hydrogels with self-assembling ordered structures and their functions. NPG Asia Mater 3:57–64
8. Lin BF et al (2012) pH-responsive branched peptide amphiphile hydrogel designed for applications in regenerative medicine with potential as injectable tissue scaffolds. J Mater Chem 22:19447
9. Kyle S, Aggeli A, Ingham E, McPherson MJ (2009) Production of self-assembling biomaterials for tissue engineering. Trends Biotechnol 27:423–433
10. El Yaagoubi M, Tewari KM, Lau KHA (2018) Peptoid self-assembly and opportunities for creating protein-mimetic biomaterials and biointerfaces. In: Self-assembling biomaterials. Elsevier. https://doi.org/10.1016/b978-0-08-102015-9.00006-x
11. Lao UL, Sun M, Matsumoto M, Mulchandani A, Chen W (2007) Genetic engineering of self-assembled protein hydrogel based on elastin-like sequences with metal binding functionality. Biomacromolecules 8:3736–3739

12. Xu C, Breedveld V, Kopeček J (2005) Reversible hydrogels from self-assembling genetically engineered protein block copolymers. Biomacromolecules 6:1739–1749
13. Riaz N, Wolden SL, Gelblum DY, Eric JA (2016) Rate insensitive linear viscoelastic model for soft tissues. Biomater 118:6072–6078. https://doi.org/10.1002/cncr.27633
14. Kopeček J, Yang J (2012) Smart self-assembled hybrid hydrogel biomaterials. Angew Chem Int Ed 51:7396–7417
15. Zhu F et al (2018a) Tough and conductive hybrid hydrogels enabling facile patterning. ACS Appl Mater Interfaces 10:13685–13692
16. Zhu S et al (2018b) Self-assembly of collagen-based biomaterials: preparation, characterizations and biomedical applications. J Mater Chem B6:2650–2676
17. Rosenblatt J, Devereux B, Wallace DG (1994) Injectable collagen as a pH-sensitive hydrogel. Biomaterials 15:985–995
18. Yonath J, Oplatka A (1968) Mechanochemical melting of collagen fibers. I. Mechanical contractions. Biopolymers 6:1129–1145
19. Oplatka A, Yonath J (1968) Mechanochemical melting of collagen fibers. II. Diffusion-controlled contractions. Biopolymers 6:1147–1158
20. Censi R, Di Martino P, Vermonden T, Hennink WE (2012) Hydrogels for protein delivery in tissue engineering. J Control Release 161:680–692
21. Mason JM, Arndt KM (2004) Coiled coil domains: stability, specificity, and biological implications. ChemBioChem 5:170–176
22. Truebestein L, Leonard TA (2016) Coiled-coils: the long and short of it. BioEssays 38:903–916
23. Nowick JS (2008) Exploring beta-sheet structure and interactions with chemical model systems. Acc Chem Res 41:1319–1330
24. Aggeli A et al (2001) Hierarchical self-assembly of chiral rod-like molecules as a model for peptide beta-sheet tapes, ribbons, fibrils, and fibers. Proc Natl Acad Sci USA 98:11857–11862
25. Clarke DE, Pashuck ET, Bertazzo S, Weaver JVM, Stevens MM (2017) Self-healing, self-assembled β-sheet peptide-poly(γ-glutamic acid) hybrid hydrogels. J Am Chem Soc 139:7250–7255
26. Clarke DE, Parmenter CDJ, Scherman OA (2018) Tunable pentapeptide self-assembled β-sheet hydrogels. Angew Chem Int Ed 57:7709–7713
27. Milner-White EJ, Poet R (1986) Four classes of beta-hairpins in proteins. Biochem J 240:289–292
28. Larini L, Shea J-E (2012) Role of β-hairpin formation in aggregation: the self-assembly of the amyloid-β(25–35) peptide. Biophys J 103:576–586
29. Rajagopal K, Lamm MS, Haines-Butterick LA, Pochan DJ, Schneider JP (2009) Tuning the pH responsiveness of β-hairpin peptide folding, self-assembly, and hydrogel material formation. Biomacromolecules 10:2619–2625
30. Miller Y, Ma B, Nussinov R (2015) Polymorphism in self-assembly of peptide-based β-hairpin contributes to network morphology and hydrogel mechanical rigidity. J Phys Chem B 119:482–490
31. Dong R, Pang Y, Su Y, Zhu X (2015) Supramolecular hydrogels: synthesis, properties and their biomedical applications. Biomater Sci 3:937–954
32. Du X, Zhou J, Shi J, Xu B (2015) Supramolecular hydrogelators and hydrogels: from soft matter to molecular biomaterials. Chem Rev 115:13165–13307
33. Zhou Y, Fan X, Zhang W, Xue D, Kong J (2014) Stimuli-induced gel-sol transition of supramolecular hydrogels based on β-cyclodextrin polymer/ferrocene-containing triblock copolymer inclusion complexes. J Polym Res 21:359
34. Hou S, Ma PX (2015) Stimuli-responsive supramolecular hydrogels with high extensibility and fast self-healing via precoordinated mussel-inspired chemistry. Chem Mater 27:7627–7635
35. Kousar A, Feng C (2019) Controlled mechanical properties and supramolecular chirality of hydrogels via pH change. Methods X6:417–423
36. Li J (2010) Self-assembled supramolecular hydrogels based on polymer-cyclodextrin inclusion complexes for drug delivery. NPG Asia Mater 2:112–118

37. Eskandari S, Guerin T, Toth I, Stephenson RJ (2017) Recent advances in self-assembled peptides: implications for targeted drug delivery and vaccine engineering. Adv Drug Delivery Rev 110–111:169–187
38. Naota T, Koori H (2005) Molecules that assemble by sound: an application to the instant gelation of stable organic fluids. https://doi.org/10.1021/JA050809H
39. Isozaki K, Takaya H, Naota T (2007) Ultrasound-induced gelation of organic fluids with metalated peptides. Angew Chem Int Ed 46:2855–2857
40. Grigoriou S et al (2012) Dipeptide hydrogel formation triggered by boronic acid–sugar recognition. Soft Matter 8:6788
41. Marchesan S et al (2012) Unzipping the role of chirality in nanoscale self-assembly of tripeptide hydrogels. Nanoscale 4:6752
42. Zhao F, Gao Y, Shi J, Browdy HM, Xu B (2011) Novel anisotropic supramolecular hydrogel with high stability over a wide pH range†. Langmuir 27:1510–1512
43. Suzuki M, Yumoto M, Shirai H, Hanabusa K (2005) l-Lysine-based supramolecular hydrogels containing various inorganic ions. Org Biomol Chem 3:3073
44. Yang Z, Liang G, Xu B (2008) Enzymatic hydrogelation of small molecules. Acc Chem Res 41:315–326
45. Yang ZM, Xu KM, Guo ZF, Guo ZH, Xu B (2007) Intracellular enzymatic formation of nanofibers results in hydrogelation and regulated cell death. Adv Mater 19:3152–3156
46. Richardson PJ, Brown SJ, Bailyes EM, Luzio JP (1987) Ectoenzymes control adenosine modulation of immunoisolated cholinergic synapses. Nature 327:232–234
47. Pospisil P, Iyer LK, Adelstein SJ, Kassis AI (2006) A combined approach to data mining of textual and structured data to identify cancer-related targets. BMC Bioinform 7:354
48. Nakashima T, Kimizuka N (2002) Light-harvesting supramolecular hydrogels assembled from short-legged cationic L-glutamate derivatives and anionic fluorophores. Adv Mater 14:1113
49. Wang H et al (2010) Enzyme-triggered self-assembly of a small molecule: a supramolecular hydrogel with leaf-like structures and an ultra-low minimum gelation concentration. Nanotechnology 21:225606
50. Milkovich R (1981) Synthesis of controlled polymer structures, pp 41–57. https://doi.org/10.1021/bk-1981-0166.ch003
51. Gao GH, Li Y, Lee DS (2012) Block copolymer hydrogels. In: Encyclopedia of polymer science and technology. https://doi.org/10.1002/0471440264.pst577
52. Jeong B, Bae YH, Lee DS, Kim SW (1997) Biodegradable block copolymers as injectable drug-delivery systems. Nature 388:860–862
53. Fu H et al (2011) Preparation and tunable temperature sensitivity of biodegradable polyurethane nanoassemblies from diisocyanate and poly(ethylene glycol). Soft Matter 7:3546
54. Li X et al (2009) Self-assembled polymeric micellar nanoparticles as nanocarriers for poorly soluble anticancer drug ethaselen. Nanoscale Res Lett 4:1502–1511
55. Hwang MJ et al (2010) Multiple sol-gel transitions of PEG-PCL-PEG triblock copolymer aqueous solution. Macromol Rapid Commun 31:2064–2069
56. Brand HR, Martinoty P, Pleiner H (2011) Physical properties of magnetic gels
57. Popov N et al (2017) Thermotropic liquid crystal-assisted chemical and biological sensors. Materials. https://doi.org/10.3390/ma11010020
58. Kaneko T, Yamaoka K, Gong JP, Osada Y (2000) Liquid-crystalline hydrogels. 1. Enhanced effects of incorporation of acrylic acid units on the liquid-crystalline ordering. https://doi.org/10.1021/MA991528V
59. Yamaoka K, Kaneko T, Gong JP, Osada Y (2001) Liquid crystalline gels. 3. Role of hydrogen bonding in the formation and stabilization of mesophase structures. Macromolecules 34:1470–1476
60. van der Asdonk P, Kouwer PHJ (2017) Liquid crystal templating as an approach to spatially and temporally organise soft matter. Chem Soc Rev 46:5935–5949
61. Haque MA et al (2018) Tough and variable-band-gap photonic hydrogel displaying programmable angle-dependent colors. ACS Omega 3:55–62

62. Wu ZL, Kurokawa T, Gong JP (2012) Hydrogels with a macroscopic-scale liquid crystal structure by self-assembly of a semi-rigid polyion complex. Polym J 44:503–511
63. Wu ZL et al (2011) Anisotropic hydrogel from complexation-driven reorientation of semirigid polyanion at Ca^{2+} diffusion flux front. Macromolecules 44:3535–3541
64. Sun T, Wu Z, Gong J (2012) Self-assembled structures of a semi-rigid polyanion in aqueous solutions and hydrogels. Sci China Chem 55:735–742
65. Shigekura Y et al (2005) Anisotropic polyion-complex gels from template polymerization. Adv Mater 17:2695–2699
66. Wu ZL, Kurokawa T, Liang S, Gong JP (2010) Dual network formation in polyelectrolyte hydrogel via viscoelastic phase separation: role of ionic strength and polymerization kinetics. Macromolecules 43:8202–8208
67. Annabi N et al (2016) Highly elastic and conductive human-based protein hybrid hydrogels. Adv Mater 28:40–49
68. Pechar M, Kopečková P, Joss L, Kopeček J (2002) Associative diblock copolymers of poly(ethylene glycol) and coiled-coil peptides. Macromol Biosci 2:199
69. Hamley IW (2014) PEG–peptide conjugates. Biomacromolecules 15:1543–1559
70. Yang J, Xu C, Kopečková P, Kopeček J (2006) Hybrid hydrogels self-assembled from HPMA copolymers containing peptide grafts. Macromol Biosci 6:201–209
71. Wang C, Stewart RJ, KopeČek J (1999) Hybrid hydrogels assembled from synthetic polymers and coiled-coil protein domains. Nature 397:417–420
72. Xia Y et al (2017) Printable fluorescent hydrogels based on self-assembling peptides. Sci Rep 7:1–10
73. Yuk H, Lu B, Zhao X (2019) Hydrogel bioelectronics. Chem Soc Rev 48:1642–1667
74. Cai G et al (2017) Extremely stretchable strain sensors based on conductive self-healing dynamic cross-links hydrogels for human-motion detection. Adv Sci 4:1600190
75. Hirst AR, Escuder B, Miravet JF, Smith DK (2008) High-tech applications of self-assembling supramolecular nanostructured gel-phase materials: from regenerative medicine to electronic devices. Angew Chem Int Ed 47:8002–8018
76. Ellis-Behnke RG et al (2006) Nano neuro knitting: peptide nanofiber scaffold for brain repair and axon regeneration with functional return of vision. Proc Natl Acad Sci 103:5054–5059
77. Kishimura A, Yamashita T, Aida T (2004) Phosphorescent organogels via "metallophilic" interactions for reversible RGB—color switching. https://doi.org/10.1021/JA0441007
78. Kishimura A, Yamashita T, Yamaguchi K, Aida T (2005) Rewritable phosphorescent paper by the control of competing kinetic and thermodynamic self-assembling events. Nat Mater 4:546–549
79. Miravet JF, Escuder B (2005) Pyridine functionalised ambidextrous gelators: towards catalytic gels. Chem Commun 5796. https://doi.org/10.1039/b510874h

Chapter 15
Synthesis, Structural Modification and Physiochemical Response of Chitosan Built Nanohydrogel for Control Drug Delivery Applications

Faheem Ullah, Fatima Javed, and Hazizan Md. Akil

Abstract The present chapter explains the progressive synthesis, structural modification and physicochemical response of chitosan built hydrogel for controlled drug delivery applications. The name chitosan built referred to the hydrogel where chitosan can be used as the main component in addition to other monomers. An overview of hydrogel classification, processing, drug loading and release mechanism is highly stressed to discover the production of in-situ gelling system and their functionalization with induced sensitivity (hydrophilicity, hydrophobicity, glucose sensing and self-assembling) for the controlled release of versatile hydrophilic and hydrophobic drugs. The detailed chemistry of various stimuli-responsive hydrogel in biomedical and pharmaceutical applications has been clarified to state of the art of physicochemical responses at physiological conditions. Particular attention is paid to stimuli, including glucose, pH, temperature, ionic strength and urea-responsive hydrogel at physiological conditions. The use of chitosan built hydrogel as a controlled drug delivery system is not only limited to structure–property–relationship but needs a fundamental understanding in terms of chemical, thermal, morphological, optical and interfacial properties. These areas are addressed in terms of synthesis of chitosan built hydrogel, the respective functionalization with induced moieties along with detailed characterization and physicochemical responses for controlled drug delivery applications.

Keywords Nanohydrogel · Chitosan · Structural modification · Physicochemical · Controlled drug delivery

F. Ullah · F. Javed · H. Md. Akil (✉)
School of Materials and Mineral Resources Engineering, Engineering Campus, Universiti Sains Malaysia, Seri Ampangan, 14300 Nibong Tebal, Pulau Pinang, Malaysia
e-mail: hazizan@usm.my

F. Ullah
Institute of Chemical Sciences, University of Peshawar, Peshawar 25120, KPK, Pakistan

F. Javed
Department of Chemistry, Shaheed Benazir Bhutto Women University, Charssada Road, Peshawar 25000, Larama, Pakistan

J. Jose et al. (eds.), *Nano Hydrogels*, Gels Horizons: From Science to Smart Materials,
https://doi.org/10.1007/978-981-15-7138-1_15

1 Chitosan Built Hydrogel

A three-dimensional network of polymers made of natural (chitosan)and synthetic materials, possessing a high degree of flexibility due to large water content is called hydrogel. Under physiological conditions, they are able to retain a large amount of water or biological fluids and are characterized by a soft rubbery consistency similar to living tissues, making them an ideal substance for a variety of applications. Hydrogel with characteristic properties such as desired functionality, reversibility, sterilizability and biocompatibility meets both material and biological requirements to treat or replace tissues, organs, function of living tissues as well as to interact with the biological system [8, 19, 29]. Hydrogels have been found in nature since life on earth. Bacterial biofilms, which are hydrated extracellular matrix components and plant structures are universal water swollen motifs in nature. Gelatine and agar were also known and used for various applications early in human history, but the modern history of hydrogel as a class of materials designed for biomedical applications can be accurately traced.

From chemistry point of view, hydrogel is a mixture with characteristic solid and liquid properties. The crosslinked network structures of hydrogel from randomly crosslinked macromolecules consist of polymeric solid phase, interstitial fluid phase and ionic phase. Polymeric chains create a three-dimensional matrix with interstitial spaces (filled up with water or biological fluids), formed by van der Waals interactions, hydrogen bonding, electrostatic interactions and physical entanglements as well as by covalent bonding [14]. The fluid phase comprises the pores which make the hydrogel wet and impart elastic properties. Due to these properties, structures of hydrogel resemble living tissue. The ionic phase consists of the ionizable groups that are bound to the polymeric counter-ions and co-ions. These phases exist normally due to the presence of electrolytic solvent. Recently, many attempts have been made to develop chitosan-based drug delivery systems, such as anticancer drug carriers, peptide carriers, antibiotic agents or steroid carriers [43]. The biodegradable polymer such as chitosan, a pH-dependent polycation, where the significant chains are able to interact with oppositely charged molecules through electrostatic interactions is highly recommended for drug delivery, wound dressing, tissue engineering and biotechnology applications due to its biocompatible and biodegradable nature. Due to its antibacterial, biofriendly, nontoxic and mucoadhesive properties, it is used to increase the time of intact for drug penetration [21]. Chitosan is known to protect the drug from hostile and antagonistic environment. Chitosan is only soluble in water at a pH below 6.5 ($\approx$pKa value of chitosan), where the protonation of the amine group will help to create positive charge cloud and the resultant electrostatic repulsion of these pendant group assists in solubilization and swelling of hydrogel matrices. Another important aspect of selecting chitosan for the proposed system is its efficient removal through renal filtration and enzymatic degradation [7, 12]. Fundamental physicochemical and electrokinetic investigations are of utmost importance in order to understand the responses of selective stimuli including glucose, pH, temperature, ionic strength, urea and drug sensitivity of the chitosan built hydrogel.

These responses govern the internal and external interaction of hydrogel entities with the biomolecules (drug, glucose, enzymes, proteins, DNA and dyes). So how and why the changes occur in the hydrogel system with the environment (glucose, pH, ionic strength, temperature, drug) depends upon the physical and chemical properties of the system. Several researchers reported the chitosan built hydrogel for drug delivery focusing on the macroscopic- and microscopic films, microspheres, effect of crosslinker and the reaction conditions, but still the effect of internal and external parameters needs to be addressed. This chapter reveals the desirable properties by inducing glucose sensitivity, self-assembling and hydrophilicity into such hydrogel, which enhanced the internal and external properties significantly. The investigation of physicochemical, electrokinetic parameters with several model drug loading versus release profiles are striking to evaluate the potential of chitosan built hydrogel for controlled drug delivery applications.

To date, there is no report of a boronic acid-based glucose sensor that fulfills all the criteria of biocompatibility, biodegradability, multi-responsiveness (toward pH, temperature, ionic strength, urea) and in vitro evaluation of loading and release profiles of model drugs at physiological conditions [38]. For a glucose sensor to be useful in a device, the sensing components must be free to allow instantaneous nursing. For in vivo practice, the device must function at physiological conditions with biocompatible and biodegradable characterizations. There is a need to address and replace unhealthy moieties containing glucose oxidase-based glucose sensors, which present random sensitivity, instability, immobilization, where the application is restricted by intrinsic nature of enzymes present in the body [23, 36]. Hence, a simple, enzyme-free glucose sensor with low cost, reproducibility, selectivity and reliably fast determination seems to be an attractive system that is free from the abovementioned drawbacks. Among the significant glucose sensors [42], the chitosan-based hydrogel is considered as the most proficient and accessible sensors with updated 3-aminophenylboronic acid (3-APBA) moieties to detect glucose in terms of simplicity, movability, controlled response, high sensitivity and selectivity at physiological conditions [6].

More than 40% new chemical entities developed in the pharmaceutical industry are hydrophobic which are practically insoluble in water [32]. So, hydrophobic drug carriers must be designed in such a way to improve the selectivity, effectiveness and safety of hydrophobic drug administration (loading and release). One class of drug delivery vehicle that has received widespread attention is micelles, formed by self-assembly of amphiphilic hydrogel in aqueous solution [15]. Chitosan is a hydrophobic biomaterial with promising features for biomedical and pharmaceutical applications due to significant swelling and mucoadhesive properties. The hydrophobic nature of chitosan can be controlled by copolymerizing with a hydrophilic entity to create a hydrophobic/hydrophilic balance regarding the administration of hydrophobic drugs. Further, chitosan built hydrogel as micelles is specified for drug delivery applications for a number of reasons. First of all, hydrophobic drugs can be physically entrapped in the core of such polymeric micelles and transported at concentration that can exceed their intrinsic water solubility. Second, the hydrophilic blocks, which are often composed of poly(ethylene glycol) PEG, have the superior ability of hydrogen bonding with the aqueous environment and form a tight shell around the micellar core. Hydrogel as micelles with a PEG corona resists protein adsorption and cellular adhesion due to the highly hydrophilic nature of PEG which is resistant to hydrophobic surfaces of protein and mucosal layers. Thus, the PEG corona easily assembles in between aqueous and cellular spaces and protects the drug from deactivation at the cellular level and contents of hydrophobic core are effectively protected against hydrolysis, deactivation and enzymatic degradation. In addition, the PEG corona prevents recognition by the endothelial system and therefore avoids the preliminary elimination of the micelles from the bloodstream. The PEG corona results in increased blood circulation and allows the drug to be administered over a prolonged period of time. A final feature that makes amphiphilic micellar block copolymer attractive for drug delivery application is the molecular weight, block length ratio and hydrophilic monomer which controls the size, morphology and association of the micelles [18, 34]. Considering the previous reports, the literature poorly characterizes chitosan in terms of various molecular weights and their effect on critical micelle concentration (CMC) and thermokinetic parameters of drug administration. Further, lack of studies associating the chitosan built hydrogel to function as self-assembled micelles and the distinct attainment methods to allow its use in hydrophobic drug delivery. The effects of varying molecular weight of chitosan on properties, particularly sol–gel transition, surface, electrokinetic and physicochemical characterization of the overall system are systematically explored. Also, the effects of pH, temperature, urea and ionic strength on physicochemical and electrokinetic parameters in terms of swelling, zeta potential, conductance and electrophoric mobility are explored in this study for hydrophobic drug delivery applications [37].

Regarding internal interactions, the carboxylate moieties present in alginic acid (AA) units interact with the protonated amines present in chitosan (CS) to form a three-dimensional interpenetrating network (IPNs) due to strong electrostatic interactions [2]. Thus, capability to modify the physicochemical properties of chitosan and alginic acid hydrogel is to control the degree of association between AA and CS moieties. Accordingly, controlling the association in such molecules requires a comprehensive understanding of the structure and introducing highly hydrophilic moieties to extend the external interactions with the surrounding environment (blood, aqueous solution, drug and cellular organelles). The tuneable properties of such a system with selective ligands to ensure the extended interactions is a very new concept for further consideration which are systematically described in this chapter [35]. Gibas et al. [10] reported that swelling of hydrogel is a complex process comprising of a number of steps. In the first step, the polar hydrophilic groups of the hydrogel matrix are hydrated by water, which appears in the form of primary bound water. In the second step, the hydrophobic pendant groups present in the polymeric hydrogel interpenetrating networks (IPNs) are also hydrated by water (due to short range Vander Wall's forces and hydrogen bonding) and thus appear in the form of secondary bound water. The primary bound water and the secondary bound water both form the total bound water. In the third step, the osmotic driving force of network toward infinite dilution is resisted by the physical or chemical crosslinks, so additional water is absorbed. The water absorbed at equilibrium swelling is called the bulk water or

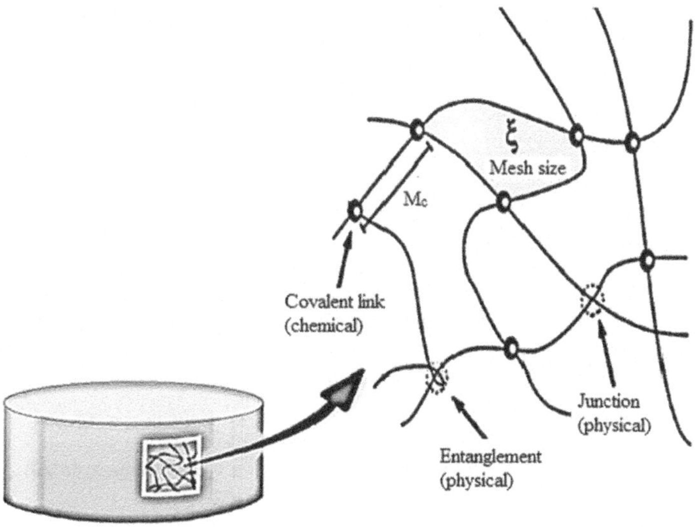

Fig. 1 Structural chemistry of hydrogel [10]

the free water, which fills the spaces between the network or chains and the centre of the larger pores. The amount of water absorbed by a hydrogel depends on the temperature and specific interaction between the water molecules and the polymer chains, which can be explained by the Flory–Huggins theory [9]. The solid portion of the hydrogel is a network of crosslinked polymer chains, a 3D network, usually referred as a mesh as shown in Fig. 1, with the spaces filled up with a fluid, normally water.

The meshes hold the fluid and impart an elastic force that can be completed by the expansion and contraction of the hydrogel and therefore are responsible for the solidity of the hydrogel. The ionic phase of hydrogel usually consists of ionizable groups bound onto the polymer chains and a number of mobile ions, including counter-ions and co-ions due to the presence of the electrolytic solvent, which surrounds the hydrogel.

2 Classification of Hydrogel

The classification of hydrogel depends on physical properties, nature of swelling, method of preparation, origin, ionic charges, sources, rate of biodegradation and observed nature of crosslinking [26]. It is clear from Fig. 2 that classification details for each type are beyond the scope of this chapter, but some of the prominent hydrogels are discussed.

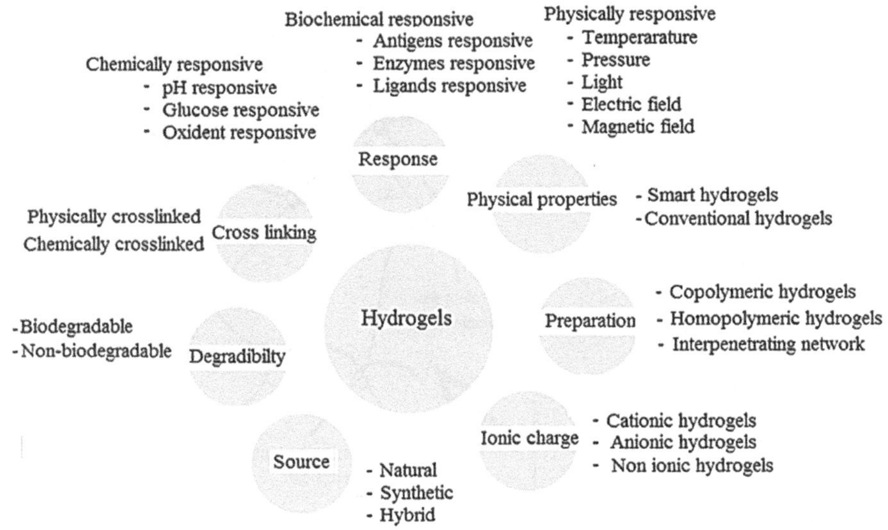

Fig. 2 Classification of hydrogel on the basis of crosslinking, responses, preparation and nature of hydrogel

3 Synthetic Strategies in Chitosan Built Hydrogel

Polymeric hydrogel is normally produced by one of two well-established schemes

- Polymerization of hydrophobic/hydrophilic monomers;
- Modification or functionalization of existing polymers (natural or synthetic).

The unique sources of hydrogel comprise of two main classes, i.e., natural, containing two main groups based on polypeptides (proteins) and polysaccharides (chitosan), and another is synthetic (petrochemical-based). Natural hydrogels are usually prepared through the addition of some synthetic parts to natural substrate, e.g., copolymerization of vinyl monomers with polysaccharides. When the term "hydrogel" is used without specifying its type, it truly means the conventional type of hydrogel [1]. The synthetic route for the production of most synthetic hydrogel is the free radical polymerization of multifunctional vinyl monomers. Each monomer contains a carbon double bond where an active centre may propagate to produce polymer chains but generating active centers also depends on solvent, reaction conditions and particular monomers which can be initiated by heat (thermal-initiators), light (photo-initiators), enzymes (bio-initiators) or electron beams [30] as shown in Fig. 3. Usually, water-soluble natural or synthetic polymers are crosslinked to form hydrogels in a number of ways, such as (1) linking polymer chains via chemical reaction, (2) using ionizing radiation to generate main chain-free radicals, which can recombine as crosslink joints and (3) interacting physically such as electrostatics,

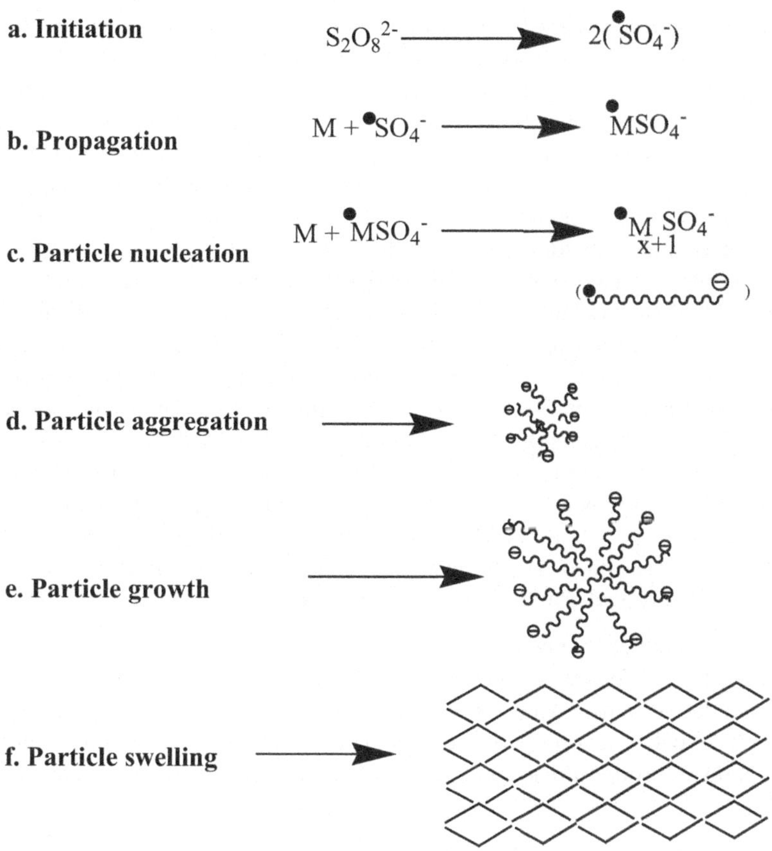

Fig. 3 Synthesis of hydrogel by free radical polymerization [40]

entanglements and crystallite interactions. Any of the various polymerization techniques can be used to form hydrogel, including bulk, solution and suspension polymerizations. The three main components of hydrogel are monomers, initiators and crosslinkers, which can be diluted in water or any solvent to control the heat of polymerization. However, its disadvantage appears in the form of impurities left from the preparation process containing unreacted monomers, initiators, crosslinkers and side products. Hydrogel is commonly prepared from monomers of both natural and synthetic origins by free radical polymerization in aqueous medium.

4 Physical and Chemical Cross-linking in Hydrogel

The reported methods to synthesize chitosan built hydrogel include physical crosslinking, chemical crosslinking and interpenetrating polymeric networks (IPNs) formation [5]. Physical crosslinking of chitosan occurs due to physical interactions like polyelectrolyte complexation, interpolymer complexation, ionic complexation and hydrophobic associations. The physically crosslinked hydrogel is produced without using any toxic chemical crosslinker, but at the same time, weak mechanical features, inconsistent in vivo behavior and shorter lifetime at physiological conditions, are considered as the key barriers in pharmaceutical applications. Consequently, physical crosslinked chitosan built hydrogels are not strong enough to establish permanent junctions in the molecular network and also lack the ability to promote the water residency in the polymeric chains [3]. Therefore, chemically crosslinked hydrogel is more favorable for pharmaceutical and biomedical applications which fulfill the above-stated features. The toxic crosslinkers are non-favorable for pharmaceutical applications, and thus, the targeted applications need biocompatible, biodegradable and non-toxic crosslinker for practical use. One of the bio-friendly crosslinker is known as methylenebisacrylamide (MBA) with reported biocompatibility and biodegradability, which is used to produce the crosslinking points by Schiff base formation where C=O double bond (from *N*-acetyl glucoseamine units) is replaced by a –C–N bond between chitosan and secondary polymer chains [11]. The advantages assigned to chemical crosslinking in chitosan built hydrogel in comparison to physical crosslinking highlighted as

- Hydrogel is obtainable below 80 °C.
- Hydrogel can stabilize the encapsulated drug.
- The pendant groups must respond to the external stimuli.
- The physicochemical properties can be improved by surface modification.
- The pendant groups are accessible to communicate with drug and cell surface.

5 Synthesis of Chitosan-co-Alginic Acid Hydrogel

The synthetic and functionalization mechanisms of chitosan built hydrogel are shown in Fig. 4. The copolymerization of chitosan (Cs) and alginic acid (AA) can be initiated by using a thermal initiator system at 75 °C to produce active radicals in both polymers as chemical crosslinking junctions points. As per reported literature, 700 mg of Cs was softened in 90 mL acidified DDH_2O (1.2% v/v) under constant magnetic stirring for 20 h at 25 °C. Further, 400 mg of AA was added to the reaction mixture and the reaction temperature was increased up to 75 °C at the rate of 3 °C/min. Exactly after 1 h of achieving the desired temperature (75 °C), 10 mL of 0.5 M APS was added drop-wise and allowed to react with the mixture for 30 min in order to produce free radicals in both the polymers, followed by the addition of 10 mL of 0.5 M MBA under constant stirring and N_2 purging. During the reaction, 0.2 mg of sodium dodecyl sulfates (SDS) was added as a surfactant in order to achieve uniform particles and particle size distribution due to the surface active properties of SDS in aqueous solution. After some time, the system became progressively thicker and was observed until it could not be stirred. The resultant hydrogel were then purified by centrifugation, decantation followed by frequently washing with DDH_2O. Finally,

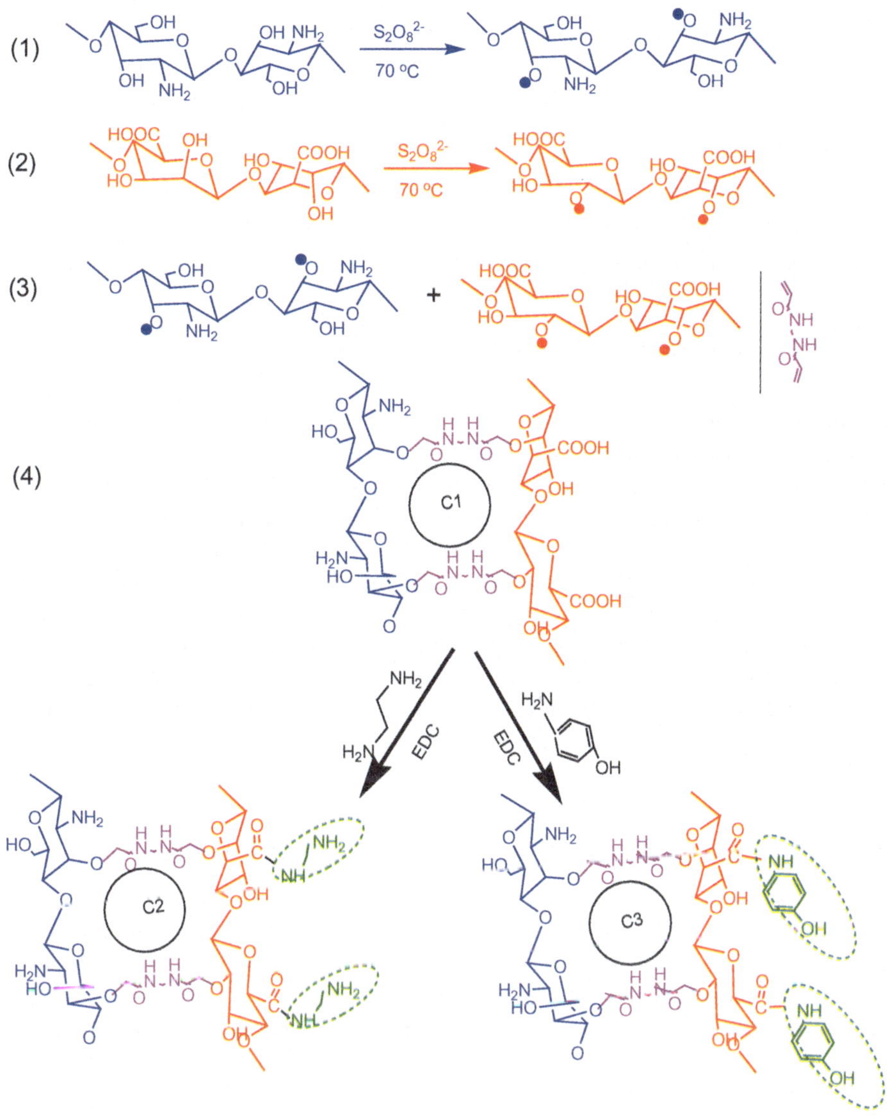

Fig. 4 Synthetic routes of native (C1) hydrogel and their functionalization with soft (C2), and hard (C3), ligands for extended interactions

the hydrogel was purified by dialysis for 07 days in membrane tubing (Spectrum laboratories, Inc., Rancho Dominguez, CA, USA; MW cutoff 12,000–14,000). The product was de-watered using ethanol for 02 h, grounded sieved and dried again at 80 °C for 72 h. The feed composition is shown in Table 1.

Table 1 Feed composition of C1, C2 and C3 hydrogel

Sample code	(Composition)[a] (mg)	SDS (mg)	APS (M)	EDA (mg)	AP (mg)	EDC (mg)	Curing time (h)	Curing temp. (°C)
C1	700:400:0.5	02	0.5	–	–	–	23	75
C2	700:400:0.5	02	0.5	150	–	150	15	25
C3	700:400:0.5	02	0.5	–	150	150	15	25

[a]Composition = (Chitosan: Alginate: MBA)

6 Functionalization CS-co-AA Hydrogel

The functionalization of CS-co-AA hydrogel termed as C1 by the respective ligand N-Ethylenediamine (EDA) and 4-Aminophenol (AP) via carbodimide (EDC) coupling was carried out as follows: stoichiometric amount of EDA (150 mL) and EDC (150 mg) was solubilized in 55 mL DDH$_2$O under constant stirring for 5 h. The solution was then placed in an ice bath followed by the addition of 200 mg dialyzed C1 hydrogel for 10 h to confirm the effective functionalization via EDC catalyzed coupling of EDA by replacing -OH groups in AA units. The functionalized hydrogel was declared as C2 and again purified by dialysis to ensure the complete removal of unlinked moieties. A similar scheme was followed for the effective functionalization of (C1) hydrogel via EDC catalyzed coupling of AP to replace -OH groups in AA units and was declared as C3 as shown in Fig. 4.

7 Choice for Controlled Drug Delivery Applications

Starting from the most classical drug delivery system, where the drug is naturally administrated by the oral, intravenous, intramuscular routes and drug distribution are governed by blood plasma. The drug is free and unable to reach the targeted site, so need several directions to show a therapeutic effect. A fast drug release also produces high plasma levels, causing adverse effects and compromising patient compliance [20]. Therefore to overcome the limitations of classical drug delivery, controlled drug delivery systems (CDDSs) have been introduced with desired characteristics at physiological conditions. Initially, many liposomes based drug delivery systems have been investigated with reported microparticles, nanoparticles, films and hydrogel formulations to substitute the classical drug delivery systems [17, 22]. Many biomaterial and synthetic strategies were applied to achieve the drug delivery system which function at physiological conditions. Thus, chitosan built hydrogel was introduced as a striking candidate with pharmacokinetics parallel to the cell activity without any side effects for targeted and controlled drug delivery applications. Chitosan built hydrogel is characterized with significant features to deliver drug to the targeted site per required level of dosage in a self-controlled manner with enhanced circulation

Table 2 Chitosan-based drug delivery system prepared by different methods

Form	Preparation method
Gel	Crosslinking
Films	Solution casting
Beads	Precipitation
Nanoparticles	Precipitation
Capsules	Emulsion/precipitation
Microspheres	Spray drying/ionic gelation
Tablets	Matrix coat

time. As many drugs and proteins are deactivated after oral and intravenous doses, thus to improve the solubility of hydrophobic drugs (e.g., paclitaxel, tamoxifen, etc.), chitosan built hydrogel is reported with odd results [31]. Nowadays, chitosan built hydrogel is under investigations to formulate the marketed drugs into new pharmaceutical arrangements. Chitosan-based hydrogel can be used in a variety of ways as controlled drug delivery system as shown in Table 2. Such hydrogel is characterized with effective role in terms of bioavailability, biodegradation, biodistribution and controlled drug administration at physiological conditions.

From physiochemical point of view, the chitosan built hydrogel has been characterized with the ability to swell and shrink in response to the external stimuli, especially pH, glucose concentration and ionic strength. Therefore, a substantial volume of research is focused on the synthesis of chitosan built hydrogel for controlled drug delivery applications as a variety of pH exist in the body. The pH sensitivity of hydrogel confirms the delivery of specified drugs to the gastrointestinal tract, stomach and colon. By controlling the physicochemical properties, chitosan built hydrogel can cover the epidermal, rectal, subcutaneous and oral drug administration without any side effects at physiological conditions. The drug administration for any polymeric hydrogel depends upon many factors like the chemical structure, hydrophilicity, hydrophobicity, reactivity, molecular weight, toxicity, nature of pendant groups and biocompatibility of polymers. Unfortunately, the natural polymers fulfilling the abovementioned properties are very few like chitosan, alginate and cellulose, so there is an urgent need to copolymerize these natural polymers with synthetic polymers in the form of interpenetrating networks (IPNs), to fabricate standard hydrogel for controlled drug delivery applications. Similarly, hydrogel with different functionalities can be prepared with effective functionalization with induced moieties to fulfill different pharmaceutical applications along with thermodynamic and thermokinetic of drug loading and release profiles. Several routes of hydrogel-based drug delivery system are presented in Fig. 5.

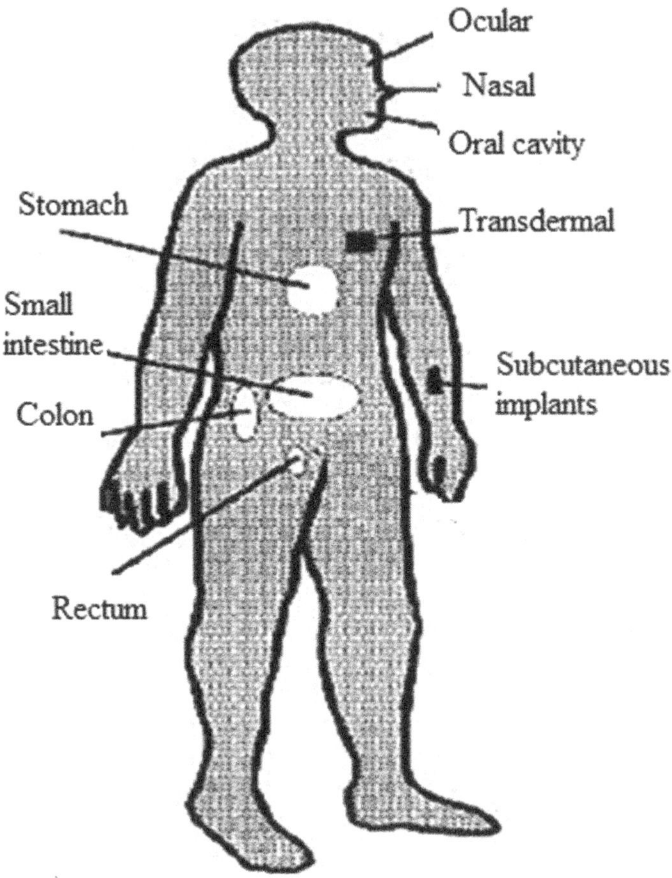

Fig. 5 Tissue locations applicable for hydrogel-based drug delivery system

8 Drug Loading Mechanismin Chitosan Built Hydrogel

There are three methods of drug loading to hydrogel matrices, namely diffusion, entrapment and tethering as shown in Fig. 6. For larger drug molecules, the drug loading is achieved by tethering of drug during the hydrogel synthesis, where a crosslinker is used to chemically attach the drug to the hydrogel. Tethering process is characterized to avoid the loss of therapeutic during administration but the main problem with tethering method is that drug is only available to tissue when the molecular tether breaks or the hydrogel degrade which mean that bioavailability of drug is negligible at the targeted site [4]. Another reported method of drug loading is entrapment, where the drug molecules are entrapped during the gelation process in hydrogel without using any crosslinker. The hydrogel work effectively in the course of entrapment, but due to free motion of drug from hydrogel matrices, initial

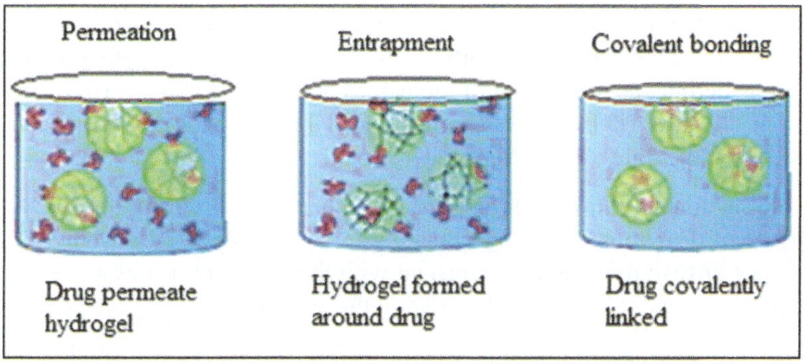

Fig. 6 Three different loading strategies in chitosan built hydrogel [4]

burst release is observed which is undesirable in controlled drug delivery system. In diffusion method, the hydrogel is allowed to interact with the saturated solution of drug, where the drug slowly diffuses into hydrogel matrices. After diffusion of drug into hydrogel, the drug-loaded hydrogel is dried for clinical use. Here the effect of hydrogel porosity, molecular weight, chemical structure and dimension of drug and hydrogel are considered as key parameters for drug administration (loading and release profiles). Diffusion of drug into hydrogel is applicable for smaller therapeutics, but larger drug molecules cannot be diffused into hydrogel matrices [39]. In overall investigations, diffusion is considered as the simplest and effective way of drug loading into hydrogel matrices. The attraction of chitosan must be addressed which is vigorously used in the synthesis of smart hydrogel for controlled drug delivery applications due to its bioavailability, biocompatibility, biodegradability and environmental (pH, temperature and ionic strength) sensitivity at physiological conditions [4, 33].

9 Drug Release Mechanism from Chitosan Built Hydrogel

In this section, a very clear picture of drug release from the hydrogel is presented. Drug release from a hydrogel is possible due to absorption of water and desorption of drug through a process known as swelling controlled mechanism [27]. As drug-loaded hydrogel particle comes in contact with water or thermodynamically stable fluid, the respective solvent penetrates into the available free spaces present on the surface of hydrogel. At this stage, the hydrodynamic radius and end-to-end distance of polymeric chains increase due to the stress produced by solvent, and this phenomena is so-called swelling [16]. Due to swelling, the water molecules penetrate into the hydrogel matrices and due to electrostatic repulsion of pendant groups, the charged entities move far away from each other and result in expulsion of entrapped drug from the hydrogel matrices to the external environment. Along with swelling, drug can also be release from the hydrogel matrices through diffusion and chemical reactions. Diffusion is the most common method for drug release from hydrogel matrices. Diffusion is defined as movement of molecules according to concentration gradient [9]. A controlled drug delivery system must fulfill the following conditions according to Higuchi steady-state assumptions [41]:

- The initial concentration of drug must be higher than solubility of drug.
- The size of drug must be smaller than pore size of drug delivery vehicle.
- The drug diffusivity should be constant with the time and position.
- Perfect sink conditions are maintained in the system.

Peppas and coworkers developed empirical equation (Eq. 1) which assumes a time-dependent power law function [25]

$$\frac{M_t}{M_O} = k \cdot t^n \tag{1}$$

where M_t/M_O is fractional release, k is structural/geometric constant, and n is known as release exponent representing the releases mechanism. Consequently, for spherical hydrogel particles, if $0.43 < n < 0.85$, refer to controlled diffusion. It is important here to mention that if drug release occurs due to polymer degradation, it is known as surface erosion, otherwise if drug release occurs through controlled diffusion, it is known as bulk erosion. According to Heller and Baker model, controlled diffusion of drug follow first order kinetic [13].

Although, hydrogel is characterized with superior controlled drug delivery applications, there are some intrinsic pharmacological limitations of hydrogel like poor mechanical strength, difficulties in processing, dissolution prior to targeted site, unpredictable homogeneity, rapid release, larger pore size and high water contents. Several strategies have been explored to minimize the burst release of drug, enhance the hydrogel-drug interactions and increase the diffusion barrier for drug release from the hydrogel matrices. The author contribution in this regard is the functionalizion of hydrogel with specified ligands which can release the drug only in response to the particular stimulus like glucose, pH, ionic strength, urea and temperature at physiological condition.

10 Photoluminescence Analysis of Drug Loading/Release from Chitosan Built Hydrogel

Fluorescein, rhodamine with diol and diamine architectures (comparative to insulin) were selected to study the drug loading and release profiles of chitosan-based hydrogel. Bromocresol green (model anionic drug) was also used as sparingly soluble drug to state the hydrogel drug loading and release trials. Fluorescein with standard absorbance of 390 nm was used as a hydrophobic model drug to study the loading and release trials of micellar hydrogel by using UV–vis spectrophotometer [35, 37, 38].

A fixed amount of dried hydrogel was allowed to mix with an aqueous solution of the drug with pre-determined concentration. Drug loading and release profiles were obtained from the hydrogel in a shaker incubator at 75 rpm at 37 °C. Each time, 4 mL of each solution was analyzed for the drug concentration/20 min delay by using a UV-Vis spectrophotometer. An equal volume of the same solution medium was added back to maintain a constant volume. The drug release study was investigated in a sophisticated dissolution apparatus by immersing 0.45 g of drug-loaded dried hydrogel beads in 250 mL of pH 6.85 solutions. After mixing, the mixture was centrifuged at 75 rpm at 37 °C. 04 mL of the solution was taken for analysis with continuously replacing by fresh buffer solution to maintain a steady volume. Thus, the concentration of the released drug was investigated in term of absorbance. The in vitro release tests of all samples were conducted in triplicate at specified time intervals [28].

11 Swelling and Degradation Analysis

Phosphate buffer solutions PBS pH = 7.45, with added NaCl (0.05 M ≈ physiological ionic strength) was used in order to state the art of hydrogel swelling gravimetrically at 37 °C. The known amount of hydrogel was immersed in DDH_2O (150 mL) and allowed to soak for several h at 37 °C. The immersion of hydrogel in the aqueous solution followed by spreading on the filter paper, and then non-stop weighing was performed for all the samples in triplicate. The swelling capacity (SC) at time t and the equilibrium swelling ratio (S_{eq}) were calculated using Eqs. 2 and 3 [24].

$$\text{Swelling ratio } (\%) = \frac{(W_t - W_d)}{W_d} \times 100 \tag{2}$$

$$S_{eq}\,(\%) = \frac{(W_e - W_d)}{W_d} \times 100 \tag{3}$$

where W_d (initial weight of the dry hydrogel), W_t (weight of the hydrogel at time t) and W_e (equilibrium weight during the swelling process).

Similarly, the introduced degradation test reflects the physiological stomach and intestinal conditions used as a guideline to explore further regarding the in vitro degradation of these biocompatible hydrogel at physiological conditions. Such tests were accomplished in phosphate buffer solution PBS pH ≈ 7.4 (simulated intestinal fluid) and pH ≈ 1.5 (simulated gastric fluid) with added 0.05 M each NaCl, NaOH, $CaCl_2$, acetic acid without any added enzymes. At specific time intervals, the loss in wet mass of hydrogel matrices was calculated by using Eq. 4.

$$\text{Wet mass change } (\%) = \left(\frac{W_t}{W_e}\right) \times 100 \tag{4}$$

where W_e (hydrogel mass in equilibrium swollen state) and W_t (hydrogel mass in at time t) in the test solutions.

12 Summary

The present chapter summarizes the literature related to hydrogel in the past 10 years, which describe the classification of hydrogel based on the different physical and chemical properties with emphasis on stimuli-responsive hydrogel for controlled drug delivery applications. The method of preparing hydrogel and the designing process influences the production of hydrogel by different techniques where a high degree of sensitivity is highlighted. The path of the research in this chapter indicates that the combination of polymers, which respond to different stimuli (physical, chemical and biochemical) must be identified and future generation of hydrogel that undergoes spontaneous swelling when in contact with the drug, cellular organelle and infected cells should be investigated. The chitosan built hydrogel is recognized with particular consideration as innovative materials that swell rapidly to a large size regardless of their original size. The materials tend to absorb much water or aqueous fluids in a relatively short period. This innovative category will receive serious attention of academic and industrial research with selective surface modification for controlled drug delivery applications. In this age of nanofabrication, there is a need for miniaturization of the hydrogel with enhanced durability, hydrophilicity, biocompatibility, mechanical and thermal properties for advanced applications. Therefore, realizing the clinical requirements and simultaneously limiting the complexity of hydrogel formulation will be the main goal for the coming decades. The role of chitosan built hydrogel is studied, especially for controlled drug delivery applications. Finally, an inclusive description of drug loading and release mechanism is provided.

Acknowledgments The authors would like to acknowledge Universiti Sains Malaysia (USM) for sponsoring this research under Grant RUI 1001/PBAHAN/8014047.

Dr. Fatima Javd also acknowledge the Higher Commission (HEC) Pakistan, for providing a platform under IPFP program to accomplish this research at Shaheed Benazir Bhutto Women Univrsity Peshawar, Pakistan.

References

1. Ahmed EM, Aggor FS, Awad AM, El-Aref AT (2013) An innovative method for preparation of nanometal hydroxide superabsorbent hydrogel. Carbohyd Polym 91:693–698
2. Allardyce CS, Dyson PJ (2016) Metal-based drugs that break the rules. Dalton Trans 45:3201–3209

3. Annabi N, Tamayol A, Uquillas JA, Akbari M, Bertassoni LE, Cha C, Camci-Unal G, Dokmeci MR, Peppas NA, Khademhosseini A (2014) 25th anniversary article: rational design and applications of hydrogels in regenerative medicine. Adv Mater 26:85–124
4. Bhattarai N, Gunn J, Zhang M (2010) Chitosan-based hydrogels for controlled, localized drug delivery. Adv Drug Deliv Rev 62:83–99
5. Buwalda SJ, Boere KW, Dijkstra PJ, Feijen J, Vermonden T, Hennink WE (2014) Hydrogels in a historical perspective: from simple networks to smart materials. J Control Rel 190:254–273
6. Chen C, Xie Q, Yang D, Xiao H, Fu Y, Tan Y, Yao S (2013) Recent advances in electrochemical glucose biosensors: a review. RSC Adv 3:4473–4491
7. Delmar K, Bianco-Peled H (2016) Composite chitosan hydrogels for extended release of hydrophobic drugs. Carbohyd Polym 136:570–580
8. El-Hefian EA, Elgannoudi ES, Mainal A, Yahaya AH (2010) Characterization of chitosan in acetic acid: rheological and thermal studies. Turk J Chem 34:47–56
9. Ganji F, Vasheghani-Farahani S, Vasheghani-Farahani E (2010) Theoretical description of hydrogel swelling: a review. Iran Polym J 19:375–398
10. Gibas I, Janik H (2010) Review: synthetic polymer hydrogels for biomedical applications. Chem Chem Technol 4:297–304
11. Giri TK, Thakur A, Alexander A, Badwaik H, Tripathi DK (2012) Modified chitosan hydrogels as drug delivery and tissue engineering systems: present status and applications. Acta Pharmaceutica Sinica B 2:439–449
12. Gorgieva S, Kokol V (2012) Preparation, characterization, and in vitro enzymatic degradation of chitosan-gelatine hydrogel scaffolds as potential biomaterials. J Biomed Mater Res Part A 100:1655–1667
13. Grassi M, Grassi G (2005) Mathematical modelling and controlled drug delivery: matrix systems. Curr Drug Deliv 2:97–116
14. Guo M, Pitet LM, Wyss HM, Vos M, Dankers PY, Meijer E (2014) Tough stimuli-responsive supramolecular hydrogels with hydrogen-bonding network junctions. J Am Chem Soc 136:6969–6977
15. Guo W, Lu CH, Orbach R, Wang F, Qi XJ, Cecconello A, Seliktar D, Willner I (2015) pH-stimulated DNA hydrogels exhibiting shape-memory properties. Adv Mater 27:73–78
16. Gupta P, Vermani K, Garg S (2002) Hydrogels: from controlled release to pH-responsive drug delivery. Drug Discov Today 7:569–579
17. Hoare TR, Kohane DS (2008) Hydrogels in drug delivery: progress and challenges. Polymer 49:1993–2007
18. Jiang G, Sun J, Ding F (2014) PEG-g-chitosan thermosensitive hydrogel for implant drug delivery: cytotoxicity, in vivo degradation and drug release. J Biomater Sci Polym Ed 25:241–256
19. Khan A, Othman MBH, Razak KA, Akil HM (2013) Synthesis and physicochemical investigation of chitosan-PMAA-based dual-responsive hydrogels. J Polym Res 20:1–8
20. Kim S, Kim J-H, Jeon O, Kwon IC, Park K (2009) Engineered polymers for advanced drug delivery. Eur J Pharm Biopharm 71:420–430
21. Klinkajon W, Supaphol P (2014) Novel copper (II) alginate hydrogels and their potential for use as anti-bacterial wound dressings. Biomed Mater 9:045008
22. Maherani B, Arab-Tehrany E, Mozafari MR, Gaiani C, Linder M (2011) Liposomes: a review of manufacturing techniques and targeting strategies. Curr Nanosci 7, 436–452
23. Ohnuki H, Saiki T, Kusakari A, Endo H, Ichihara M, Izumi M (2007) Incorporation of glucose oxidase into langmuir–blodgett films based on prussian blue applied to amperometric glucose biosensor. Langmuir 23:4675–4681
24. Peng Z, Peng Z, Shen Y (2011) Fabrication and properties of gelatin/chitosan composite hydrogel. Polymer-Plastics Technol Eng 50:1160–1164
25. Peppas N, Bures P, Leobandung W, Ichikawa H (2000) Hydrogels in pharmaceutical formulations. Eur J Pharm Biopharm 50:27–46
26. Qiu Y, Park K (2001) Environment-sensitive hydrogels for drug delivery. Adv Drug Deliv Rev 53:321–339

27. Rao KR, Devi KP (1988) Swelling controlled-release systems: recent developments and applications. Int J Pharm 48:1–13
28. Rasib S, Ahmad Z, Khan A, Akil H, Othman M, Hamid Z, Ullah F (2018) Synthesis and evaluation on pH-and temperature-responsive chitosan-p (MAA-co-NIPAM) hydrogels. Int J Biol Macromol 108:367–375
29. Rosiak JM, Yoshii F (1999) Hydrogels and their medical applications. Nucl Instrum Methods Phys Res, Sect B 151:56–64
30. Saxena AK (2010) Synthetic biodegradable hydrogel (PleuraSeal) sealant for sealing of lung tissue after thoracoscopic resection. J Thoracic Cardiovasc Surg 139:496–497
31. Shi J, Votruba AR, Farokhzad OC, Langer R (2010) Nanotechnology in drug delivery and tissue engineering: from discovery to applications. Nano Lett 10:3223–3230
32. Smith AM, Miri T (2010) 6 alginates in foods. Pract Food Rheol Interpret Appr 113
33. Taleb MFA, Alkahtani A, Mohamed SK (2015) Radiation synthesis and characterization of sodium alginate/chitosan/hydroxyapatite nanocomposite hydrogels: a drug delivery system for liver cancer. Polym Bull 72:725–742
34. Tsao CT, Hsiao MH, Zhang MY, Levengood SL, Zhang M (2015) Chitosan-PEG hydrogel with sol-gel transition triggerable by multiple external stimuli. Macromol Rapid Commun 36:332–338
35. Ullah F, Javed F, Othman M, Khan A, Gul R, Ahmad Z, Akil Md H (2018) Synthesis and functionalization of chitosan built hydrogel with induced hydrophilicity for extended release of sparingly soluble drugs. J Biomater Sci Polym Ed 29:376–396
36. Ullah F, Javed F, Othman MBH, Ahmad Z, Akil Md H (2017) Synthesis and physicochemical investigation of chitosan-built hydrogel with induced glucose sensitivity. Int J Polymer Mater Polym Biomater 66:824–834
37. Ullah F, Javed F, Othman MBH, Rehman SU, Ahmad Z, Akil HM (2018) Star-shaped self-assembled micelles of block copolymer [chitosan-co-poly (ethylene glycol) methyl ether methacrylate] hydrogel for hydrophobic drug delivery. Polym Bull 75:2243–2264
38. Ullah F, Othman MBH, Javed F, Ahmad Z, Akil HM, Rasib SZM (2016) Functional properties of chitosan built nanohydrogel with enhanced glucose-sensitivity. Int J Biol Macromol 83:376–384
39. Ur-Rehman T, Tavelin S, Gröbner G (2011) Chitosan in situ gelation for improved drug loading and retention in poloxamer 407 gels. Int J Pharm 409:19–29
40. Washington RP, Steinbock O (2001) Frontal polymerization synthesis of temperature-sensitive hydrogels. J Am Chem Soc 123:7933–7934
41. Zarzycki R, Modrzejewska Z, Nawrotek K (2010) Drug release from hydrogel matrices. Ecol Chem Eng S 17:117–136
42. Zhai D, Liu B, Shi Y, Pan L, Wang Y, Li W, Zhang R, Yu G (2013) Highly sensitive glucose sensor based on Pt nanoparticle/polyaniline hydrogel heterostructures. ACS Nano 7:3540–3546
43. Zhou C, Wang M, Zou K, Chen J, Zhu Y, Du J (2013) Antibacterial polypeptide-grafted chitosan-based nanocapsules as an "armed" carrier of anticancer and antiepileptic Drugs. ACS Macro Lett 2:1021–1025

Chapter 16
Novel Biocompatible Hydrogels via Click Chemistry

Manne Madhava Reddy, T. Boominathan, A. S. Vijai Anand, Rakesh R. Panicker, Varun Kaushal, Arinjoy Das, Nandini Jain, Ivaturi Sai Vighnesh, Rajagopal Desikan, Kari Vijayakrishna, Kishor Padala, C. V. S. Brahmmananda Rao, Gregory S. Smith, and Akella Sivaramakrishna

Abstract Currently, the designing and development of advanced hydrogel platforms is one of the important research areas due to their applications in the fabrication of functionalized materials useful in biomedical sciences. The rich literature reveals that most of these advanced materials are derived from the utilization of click reaction-based approaches through arranging the appropriate building blocks together in order to fabricate the desirable hydrogel architectures useful mainly in tissue engineering and drug delivery including the stem cell differentiation. Among the limitations of these materials, the non-degradability of synthetic polymers is responsible for the restricted usage in biomedical fields. Therefore, there is a constant demand to develop systematic methodologies for the synthesis of novel hydrogel materials to improve the degradability of the hydrogels by fine-tuning the functional groups and by incorporating more hydrophilicity for the ready hydrolysis.

Keywords Biocompatible polymers · Synthetic routes · Click chemistry · Cross-linking networks · Applications

---

M. M. Reddy · T. Boominathan · A. S. Vijai Anand · R. R. Panicker · V. Kaushal · A. Das · N. Jain · I. S. Vighnesh · R. Desikan · K. Vijayakrishna · K. Padala · A. Sivaramakrishna (✉)
Department of Chemistry, School of Advanced Sciences, Vellore Institute of Technology, Vellore, Tamil Nadu 632014, India
e-mail: asrkrishna@vit.ac.in

K. Vijayakrishna
Department of Chemistry, School of Basic Sciences, Indian Institute of Technology Bhubaneswar, Argul, Khordha, Odisha 752050, India

C. V. S. Brahmmananda Rao
Chemistry Group, Indira Gandhi Centre for Atomic Research, HBNI, Kalpakkam, Tamil Nadu 603102, India

G. S. Smith
Department of Chemistry, University of Cape Town, Rondebosch, Cape Town 8801, South Africa

J. Jose et al. (eds.), *Nano Hydrogels*, Gels Horizons: From Science to Smart Materials, https://doi.org/10.1007/978-981-15-7138-1_16

Abbreviations

PAA	Polyacryliccacid
PEO	Polyethylene oxide
PVA	Polyvinyl alcohol
DMSO	Dimethyl sulfoxide
EDC	1-Ethyl-3-(3-dimethylaminopropyl)carbodiimide
NHS	N-Hydroxysuccinimide
PBS	Phosphate-buffered saline
TEMPO	2,2,6,6-Tetramethylpiperidin-1-yl)oxyl or (2,2,6,6-tetramethylpiperidin-1-yl)oxidanyl
AS	Ally starch
CS	Chitosan
St	Starch
CS–Fu	Furan–functionalized chitosan
CS–AMI	Themaleimide–functionalized chitosan
Py–SA	TOMFC
MES	2-(N-morpholino)ethanesulfonic acid
HA	Hyaluronic acid
HAAA	Hyaluronic acid-11-azido-3,6,9-trioxaundecan-1-amine
AA	11-Azido-3,6,9-trooxaundecan-1-amine
BH_3NH_3	Boranemonoammoniate
4-AC-TEMPO	4-Acetamido-2,2,6,6-tetramethylpiperidin-1-yl)oxyl
NaBr	Sodium bromide
NaClO	Sodium-hypochloride
$NaIO_4$	Sodium metaperiodate
CuCl	Copper(I) chloride
$CuSO_4$	Copper(II) sulfate
BMI	Bismaleimide
CuAAC	Copper(I)-catalyzed azide-alkyne cycloaddition
Cu(I)	Copper (I)-iodide
DNA	Deoxyribonucleic acid
$NaBH_4$	Sodium borohydride
CS-Fu-BMI	Chitosan-furfural-bismaleimide
PEG MA	Poly(ethylene glycol) methacrylate
PEG TMA	Trimethylamine polyethylene glycol
DMF	Dimethylformamide
AIBN	Azobisisobutyronitrile
DMAP	4-Dimethylaminopyridine
DCC	N,N′-Dicyclohexylcarbodiimide
P(NIPAAm-co-HEMA)	Poly(N-isopropylacrylamide-co-hydroxylethyl methacrylate)
HA/PEG	Hyaluronic acid/polyethylene glycol
ATRP	Atom transfer radical polymerization

PEG TMC	Polyethylene glycol-trimethylene carbonate
PHEA	Poly(2-hydroxyethyl acrylate)
HEP	1,4-Di(2-hydroxyethyl)piperazine
HDI	1,1-Diisocyanatoethane
DBTDL	Dibutyltindilaurate
FGE	Furfurylglycidyl ether
PAH	Polycyclic aromatic hydrocarbon

1 Introduction

The term "click chemistry" introduced by Sharpless in 2001 describes the high yield coupling of two molecules A and B which are versatile, stereospecific, simple to perform, and can be performed in easily removable or benign solvent systems [1, 2]. In addition to this, these reactions produce by-products that can be removed without any chromatographic technique. Also, these reactions found high significance in synthetic organic chemistry of therapeutic applications [3]. In general, the first step of mechanism embraces the activation of biomolecules (via compatible "click" functional groups) and the subsequent step involves the coupling of activated molecules to arrange a stable conjugate. The key advantages of this click chemistry are: (i) facile reactions in nature, (ii) excellent yields, (iii) easily separable by-products, (iv) stereospecificity, (v) the usage of environmentally benign solvents, (vi) to support both in vitro and in vivo of enzymatic activities with non-radioactive analysis, and (vii) high selective, etc. The "click" reactions are of several types including [4] (i) "one-pot" synthesis with thermodynamically feasible reactions, e.g. nucleophilic ring opening of aziridines and epoxides, (ii) reactions of carbonyl groups (non-aldol type), e.g. formation of heterocycles, (iii) formation of carbon–carbon multiple bonds, e.g. reactions from Michael addition and epoxides, and (iv) reactions through alkyne–azide cycloaddition. One of the best examples for a click reaction is the copper(I)-catalyzed 1,3-dipolar cycloaddition between azides and alkynes. Azide and alkyne groups are stable to aqueous solutions and have almost no reaction with biomolecules. This allows further achieving the target-guided synthesis and further activity-based protein profiling [5]. In addition to this, Bertozzi et al. established a route to the [3 + 2] azide–alkyne cycloaddition reaction due to the ring strain in the absence of copper(I) as this method avoids the cytotoxicity due to the presence of copper(I) [6].

In general, hydrogels are polymeric materials and exhibit the ability to swell and hold a significant fraction of water within the structure without dissolving in water. Due to this, hydrogels also possess a definite degree of flexibility similar to the natural tissues [7]. Consequently, these hydrogels function as delivery vehicles in cell transplantation efficiently in a controlled manner and tolerate the culture of stem cells under different environments. Due to their biocompatible nature, the research on the development of new hydrogel polymers has been gained high significance for their prospective applications in the construction of devices for drug delivery [8, 9], tissue engineering [10, 11], coating [12, 13], cell culture [14, 15] and so on. In view of this, click chemistry appears as a suitable alternative for the fabrication of chemically cross-linked and polysaccharide-based hydrogel materials [16]. Among all these click reactions reported, the Diels–Alder reaction has received huge demand as this reaction has been carried out under mild reaction conditions without any side products [17] and the biocompatibility of the material in the absence of catalysts or initiators [18]. Further, this reaction has been used in synthesis of chitosan-based hydrogels [19] and other types of polymeric hydrogels [20, 21]. The remarkable impact of click chemistry on extraordinary efficiency and reliability of these reactions which enabled rapid synthesis of hydrogel materials with appropriate network structures has been highlighted. Also, the peptide sequences of biomolecular building blocks have been incorporated efficiently through various click reactions either during or after the synthesis of hydrogels. Further, this has led to the fabrication of many stimuli responsive or "smart" hydrogels in recent years [22]. Natural polymers such as collagen, gelatin or hyaluronate and synthetic polymers (e.g. PAA, PEO and PVA) are the right choice to design the biocompatible hydrogel architectures having large surface area. As the entire polymer support of these hydrogels is exposed to aqueous solutions and enzymes, this can probably lead to quick hydrolysis [23]. Interestingly, these unique properties including great water absorption capacity and water preservation ability make hydrogels remarkable candidates in contact lenses, diapers and drug reservoirs [24].

2 Synthesis of Biocompatible Hydrogels via Click Chemistry

Li et al. reported the synthesis of thiolene-based hydrogel material as shown in Scheme 1 [25]. The analysis revealed that the hydrogel displays adjustable swelling capacity and good mechanical properties. The degradation was due to the combination of both diffusion and surface erosion.

A chemically cross-linked hydrogel derived from chitosan was successfully synthesized through Diels–Alder reaction [26]. Further, chitosan derivatives for example furan-modified chitosan (Cs–Fu) resulted from the reaction of furfural and free amino groups of chitosan. The maleimide–functionalized chitosan (Cs–AMI) was prepared from the reaction of a maleimide-modified aminoacid with the amino groups of chitosan (Scheme 2). These hydrogel materials were found to be pH-sensitive, biocompatible and anti-bacterial.

Lueckgen and the co-workers fabricated a flexible and degradable cross-linked alginate-based polymer with tunable material properties by introducing either tetrazine or norbornene functional groups for cross-linking (Scheme 3) [27]. The degradation behaviour, swelling ability and the cell compatibility were assessed to determine the in vivo functionality of the materials. Further, the biomaterial was

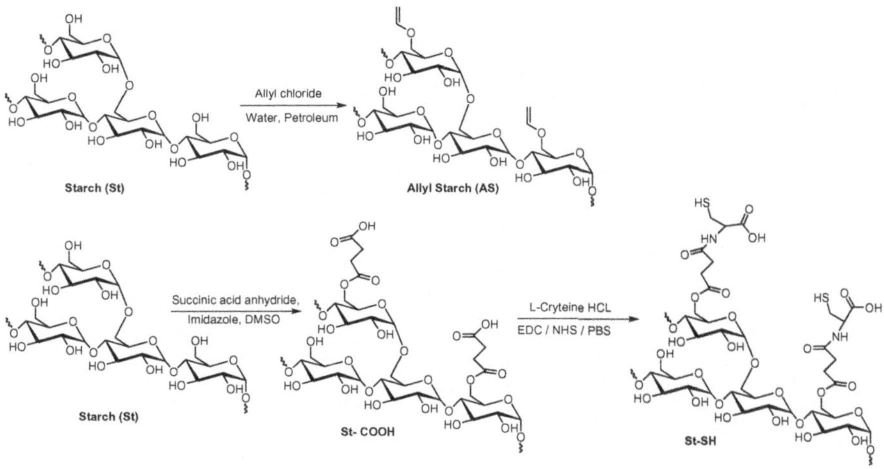

Scheme 1 The chemical structure of AS, St-SH and schematic illustration of thiolene click hydrogel

implanted internally into the mice, and further, the degradation and cytocompatibility were determined via histological staining.

Alginate-based hydrogels have been fabricated by introducing micro-fibrillated cellulose oxidized by TEMPO into the in situ polymerization of pyrrole to build PPy/SA/TOMFC conductive hydrogels [28]. Interestingly, the incorporation of TOMFC resulted in the significant improvement of structural integrity, enhanced electrical conductivity and mechanical properties of the composite hydrogels. The preparation of Cu(I)) catalyzed water-soluble polysaccharide derivatives bearing side chains endowed with either azide or alkyne terminal functionality was carried out by mixing together in aqueous solution through a 1,3-dipolar cycloaddition reaction [29] as shown in Scheme 4.

Hyaluronic acid was effectively modified structurally through chemical reactions like oxidation/reductive amination and cross-linking via click chemistry (Scheme 5) [30]. The combination of 4-acetamido-TEMPO/sodium hypochlorite/NaBr was found as good alternative towards the modifications of the C-6 of hyaluronic acid. These modified hydrogel materials were found as biocompatible.

Starch-based hydrogels were prepared by cross-linking through Diels–Alder reactions between furan-modified starch and bismaleimide as given in Scheme 6. The conducting properties of these materials were remarkably improved by graphene layers as active nanofillers [31]. The effect of increasing the furan/maleimide ratio on the structural, morphological, rheological and swelling properties of hydrogels was evaluated. The pore size decreases up on increasing the cross-linker content and this leads to an effective network structure. As the presence of bismaleimide imparts the hydrophilic character, graphene nanosheets produce nanocomposite hydrogel with better rheologic al properties, electrical conductivity and antimicrobial activity.

The azide-alkyne cycloaddition (CuAAC) click reaction catalyzed by Cu(I) yields cross-linked functional polymer chains having a sieving gel which was useful for

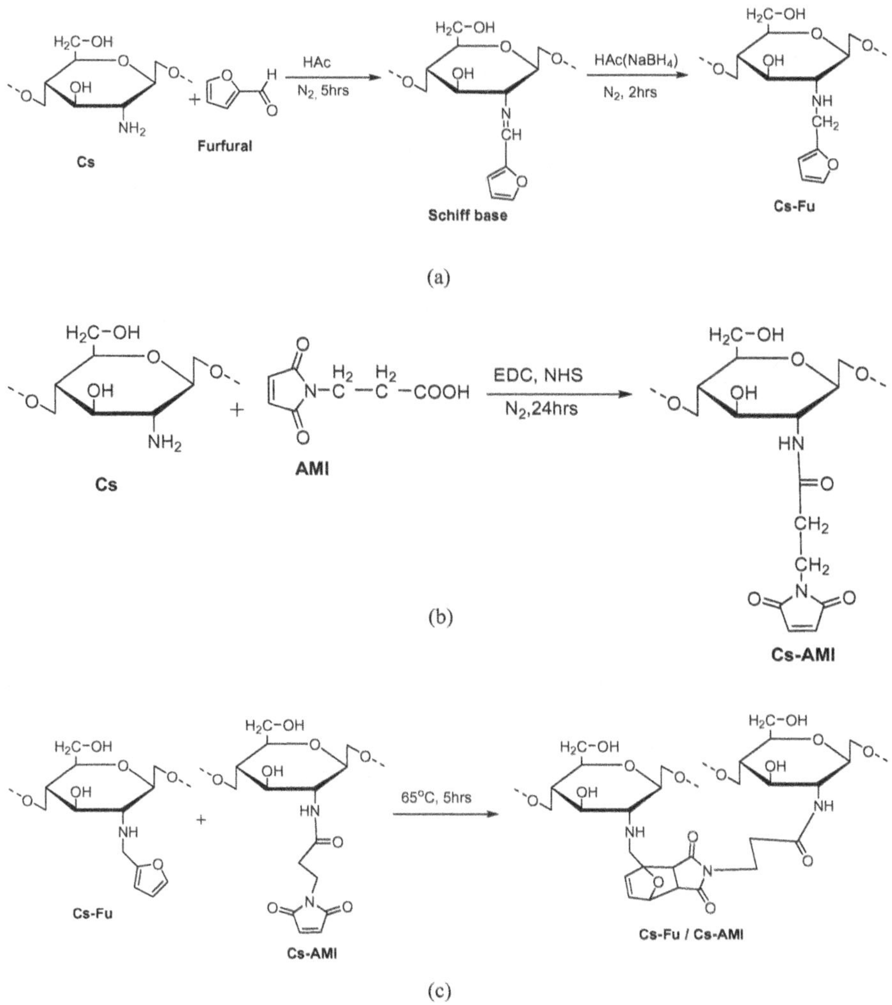

Scheme 2 **a** Synthesis of Cs–Fu through the reaction of chitosan and furfural; **b** synthesis of Cs–AMI through the reaction of chitosan and AMI modifier; **c** Diels–Alder reaction between furan-functionalized chitosan (Cs–Fu) and maleimide-functionalized chitosan (Cs–AMI)

DNA electrophoresis [32]. The competence of this reaction offers hydrogels with near-ideal linkage connectivity with improved physical properties under mild conditions. The sieving environment was formed by reacting two polymers holding reactive functional groups like poly(dimethylacrylamide) with an alkyne moiety in the presence of poly(ethylene glycol) functionalized bis-azideazido groups at both ends. In addition to this, the Diels–Alder reaction (Scheme 7) was employed in the fabrication of stimuli-responsive chitosan-based cross-linked hydrogels for biomedical applications by reacting furan-modified chitosan (Cs–Fu) with polyetheramine derived

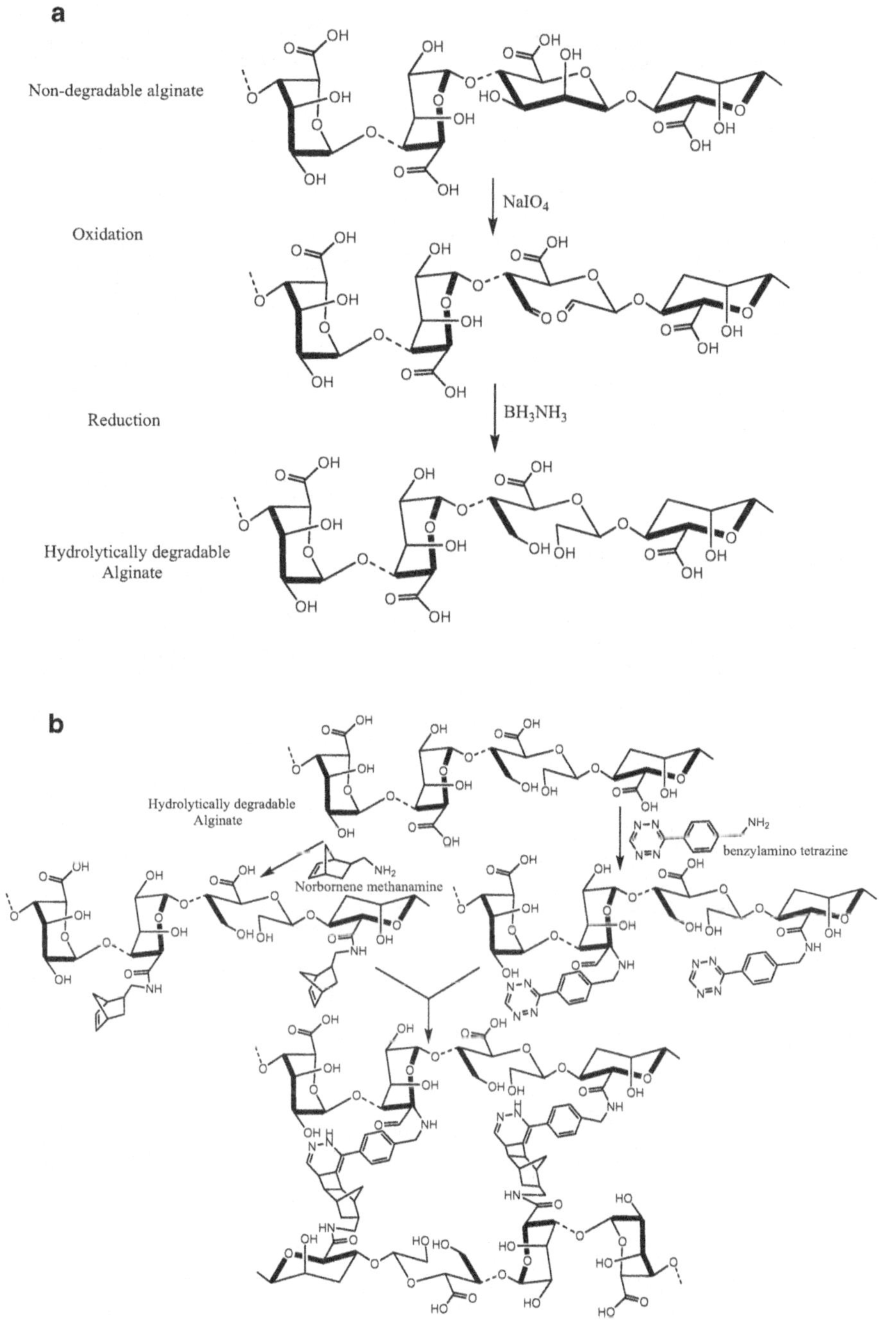

Scheme 3 Synthesis of hydrolytically degradable click cross-linked alginate gels. Oxidation of non-degradable base material by sodium periodate and then reduction through ammonia borane (**a**). Dashed boxes represent reacting groups. Spontaneous covalent cross-linking by Diels–Alder reactions (**b**). Fine-tuning the properties

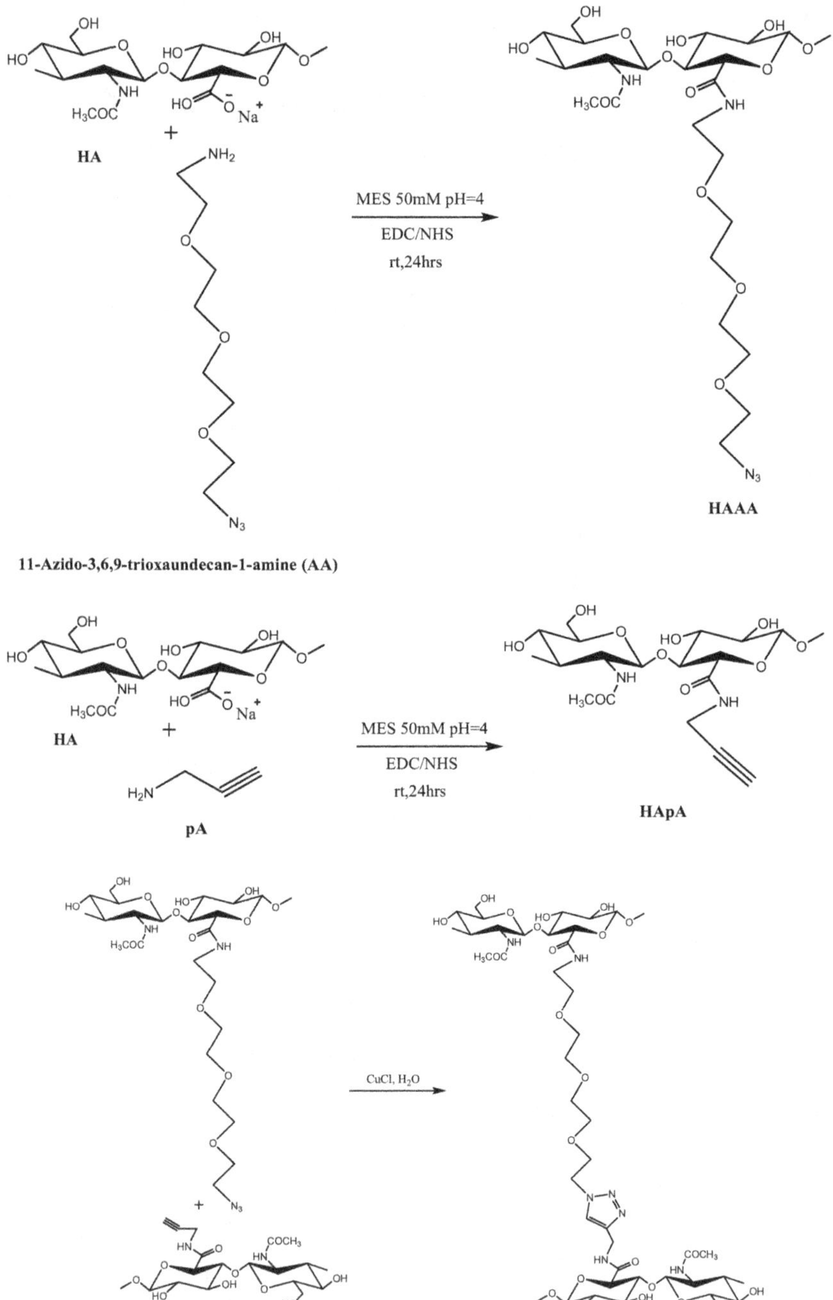

Scheme 4 Preparation of polysaccharide derivatives bearing side chains functionalized with either azides or alkynes

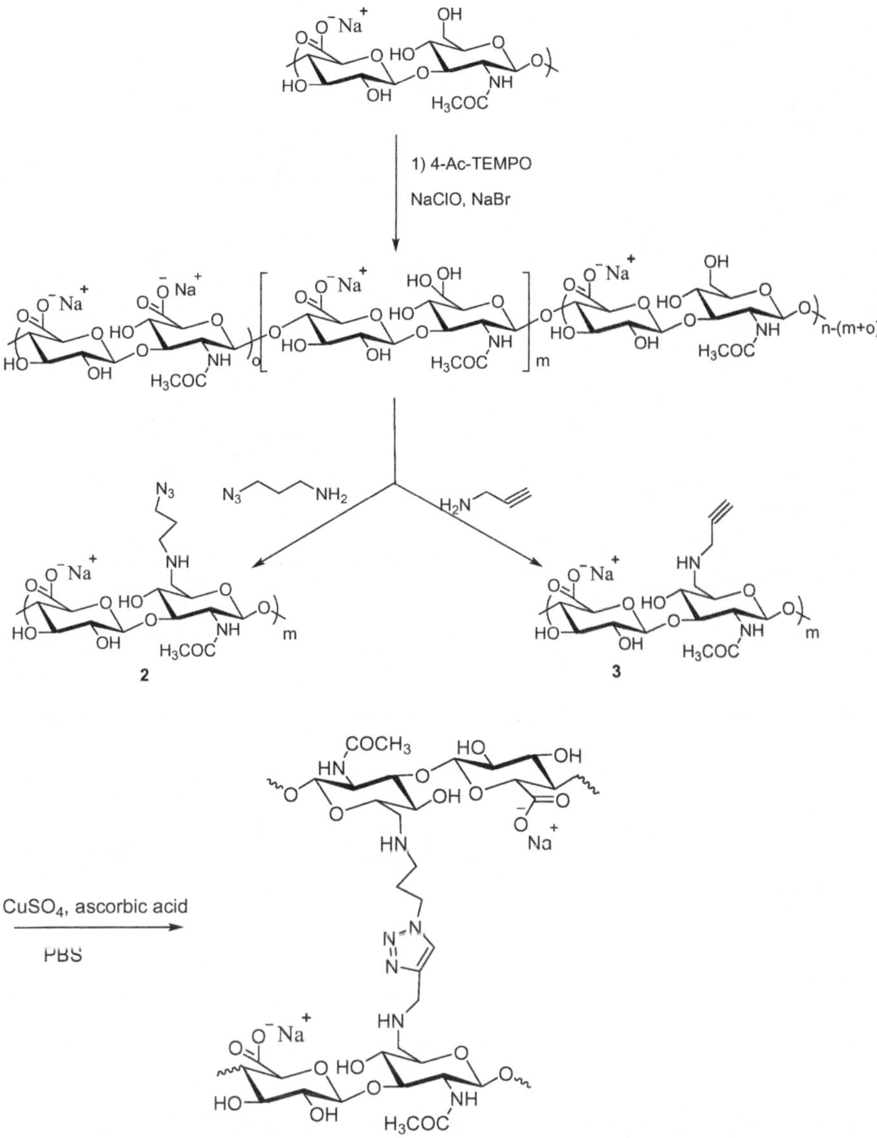

Scheme 5 Structural modification by xidation/reductive amination and cross-linking reactions via click chemistry

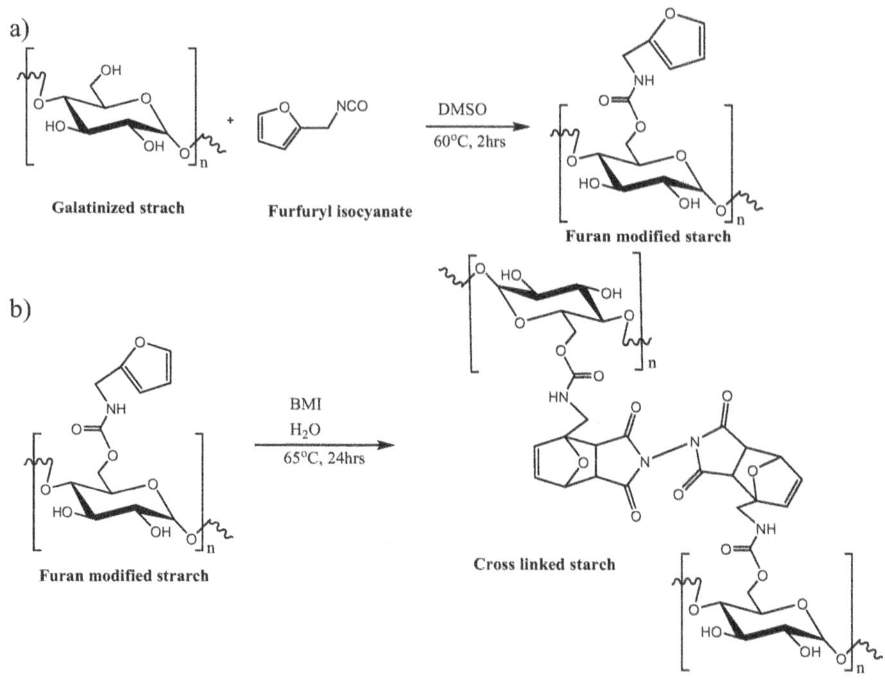

Scheme 6 Preparation of starch-based cross-linked hydrogels through Diels–Alder reactions

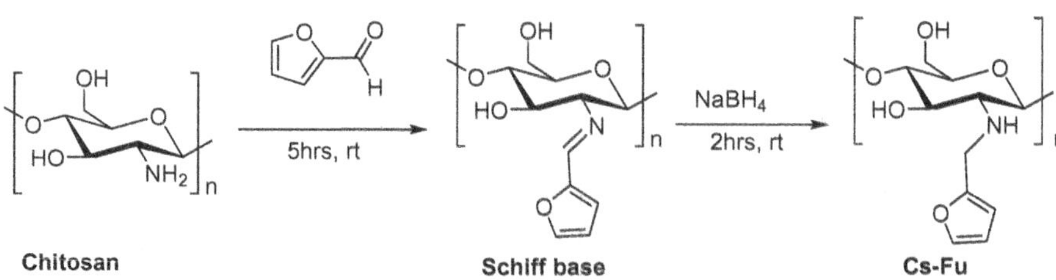

Scheme 7 Synthesis of Cs–Fu through the reaction of chitosan and furfural

from bismaleimide (Scheme 8) [33]. Both the final storage modulus and the sol–gel transition value for the different formulations were almost similar and close to 40 min and 400 Pa, respectively. Studies on the influence of the quantity and the behaviour of the cross-linker in the properties of these polymers were investigated by varying the furan to maleimide ratio.

Several strategies were used to produce 3D-hydrogel networks by joining functional polymers or polymeric fragments for various applications including tissue engineering [34]. The development of junctions between each polymer segments is important in altering the stability and mechanical strength of these gels. This was recognized via formation of covalent and non-covalent bonds with different

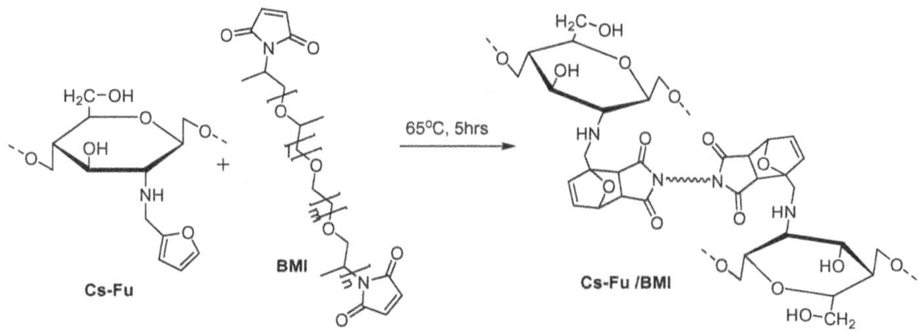

Scheme 8 Hydrogel formation through DA reaction between Cs–Fu and BMI

strengths and density [35, 36]. Even though the physical hydrogels were formed by the transient cross-linking between polymer chains through various kinds of physical interactions [36], these weak physical cross-linking generally provides to low mechanical strength. Nevertheless, these interactions play a vital role in the generation of self-healing properties via dynamic self-assembly/disassembly features. A typical example for this is a combination of clay and the dendritic molecular binder to fabricate self-healing hydrogels as reported by Aida and co-workers [37]. In contrast, chemical hydrogels usually hold networks produced by cross-linked covalent bonds, and their mechanical properties can be controlled with the cross-linking density. In this connection, Anseth et al. reported the fabrication of photo-controlled degradable hydrogel by sequentially performed CuAAC and thiolene reactions with variable architecture and functionality [38].

In general, the Michael-type thiolene "click" reaction was reported by carrying out under mild conditions which are similar to human physiological conditions [39]. The gelation of PEG–MA and PEG–TMA was carried out to prepare two biodegradable and biocompatible PEG hydrogel derivatives with multienes or multithiols by polycondensation employing scandium trifluoromethane sulfonate ($Sc(OTf)_3$) as a chemo selective catalyst and further the influence of concentration and pH values was evaluated [39]. Zhang and co-workers have reported a series of thermosensitive hydrogels derived from the chemoselective cross-linking reaction between two different types of polymer backbones with cellulose modified by azide and alkyne-modified poly(N-isopropylacrylamide-co-hydroxylethyl methacrylate) P(NIPAAm-co-HEMA) in the presence of Cu(I) catalyst [40]. Also, alkyne-modified P(NIPAAm-co-HEMA) and azide-modified cellulose were produced to investigate the formation of in situ hydrogel through "click" chemistry by Zhou and co-workers [41]. The synthesis routes of the two polymers were given in Scheme 9.

A double cross-linked network was designed and further prepared by Diels–Alder click reaction, followed by the incorporation of acylhydrazone bond (Schemes 10 and 11). As the Diels–Alder reaction preserved the structural integrity and mechanical strength of hydrogel under physiological environment, the flexible covalent acylhydrazone bond leads to the development of hydrogel's self-healing property and

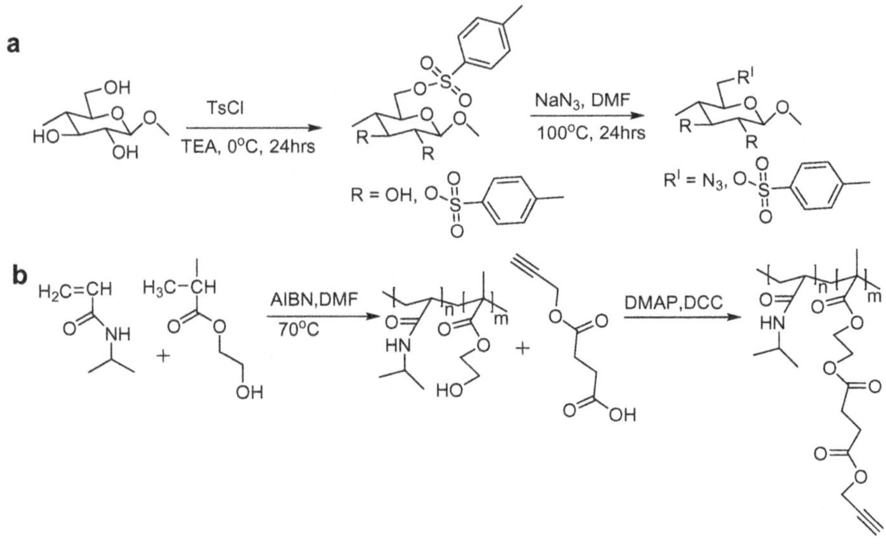

Scheme 9 The synthesis of the azide-modified cellulose (**a**) and alkyne-modified P(NIPAAm-co-HEMA) (**b**)

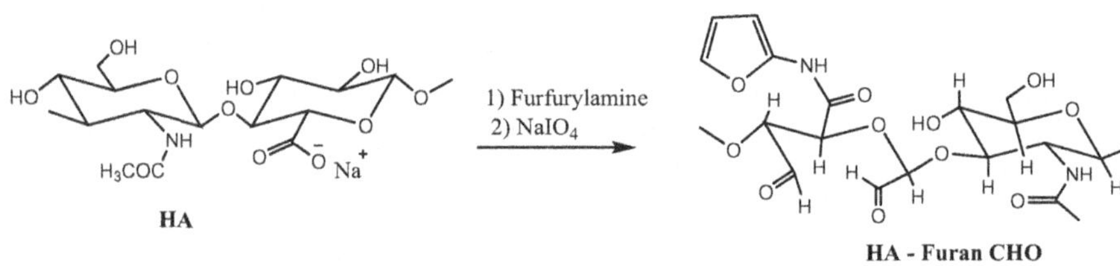

Scheme 10 The preparation of HA-furan-CHO

controlled the on–off switch of network cross-link density. At the same time, the aldehyde groups present in hydrogel further support the integration of hydrogel based on the formation of imine from the aldehyde–amine Schiff-base reaction [42].

HA/PEG hydrogels formed by Diels–Alder reaction showed with short gelation times and appropriate mechanical properties [43]. Unlike traditional Diels–Alder hydrogels, the series of HA/PEG hydrogels, i.e. DS1 (1:1), DS1 (3:1) and DS2 (1:1) exhibited the required gelation times for cell encapsulation, survival and proliferation. Among these hydrogels, DS1 (3:1) was effective with fatigue resistance and high elasticity even after 2000 loading cycles. Studies on the use of propargyl acrylamide (PAm) as a comonomer along with acrylamide (AAm) and N,N′-methylene bisacrylamide (BAAm) as cross-linkers in photoinitiated polymerization were carried out [44]. Hydrogels with clickable acetylene groups can be prepared photochemically in a single step to achieve the selectivity by generation of free radicals towards acrylic function of PAm. Based on the acetylene functionality, the molecules

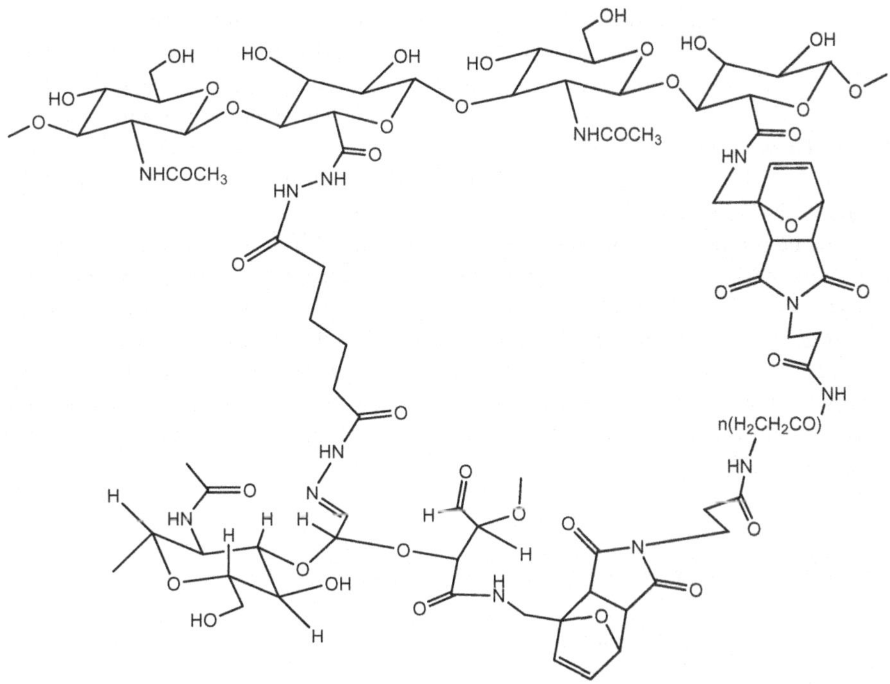

Scheme 11 The scheme of double cross-linked processes

possessing azide groups can be conjugated onto hydrogel easily. The preparation of distinct sliding-graft semi-IPN of PEG and poly(2-hydroxyethyl methacrylate) (s-IPNPEG/R-CD-sg-PHEMAs)with grafted linear poly-2-hydroxyethyl methacrylate (PHEMA) on the grids of PEG linkages was possible via simultaneous CuAAC and ATRP [45] to achieve the biocompatible hydrogels having very good physical and mechanical properties. Further, the reaction of azide-terminated PEGs having 4-arms with dialkyne flanked peptides in the presence of CuBr/L-ascorbic acid/DMF yielded the hydrogels of the required template [46].

A click reaction was carried out to prepare zwitterionic antifouling hydrogels such as poly(2-hydroxyethyl methacrylate-co-glycidyl methacrylate) (poly(HEMA-co-GMA)) by implanting amino acids onto polymer chains through ring opening reaction (i.e. primary amino groups of amino acid and epoxy groups of polymer chains) in weakly alkaline aqueous solution. Further, the protonation of secondary amino groups and deprotonation of carboxyl groups at pH 7 were carried out [47, 48]. This zwitterionic structure possesses protonated secondary amino cations (PSA, –NH_2^+–) and deprotonated carboxyl anions (DPC, –COO–). Recently, thiol-ene "click" reactions (Michael addition type) between electron-deficient enes and thiols have been widely used over the well-known traditional polymer networks and they do not require light irradiation or a metal catalyst [49]. In this connection, a series of polyethylene glycol (PEG)-based derivatives containing multiple "clickable" groups by the polycondensation of dihydroxyloligo (ethylene glycol) with maleic anhydride/thiolmalic were prepared for biomedical applications [50, 51].

A series of PEG-TMC networks were prepared by Huisgen's 1,3-dipolar cycloaddition of azides with alkynes catalyzed by Cu(I) to yield completely hydrophilic PEG hydrogels, as well as PEG-poly(TMC) (PTMC) hydrogels with amphiphilic behaviour [52] (Scheme 12).

A facile preparation of poly(ethylene glycol) (PEG)-cyclodextrin containing hydrogels by radical thiol-ene reaction was reported using the hydrophilic matrix of the type alkene end-functionalized poly(ethylene glycol)s and thiol functionalized β-cyclodextrin as multifunctional cross-linker [53]. Two bis-alkyne reagents (iso-propargyl succinate and bis-propargyl hexane urethane) were employed as cross-linkers to fabricate the click gels containing degradable ester or urethane groups based on azido-functional PHEA (PHEA-N3) and di-alkyne cross-linkers as shown in Scheme 13 [54].

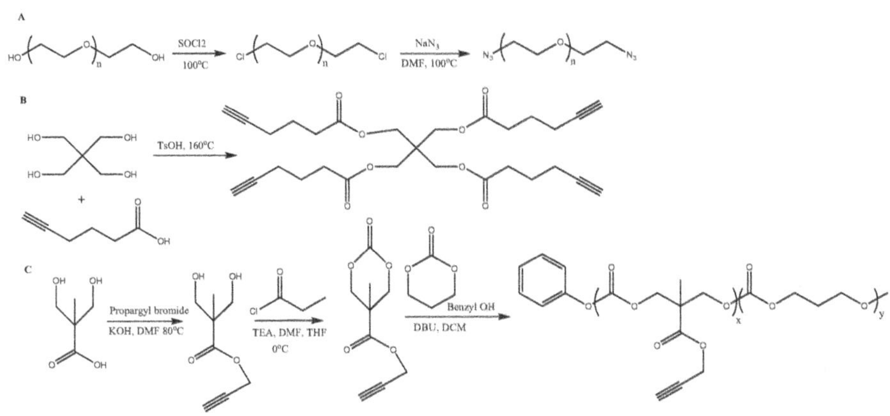

Scheme 12 Preparation of hydrophilic PEG hydrogels by Huisgen's 1,3-dipolar cycloaddition of azides with alkynes

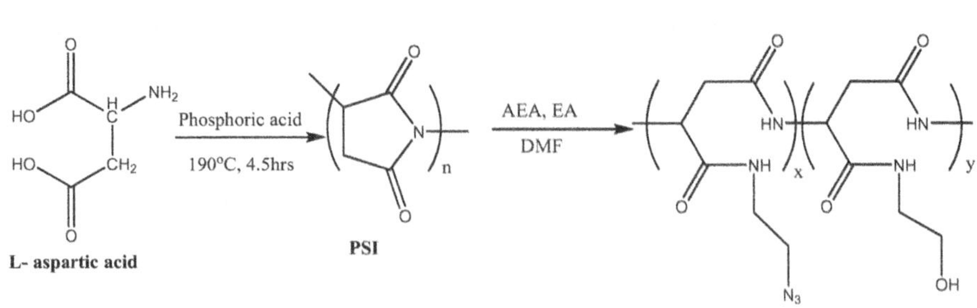

Scheme 13 Synthesis of PHEA-N_3

A series of click hydrogels were obtained by the reactions of functionalized alkyne groups with azido-terminal cross-linkers of the types 3-arms poly(ethylene glycol) (PEG) and 3-arms poly(ethylene glycol)-poly(amino urethane) (PEG-$(PAU)_3$) with 3-azido-1-propionic acid (APrA). Then the "click" hydrogels can be obtained with cross-linkers (Schemes 14 and 15) [55].

As showed in Scheme 15, poly(ethylene glycol)-block-poly(γ-propargyl-L-glutamate) (PEG-PPLG) with pendent alkynyl groups derived by click chemistry displayed good cytocompatibility in vitro and acceptable in vivo biocompatibility [56]. A bactericidal poly(ethylene glycol)-based (PEG) hydrogel was synthesized and utilized as a layer with covalently attached antimicrobial peptides (AMP) stabilized against proteolytic degradation [57]. New hydrogels were developed based on furan-modified gelatine using bismaleimide cross-linker [58]. The furan groups were grafted on to gelatin by the reaction of epoxy-amine with furfuryl glycidyl ether, and then further cross-linked with Jeffamine®-based bismaleimides (Schemes 16 and 17). Attempts were also made to prepare the hydrogels with polyampholyte based on dextran with cryoprotective properties for tissue engineering applications [59].

A facile synthesis of PAH from PMA with quantitative conversion of carboxylates to carbonyl hydrazides was carried out using various hydrazide based click reactions

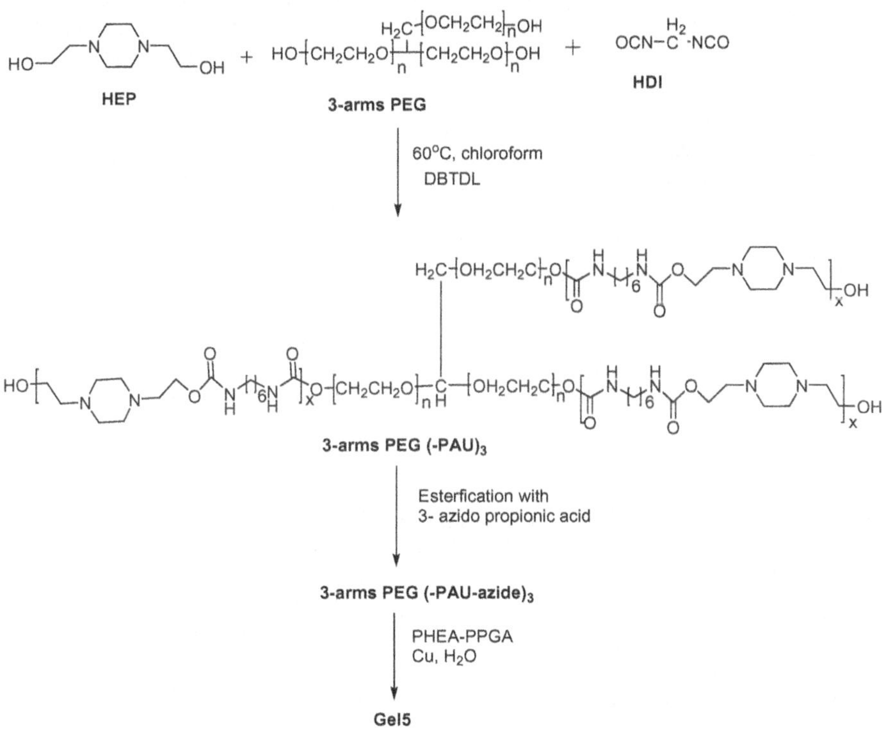

Scheme 14 Synthesis of 3-arms based poly(ethylene glycol)-poly(amino urethane)

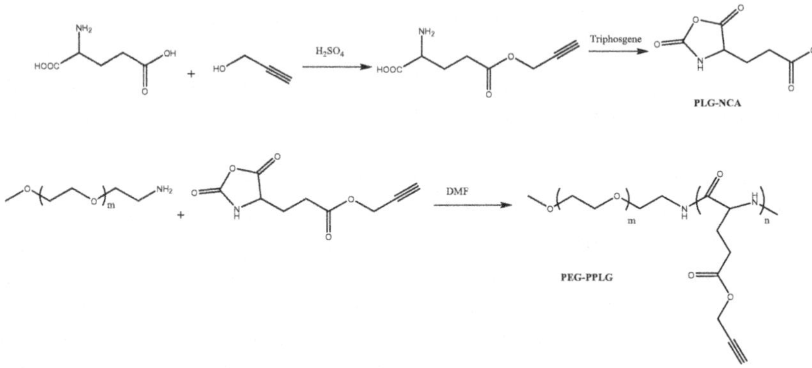

Scheme 15 Synthesis of poly(ethylene glycol)-block-poly(γ-propargyl-L-glutamate) (PEG-PPLG) with pendent alkynyl groups

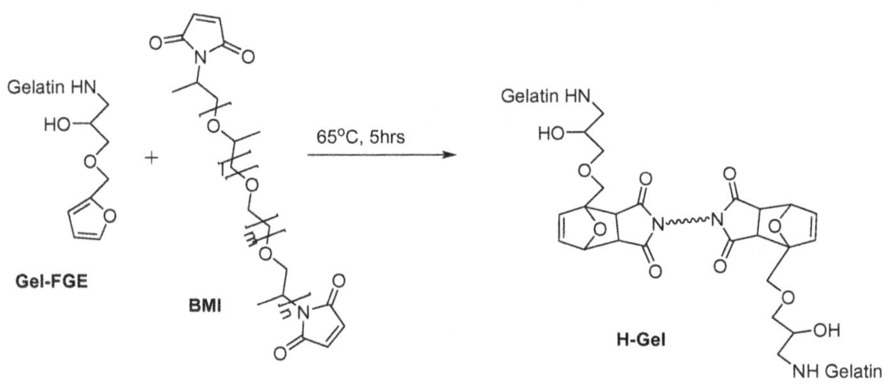

Scheme 16 Synthesis of furan-grafted gelatin by the reaction of epoxy-amine with furfuryl glycidyl ether

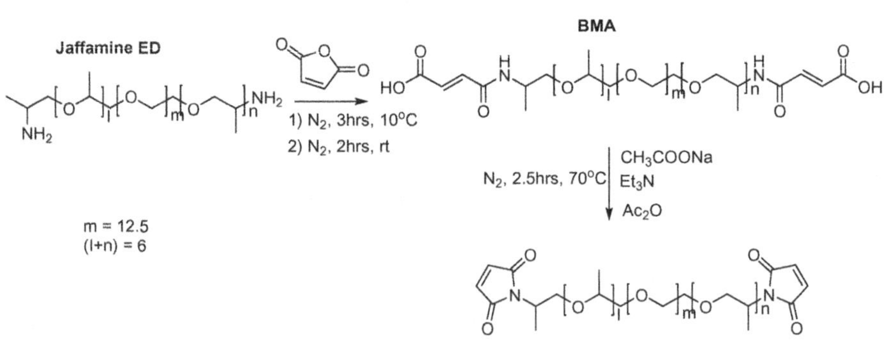

Scheme 17 Preparation of cross-linked Jeffamine-based bismaleimides

to produce a range of useful materials like pH sensors, stimuli responsive hydrogels, ion exchange epoxy resins, and polymer–dye conjugates as outlined in Scheme 18 [60].

Ossipov and Hilborn investigated a click reaction by grafting the azide and alkyne pendant groups onto poly(ethylene glycol) (PEG) and poly(vinyl alcohol) (PVA) in the formation of hydrogel in order to derive structure–property relationships as shown in Scheme 19 [61]. The first approach describes the telechelic PEG-diazide as a cross-linker for the PVA functionalized with alkyne groups, whereas the second approach deals with the functionalization of two PVA components with azide and alkyne groups.

PEG-based hydrogels were synthesized in well-defined networks with significantly improved mechanical properties and the selectivity of the azide/acetylene coupling reaction allows the incorporation of functional groups into the hydrogel architectures as described in Scheme 20 [62].

Interestingly, the single-walled carbon nanotubes (SWNTs) were fused into hydrogel networks to encourage the electron transport leading to the formation of

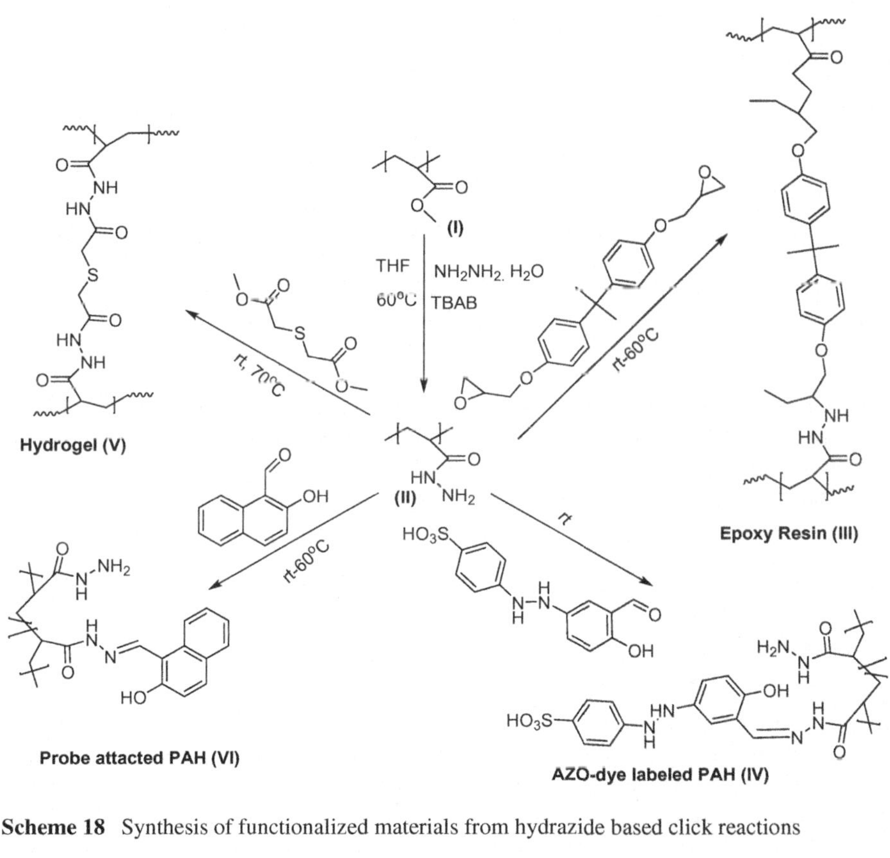

Scheme 18 Synthesis of functionalized materials from hydrazide based click reactions

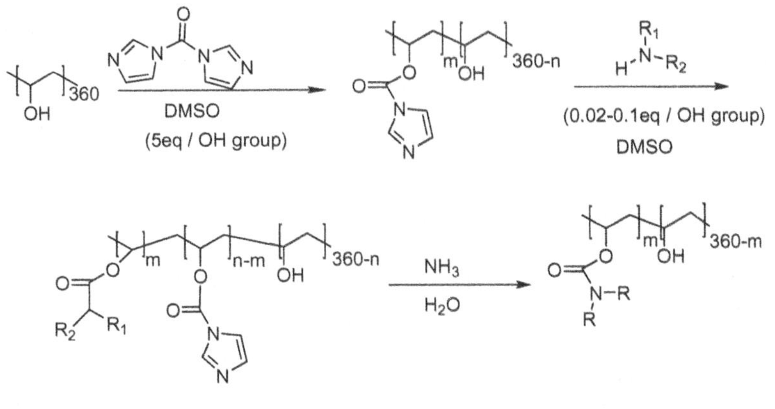

Compounds	R_1	R_2
1	H	$-\overset{H_2}{C}-\equiv$
2	Me	$-\overset{H_2}{C}-\equiv$
3	H	$-\overset{H_2}{C}-\overset{H_2}{C}-N_3$
4	H	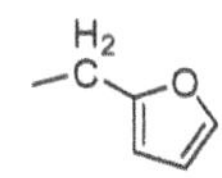
5	H	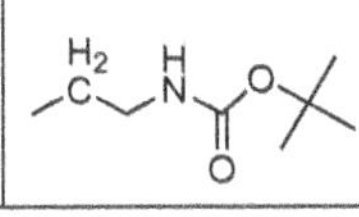

Scheme 19 Synthesis of grafted azide and alkyne based PEG and PVA hydrogels

well-dispersed co-networks of electroactive polymers [63]. The fabrication of PEG–CMC hydrogel was carried out via thiol-ene photo polymerization using thiol groups anchored CMC and by norbornene immobilized tetra-arm poly(ethylene glycol) (PEG4NB). The properties of PEG–CMC hydrogel materials allow these materials towards a pH-responsive drug release carriers (Fig. 1) [64].

3 Conclusion

Recently, there has been a tremendous development in the growth of functional hydrogel platforms due to their applications in the fabrication of advanced materials and in biomedical sciences. Certainly, this has largely originated from the utilization of click reaction-based approaches toward the construction and functionalization of these hydrogel materials. The impact of these chemical reactions to arrange the

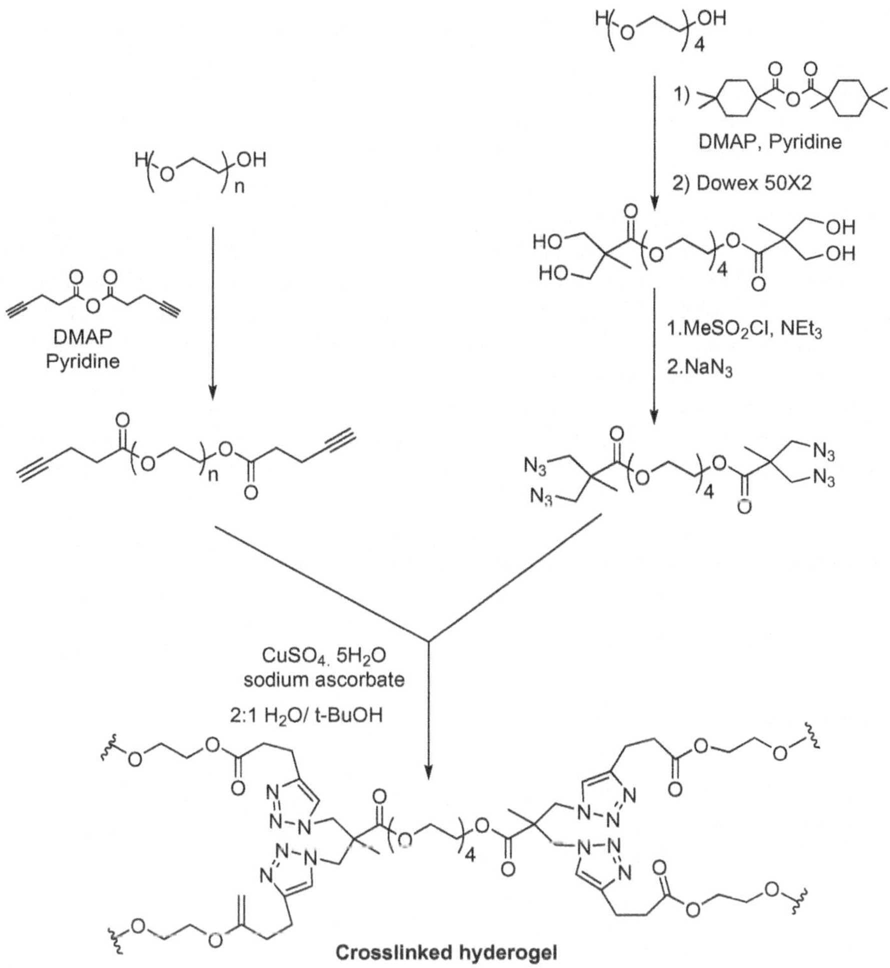

Scheme 20 Construction of hydrogel materials based on click chemistry

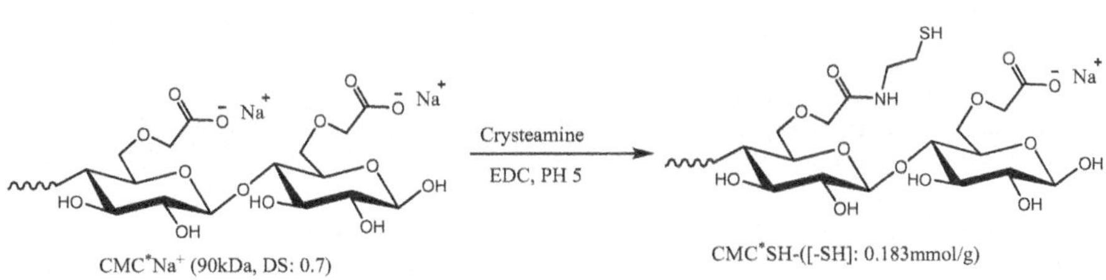

Fig. 1 Synthesis of CMC-SH materials

building blocks together has been established in the design of numerous hydrogel materials within the past few years. The literature witnesses the reports on a wide range of materials based on HA and their potential claims in tissue engineering and drug delivery. In addition to this, HA-based hydrogels can also exhibit biological activity to cells up on interaction with biomaterials, as evident in cellular behaviour and stem cell differentiation. Similar to HA-based materials, a significant progress has been observed for thiolene hydrogels towards the controlled delivery of therapeutics. However, there are some challenges regarding the broad clinical translation of thiolene hydrogels that the retaining of bioactivity of cargomolecules when they are exposed to the hydrogel environment during formation or degradation. Maintaining the controlled drug cargo release is another challenge. One of the other challenges of these hydrogels is the non-degradability of synthetic polymers which is responsible for the restricted usage in biomedical fields. Therefore, there is a constant demand to develop systematic methodologies for the synthesis of novel hydrogel materials to improve the degradability of the hydrogels by fine-tuning the functional groups and by incorporating more hydrophilicity for the ready hydrolysis.

Acknowledgements Dr. ASRK thanks VIT-RGEMS and VIT–Vellore for the encouragement and support.

References

1. (a) Kolb HC, Finn MG, Sharpless KB (2001) Click chemistry: diverse chemical function from a few good reactions. Angew Chem Int Ed 40(11):2004–2021; (b) Best MD (2009) Click chemistry and bioorthogonal reactions: unprecedented selectivity in the labeling of biological molecules. Biochemistry 8(28):6571–6584
2. (a) Sletten EM, Bertozzi CR (2009) Bioorthogonal chemistry: fishing for selectivity in a sea of functionality. Angew Chem Int Ed 48(38):6974–6998; (b) Jewett JC, Bertozzi CR (2010) Cu-free click cycloaddition reactions in chemical biology. Chem Soc Rev 39(4):1272–1279; (c) Lallana E, Riguera R, Fernandez-Megia E (2011) Reliable and efficient procedures for the conjugation of biomolecules through Huisgen azide–alkyne cycloadditions. Angew Chem Int Ed 50(38):8794–8804
3. Himo F, Lovell T, Hilgraf R, Rostovtsev VV, Noodleman L, Sharpless KB, Fokin VV (2005) Copper (I)-catalyzed synthesis of azoles. DFT study predicts unprecedented reactivity and intermediates. J Am Chem Soc 127:210–216
4. (a) Demko ZP, Sharpless KB (2002) A click chemistry approach to tetrazoles by Huisgen 1, 3-dipolar cycloaddition: synthesis of 5-sulfonyl tetrazoles from azides and sulfonyl cyanides. Angew Chem Int Ed 41(12):2110–2113; (b) Christopher DH, Xin-Ming L, Dong W (2008) Click chemistry, a powerful tool for pharmaceutical sciences. Pharm Res 25:2216–2230
5. (a) Rostovtsev VV, Green LG, Fokin VV, Sharpless KB (2002) A stepwise Huisgen cycloaddition process: copper(I)-catalyzed regioselective "ligation" of azides and terminal alkynes. Angew Chem Int Ed 41:2596–2599; (b) Tornøe CW, Christensen C, Meldal M (2002) Peptidotriazoles on solid phase: [1,2,3]-triazoles by regiospecific copper(I)-catalyzed 1,3-dipolar cycloadditions of terminal alkynes to azides. J Org Chem 67:3057–3064; (c) Manetsch R, Krasiński A, Radić Z, Raushel J, Taylor P, Sharpless KB, Kolb HC (2004) In situ click chemistry: enzyme inhibitors made to their own specifications. J Am Chem Soc 126:12809–12818; (d) Speers AE, Adam GC, Cravatt BF (2003) Activity-based protein profiling in vivo using

a copper (I)-catalyzed azide-alkyne [3+2] cycloaddition. J Am Chem Soc 125:4686–4687; (e) Lewis WG, Green LG, Grynszpan F, Radić Z, Carlier PR, Taylor P, Finn MG, Sharpless KB (2002) Click chemistry in situ: acetylcholinesterase as a reaction vessel for the selective assembly of a femtomolar inhibitor from an array of building blocks. Angew Chem Int Ed 41:1053–1057

6. Agard NJ, Prescher JA, Bertozzi CR (2004) A strain-promoted [3+2] azide–alkyne cycloaddition for covalent modification of biomolecules in living systems. J Am Chem Soc 126:15046–15047
7. (a) Peak C, Wilker J, Schmidt G (2013) A review on tough and sticky hydrogels. Colloid Polym Sci 291:2031; (b) Billiet T, Vandenhaute M, Schelfhout J, Vlierberghe SV, Dubruel P (2012) A review of trends and limitations in hydrogel-rapid prototyping for tissue engineering. Biomaterials 33:6020; (c) Kabiri K, Omidian H, Zohuriaan-Mehr MJ, Doroudiani S (2011) Superabsorbent hydrogel composites and nanocomposites: a review. Polym Compos 32:277
8. (a) Torre IG, Wolf F, Santos M, Rongen L, Alonso M, Jockenhoevel S, Cabello JR, Mela P (2015) Elastin-like recombinamer-covered stents: towards a fully biocompatible and non-thrombogenic device for cardiovascular diseases. Acta Biomater 12:146–155; (b) Burdick JA, Prestwich GD (2011) Hyaluronic acid hydrogels for biomedical applications. J Adv Mater 23:H41–H56; (c) DeForest CA, Anseth KS (2012) Photoreversible patterning of biomolecules within click-based hydrogels. Angew Chem Int Ed 51:1816–1819
9. (a) Du H, Wang Y, Yao X, Luo Q, Zhu W, Li X, Shen Z (2016) Injectable cationic hydrogels with high antibacterial activity and low toxicity. Polym Chem 7:5620–5624; (b) Kharkar PM, Rehmann MS, Skeens KM, Maverakis E, Kloxin AM (2016) Thiol–ene click hydrogels for therapeutic delivery. ACS Biomater Sci Eng 2:165–179; (c) Jiang Y, Chen J, Deng C, Suuronen EJ, Zhong Z (2014) Click hydrogels, microgels and nanogels: emerging platforms for drug delivery and tissue engineering. Biomaterials 35:4969–4985
10. Choi YC, Choi JS, Jung YJ, Cho YW (2014) Human gelatin tissue-adhesive hydrogels prepared by enzyme-mediated biosynthesis of DOPA and Fe^{3+} ion crosslinking. J Mater Chem B 2:201
11. Vulic K, Shoichet MS (2012) Tunable growth factor delivery from injectable hydrogels for tissue engineering. J Am Chem Soc 134:882
12. Choi J, Konno T, Takai M, Ishihara K (2012) Controlled drug release from multilayered phospholipid polymer hydrogel on titanium alloy surface. Biomaterials 33:954
13. Yang J, Zhao JJ, Han CR, Duan JF, Xu F, Sun RC (2014) Tough nanocomposite hydrogels from cellulose nanocrystals/poly (acrylamide) clusters: influence of the charge density, aspect ratio and surface coating with PEG. Cellulose 21:541
14. (a) Bhattacharya M, Malinen MM, Lauren P, Lou YR, Kuisma SW, Kanninen L, Lille M, Corlu A, GuGuen-Guillouzo C, Ikkala O, Laukkanen A, Urtti A, Yliperttula M (2012) Nanofibrillar cellulose hydrogel promotes three-dimensional liver cell culture. J Control Release 164:291; (b) Jeon O, Wolfson DW, Alsberg E (2015) In-situ formation of growth-factor-loaded coacervate microparticle-embedded hydrogels for directing encapsulated stem cell fate. Adv Mater 27:2216
15. Yang X, Bakaic E, Hoare T, Cranston ED (2013) Injectable polysaccharide hydrogels reinforced with cellulose nanocrystals: morphology, rheology, degradation, and cytotoxicity. Biomacromolecules 14:4447
16. Koschella A, Hartlieb M, Heinze T (2011) A 'click–chemistry' approach to cellulose-based hydrogels. Carbohydr Polym 86:154–161
17. (a) Gregoritza M, Brandl FP (2015) The Diels–Alder reaction: a powerful tool for the design of drug delivery systems and biomaterials. Eur J Pharm Biopharm 97:438–453; (b) García–Astrain C, Gandini A, Coelho D, Mondragon I, Retegi A, Eceiza A, Corcuera MA, Gabilondo N (2013) Green chemistry for the synthesis of methacrylate-based hydrogels cross-linked through Diels–Alder reaction. Eur Polym J 49:3998–4007
18. Nimmo CM, Owen SC, Shoichet MS (2013) Diels–Alder click cross-linked hyaluronic acid hydrogels for tissue engineering. Biomacromolecules 12:824–830
19. (a) Gandini A, Hariri S, Le Nest J (2003) Furan–polyether-modified chitosans as photosensitive polymer electrolytes. Polymer 44:7565–7572; (b) Montiel–Herrera M, Gandini A, Goycoolea

FM, Jacobsen NE, Lizardi–Mendoza J, Recillas–Mota M, Argüelles–Monal WM (2015) N–(furfural) chitosan hydrogels based on Diels–Alder cycloadditions and application as microspheres for controlled drug release. Carbohydr Polym 128:220–227; (c) Bilal M, Rasheed T, Zhao Y, Iqbal HMN, Cui J (2018) "Smart" chemistry and its application in peroxidase immobilization using different support materials. Int J Biol Macromol 119:278–290; (d) Yuan Y, Liang G (2014) A biocompatible, highly efficient click reaction and its applications. Org Biomol Chem 12:865; (e) Yigit S, Sanyal R, Sanyal A (2011) Fabrication and functionalization of hydrogels through "click" chemistry. Chem Asian J 6:2648–2659

20. (a) García–Astrain C, Gandini A, Peña C, Algar I, Retegi A, Eceiza A, Corcuera MA, Gabilondo N (2014) Diels–Alder "click" chemistry for the cross-linking of furfuryl–gelatin–polyetheramine hydrogels. RSC Adv 4:35578–35587; (b) García–Astrain C, Ahmed I, Kendziora D, Guaresti O, Eceiza A, Fruk L, Corcuera MA, Gabilondo N (2015) Effect of maleimide–functionalized gold nanoparticles on hybrid biohydrogels properties. RSC Adv 5:50268–50277; (c) García–Astrain C, Chen C, Burón M, Palomares T, Eceiza A, Fruk L, Corcuera MA, Gabilondo N (2015) Biocompatible hydrogel nanocomposite with covalently embedded silver nanoparticles. Biomacromolecules 16:1301–1310; (d) García–Astrain C, Peña–Rodriguez C, Retegi A, Eceiza A, Corcuera MA, Gabilondo N (2015) Green chemistry for the cross-linking of photo sensitive furan-modified gelatine. Mater Lett 160:142–145
21. (a) Tan H, Rubin JP, Marra KG (2011) Direct synthesis of biodegradable polysaccharide derivative hydrogels through aqueous Diels–Alder chemistry. Macromol Rapid Commun 32:905–911; (b) Wei HL, Yao K, Chu HJ, Li ZC, Zhu J, Shen YM, Zhao ZX, Feng YL (2012) Click synthesis of the thermo- and pH-sensitive hydrogels containing β-cyclodextrins. J Mater Sci 47332–47340; (c) Stewart SA, Backholm M, Burke NAD, Stöver HDH (2016) Cross-linked hydrogels formed through Diels–Alder coupling of furan- and maleimide-modified poly(methyl vinyl ether-alt-maleic acid). Langmuir 32:1863–1870; (d) Fan M, Ma Y, Zhang Z, Mao J, Tan H, Hu X (2015) Biodegradable hyaluronic acid hydrogels to control release of dexamethasone through aqueous Diels–Alder chemistry for adipose tissue engineering. Mater Sci Eng C 56:311–317
22. (a) Yigit S, Sanyal R, Sanyal A (2011) Fabrication and functionalization of hydrogels through "click" chemistry. Chem Asian J 6:2648–2659; (b) Imran AB, Seki T, Takeoka Y (2010) Recent advances in hydrogels in terms of fast stimuli responsiveness and superior mechanical performance. Polym J 42:839–851
23. (a) Lee KY, Mooney DJ (2001) Hydrogels for tissue engineering. Chem Rev 101:1869–1880; (b) Landers R, Hübner U, Schmelzeisen R, Mülhaupt R (2002) Rapid prototyping of scaffolds derived from thermoreversible hydrogels and tailored for applications in tissue engineering. Biomaterials 23:4437–4447; (c) Ahmed EM, Aggor FS, Awad AM, El-Aref AT (2013) An innovative method for preparation of nanometal hydroxide superabsorbent hydrogel. Carbohydr Polym 91:693–698
24. (a) Sakai T, Matsunaga T, Yamamoto Y, Ito C, Yoshida R, Suzuki S, Sasaki N, Shibayama M, Chung U (2008) Design and fabrication of a high-strength hydrogel with ideally homogeneous network structure from tetrahedron-like macromonomers. Macromolecules 41:5379–5384; (b) Hunt NC, Grover LM (2010) Cell encapsulation using biopolymer gels for regenerative medicine. Biotechnol Lett 32:733–742
25. Li Y, Tan Y, Xu K, Lu C, Wang P (2017) A biodegradable starch hydrogel synthesized via thiol-ene click chemistry. Polym Degrad Stab 137:75–82
26. Guaresti O, García-Astrain C, Palomares T, Alonso-Varona A, Eceiza A, Gabilondo N (2018) Synthesis and characterization of a biocompatible chitosan-based hydrogel cross-linked via 'click' chemistry for controlled drug release. Int J Biol Macromol 102:1–9
27. Lueckgen A, Garske DS, Ellinghaus A, Desai RM, Stafford AG, Mooney DJ, Duda GN, Cipitria A (2018) Hydrolytically-degradable click-crosslinked alginate hydrogels. Biomaterials 181:189–198
28. Lin F, Zheng R, Chen J, Su W, Dong B, Lin C, Huang B, Lu B (2019) Microfibrillated cellulose enhancement to mechanical and conductive properties of biocompatible hydrogels. Carbohydr Polym 205:244–254

29. Crescenzi V, Cornelio L, Meo CD, Nardecchia S, Lamanna R (2007) Novel hydrogels via click chemistry: synthesis and potential biomedical applications. Biomacromolecules 8:1844–1850
30. Angeles GH, Nêmcová M, Příkopová E, Smejkalová D, Pravda M, Kucera L, Velebny V (2012) Reductive alkylation of hyaluronic acid for the synthesis of biocompatible hydrogels by click chemistry. Carbohydr Polym 90:1704–1711
31. González K, García-Astrain C, Santamaria-Echart A, Ugarte L, Avérous L, Eceiza A, Gabilondo N (2018) Starch/graphene hydrogels via click chemistry with relevant electrical and antibacterial properties. Carbohydr Polym 202:372–381
32. Finetti C, Sola L, Elliott J, Chiari M (2017) Synthesis of hydrogel via click chemistry for DNA electrophoresis. J Chromatogr A 1513:226–234
33. Guaresti O, Astrain G, Aguirresarobe RH, Eceiza A, Gabilondo N (2018) Synthesis of stimuli-responsive chitosan-based hydrogels by Diels–Alder cross-linking 'click' reaction as potential carriers for drug administration. Carbohydr Polym 183:278–286
34. Zou Y, Zhang L, Yang L, Zhu F, Ding M, Linc F, Wang Z, Li Y (2018) "Click" chemistry in polymeric scaffolds: bioactive materials for tissue engineering. J Control Release 273:160–179
35. Dong R, Pang Y, Su Y, Zhu X (2015) Supramolecular hydrogels: synthesis, properties and their biomedical applications. Biomater Sci 3:937–954
36. Hoffman AS (2012) Hydrogels for biomedical applications. Adv Drug Deliv Rev 64:18–23
37. Wang Q, Mynar JL, Yoshida M, Lee E, Lee M, Okuro K, Kinbara K, Aida T (2010) High-water-content mouldable hydrogels by mixing clay and a dendritic molecular binder. Nature 463:339–343
38. DeForest CA, Anseth KS (2011) Cytocompatible click-based hydrogels with dynamically tunable properties through orthogonal photoconjugation and photocleavage reactions. Nat Chem 3:925–931
39. Zhu W, Gao L, Luo Q, Gao C, Zha G, Shen Z, Li X (2014) Metal and light free "click" hydrogels for prevention of post-operative peritoneal adhesions. Polym Chem 5(6):2018–2026
40. Zhang J, Xu XD, Wu DQ, Zhang XZ, Zhuo RX (2009) Synthesis of thermosensitive P(NIPAAm-co-HEMA)/cellulose hydrogels via "click" chemistry. Carbohydr Polym 77:583–589
41. Zhou JP, Chang CC, Zhang RP, Zhang LN (2007) Hydrogels prepared from unsubstituted cellulose in NaOH/urea aqueous solution. Macromol Biosci 7:804–810
42. Feng Y, Xiaodong C, Jie D, Gang W, Xiaofeng CA (2015) Multi-functional hydrogel with good structure integrity, self-healing and tissue-adhesive property formed by combining Diels–Alder click reaction and acylhydrazone bond. ACS Appl Mater Interfaces 7(43):24023–24031
43. Feng Y, Xiaodong C, Yuli L, Lei Z, Jiehua Z, Gang W, Xiaofeng C (2014) Diels–Alder crosslinked HA/PEG hydrogels with high elasticity and fatigue resistance for cell encapsulation and articular cartilage tissue repair. Polym Chem 5:5116
44. Gorkem Y, Muhammet UK Yusuf Y (2011) A one pot, one step method for the preparation of clickable hydrogels by photoinitiated polymerization. Macromol Rapid Commun 32:1906–1909
45. Fang Y, LiQun X, Guo-Dong F, BaoPing L (2010) Sliding-graft interpenetrating polymer networks from simultaneous "click chemistry" and atom transfer radical polymerization. Macromolecules 43:9761–9770
46. Jiyuan Y, Michael TJ, Huaizhong P, Jindřich K (2010) Synthesis and characterization of enzymatically degradable PEG-based peptide-containing hydrogels. Macromol Biosci 10:445–454
47. Chen X, Xin H, Jie W, Ye-Min Z, Xiao-Jiu L, Bin-Bin X, Chen Y, Li Y-S (2015) Library of antifouling surfaces derived from natural amino acids by click reaction. ACS Appl Mater Interfaces 7(31):17337–17345
48. (a) GhavamiNejad A, Park CH, Kim CS (2016) In situ synthesis of antimicrobial silver nanoparticles within antifouling zwitterionic hydrogels by catecholic redox chemistry for wound healing application. Biomacromolecules 17(3):1213–1223; (b) Banerjee SL, Bhattacharya K, Samanta S, Singha NK (2018) Self-healable antifouling zwitterionic hydrogel

based on synergistic phototriggered dynamic disulfide metathesis reaction and ionic interaction. ACS Appl Mater Interfaces 10(32):27391–27406; (c) Huang H, Tan Y, Ayers DC, Song J (2018) Anionic and zwitterionic residues modulate stiffness of photo-cross-linked hydrogels and cellular behavior of encapsulated chondrocytes. ACS Biomater Sci Eng 4(5):1843–1851
49. (a) Hoyle CE, Bowman CN (2010) Thiol-ene click chemistry. Angew Chem Int Ed 49(9):1540–1573; (b) DeForest CA, Polizzotti BD, Anseth KS (2009) Sequential click reactions for synthesizing and patterning three-dimensional cell microenvironments. Nat Mater 8(8):659–664
50. Gao LL, Luo QJ, Wang Y, Du H, Li XD, Shen ZQ, Zhu WP (2014) Facile preparation of shell crosslinked micelles for redox-responsive anticancer drug release. RSC Adv 4:4177–4180
51. Sun R, Luo Q, Gao C, Wang Y, Gao L, Du H, Zhu W (2014) Facile fabrication of reduction-responsive nanocarriers for controlled drug release. Polym Chem 5(17):4879–4883
52. Truong V, Blakey I, Whittaker AK (2012) Hydrophilic and amphiphilic polyethylene glycol-based hydrogels with tunable degradability prepared by "click" chemistry. Biomacromolecules 13(12):4012–4021
53. Arslan M, Aydin D, Degirmenci A, Sanyal A, Sanyal R (2017) Embedding well-defined responsive hydrogels with nanocontainers: tunable materials from telechelic polymers and cyclodextrins. ACS Omega 2(10):6658–6667
54. Bui QT, Jeon Y, Kim J, Kim JH (2017) Stabilized polymeric nanoparticle from amphiphilic mPEG-b-polyaspartamides containing "click" functional groups. Int J Polym Mater Polym Biomater 66(15):798–804
55. Huynh NT, Jeon YS, Kim D, Kim JH (2013) Preparation and swelling properties of "click" hydrogel from polyaspartamide derivatives using tri-arm PEG and PEG-co-poly(amino urethane) azides as crosslinking agents. Polymer 54(4):1341–1349
56. Cheng Y, He C, Xiao C, Ding J, Cui H, Zhuang X, Chen X (2013) Versatile biofunctionalization of polypeptide-based thermosensitive hydrogels via click chemistry. Biomacromolecules 14(2):468–475
57. Rik TCC, Jelmer S, Henk JB, John AWK, Rob MJL (2014) Characterization and activity of an immobilized antimicrobial peptide containing bactericidal PEG-hydrogel. Biomacromolecules 15(9):3390–3395
58. García-Astrain C, Algar I, Gandini A, Eceiza A, Corcuera MÁ, Gabilondo N (2014) Hydrogel synthesis by aqueous Diels–Alder reaction between furan modified methacrylate and polyetheramine-based bismaleimides. J Polym Sci Part A Polym Chem 53(5):699–708
59. Minkle J, Robin R, Suong-Hyu H, Kazuaki M (2014) Hydrogelation of dextran-based polyampholytes with cryoprotective properties via click chemistry. Biomater Sci 2:308–317
60. Kumar A, Ujjwal RR, Mittal A, Bansal A, Ojha U (2014) Polyacryloyl hydrazide: an efficient, simple, and cost effective precursor to a range of functional materials through hydrazide based click reactions. ACS Appl Mater Interfaces 6(3):1855–1865
61. Ossipov DA, Hilborn J (2006) Poly(vinyl alcohol)-based hydrogels formed by "click chemistry." Macromolecules 39:1709–1718
62. Malkoch M, Vestberg R, Gupta N, Mespouille L, Dubois P, Mason AF, Hawker CJ (2006) Synthesis of well-defined hydrogel networks using click chemistry. Chem Commun 26:2774
63. Lee E, Park J, Im SG, Song C (2012) Synthesis of single-walled carbon nanotube-incorporated polymer hydrogels via click chemistry. Polym Chem 3(9):2451
64. Nair DP, Podgórski M, Chatani S, Gong T, Xi W, Fenoli CR, Bowman CN (2013) The thiol-Michael addition click reaction: a powerful and widely used tool in materials chemistry. Chem Mater 26(1):724–744

The manufacturer's authorised representative in the EU is Springer Nature Customer Service Centre GmbH, Europaplatz 3, 69115 Heidelberg, Germany. If you have any concerns regarding our products, please contact ProductSafety@springernature.com

Printed and bound by CPI Group (UK) Ltd, Croydon, CR0 4YY
30/09/2026
02225291-0009